Antidepressants:
Science, Magic or Marketing?

by
Les Ruthven, Ph.D.
President/CEO Preferred Mental Health Management, Inc.
Wichita, Kansas

Foreword by
David Antonuccio, Ph.D.
Professor of Psychiatry and Behavioral Sciences
University of Nevada School of Medicine

PMHM Publishing
Wichita, Kansas

Cover design by Jim Simpson, Simpson Design, Inc.
Cover photograph of John Carrol, N.A. lithograph by Rick Luther
Back cover photograph by Rick Luther

First paperback edition March 2005

Manufactured in the United States of America

ISBN 0-9765807-0-5

Library of Congress Control Number: 2005920742

DEDICATION

I dedicate this book to my wife-colleague, Courtney L. Ruthven, Ph.D., also a psychologist, and to the dedicated psychologist and non-psychologist staff at our company, Preferred Mental Health Management, Inc. (www.pmhm.com).

Courtney, this Tennessee country gal with a giant intellect, among other assets, and this transplanted New Yorker began a very good thing together in the 1960s. We have shared much together since, probably more than many couples since we share a career in common. I have been the visionary and Courtney has helped to keep us firmly grounded to terra firma. This book is a recent example of a long line of projects we have shared together. With this book my thanks to Courtney for doing most of the editorial work, especially the task of reducing my complex sentences to simple sentences. For these and other contributions my love and deeply felt thanks. Kiddingly, I tell couples we meet that Courtney and I share a division of labor. I do the division and Courtney does the labor.

My thanks also to Lois Bailey for editorial assistance, especially for her advice in reorganizing its contents. Thanks also to PMHM staff members Cynthia Erker for typing the manuscript and Jeannie Wayne for taking care of many details prior to publishing.

My thanks and appreciation also to PMHM's dedicated staff, some of whom have been with us from the start in 1987. I thank them for taking my vision as their own, the mission to improve the quality of behavioral health services by changing the way in which these services are delivered. I doubt that any company has a more loyal, dedicated and competent staff than PMHM, nor one that achieves a higher level of customer service for all of our clients — those calling for services, PMHM's network of providers, and our employer clients who pay for the services. My special thanks go to the latter, PMHM's employer clients who had the intelligence and courage not to do the "safe" thing but to do the right thing when a better way was offered.

TABLE OF CONTENTS

ABOUT THE AUTHOR

Dr. Les Ruthven's credentials include a Ph.D. in clinical Psychology from the University of Tennessee with a clinical internship at the V.A. Psychiatric Hospital in Salisbury, North Carolina. The program was approved by the American Psychological Association and designed after the Boulder Model, which viewed the training of psychologists in the scientist/practitioner model.

He was a staff psychologist in the Department of Psychiatry of the Medical College of South Carolina until he began a private practice in Wichita, Kansas in 1966, providing inpatient and outpatient psychodiagnostic and psychotherapy services to a wide range of patients.

While in private practice, Dr. Les developed a specialty in the field of clinical neuropsychology and was Principal Investigator of a National Institute of Mental Health research grant, which resulted in the book, Rehabilitation of the Brain-Damaged Adult, Plenum Press, 1983.

During the forty years of experience in his field, Dr. Les has diagnosed and treated many thousands of patients with depression and other mental health problems.

However, he has not been content to simply lean on his wide clinical experience and, for the past six years, he has been reviewing the scientific literature on depression and its treatment, especially the placebo-controlled, double-blind depression outcome studies.

His conclusions about depression, based upon the scientific evidence and his clinical experience, are 180 degrees from the current model of drug treatment for depression by family physicians and psychiatrists. Founder and president/CEO of a national behavioral health management firm (PMHM), he is no stranger to going against what is momentarily popular in the profession and looks to science and not propaganda to guide clinical practice.

Dr. Les's latest innovations at his company include HealthPromotions™, in which PMHM staff psychologists help callers to change their behavior for better health.

In combining his aviation and psychology interests, Dr. Les has developed for the airlines and corporate flight departments a program in which psychologists apply the science of human behavior to pilot training for improved aviation safety.

ABOUT PMHM

- Preferred Mental Health Management (**PMHM**) is a managed behavioral health organization (MBHO) that Dr. Les Ruthven founded in 1987, which he and his wife, Dr. Courtney L. Ruthven, also a psychologist, co-manage in Wichita, Kansas.
- **PMHM** is a privately held corporation which has arranged a full scope of behavioral health services (employee assistance and mental health benefit plan services) for employees of several Fortune 500 as well as smaller companies with employees and dependents in all fifty states and Puerto Rico. **PMHM** has an extensive national network of the most highly credentialed providers in the industry.
- The guiding principle at **PMHM** is to arrange and authorize the most effective treatment of the patient's problems through focused treatment, which ensures not only the highest quality care but also cost effective treatment.
- At **PMHM** care is initiated by the unique use of *doctorate psychologists.* These psychologists conduct telephonic assessment, consultation and referral for those accessing **PMHM** for help with a variety of mental health problems and human concerns. By using a broadly trained expert in human behavior and mental disorder at the point of access to care, **PMHM** is often able to initiate problem resolution with the first call. The psychologist initiating care at **PMHM** also manages all subsequent care.
- The **PMHM** psychologist can, when needed, refer the patient to its national panel of 8,000 psychologists and clinical social workers for behavioral intervention and, when needed, 1500 psychiatrists for drug treatment and hospitalization in about 900 acute care facilities across the country.
- The provider and **PMHM** psychologist manager are able to share their diagnostic expertise to ensure that the patient receives the best and most effective care available.

FOREWORD

By David Antonuccio, Ph.D.
Professor of Psychiatry and Behavioral Sciences
University of Nevada School of Medicine

It is important to understand why a book like this is necessary. First of all depression is a highly prevalent condition, with major depression affecting as many as 24% of Americans at some time during their lives (Kessler et al., 2003). Depression has a number of debilitating symptoms including an overwhelming sadness, reduced rate of behavior (particularly pleasant activities), social interaction problems, guilt, a feeling of being weighted down, and numerous somatic complaints. Severe role impairment associated with depression has been documented in a variety of domains, including social and work roles (Kessler et al, 2003). The primary care medical setting is where many if not most patients are seeking and receiving treatment for depression (Cummings, 2003). Up to one third of patients in waiting rooms of primary care settings may be experiencing clinically significant symptoms of depression (Robinson, 2003). Furthermore, approximately 44% of depressed patients are receiving treatment for their problems in the medical setting (Greenberg et al., 2003), an increase from 28% in 1990 (Greenberg et al, 1993).

Although the prevalence of depression has remained fairly stable at 18 million Americans (Greenberg et al., 2003), the costs in the U.S. associated with depression have increased at an alarming rate; from 44 billion dollars in 1990 (Greenberg et. al, 1993) to 83 billion dollars in 2000 (Greenberg et al., 2003). The cost increases appear to be fueled primarily by pharmaceutical costs. Pharmaceutical interventions prevail as the predominant treatment delivered in primary care medical settings (Moore, 2004). Among adults 18-years-old and older, office visits where an antidepressant was mentioned in progress notes increased from 45.1 million in 1998 to 60 million in 2001. By 2001, antidepressants were mentioned in 7.1% of all office visits in outpatient settings (Moore, 2004).

While psychotropic medications have been helpful in ameliorating some mental and behavioral problems, all medical interventions carry with them certain risks and side effects (Antonuccio et al, 1999). As patients age and develop multiple health problems, the risks associated with combining medications also multiply.

Consistent with the Hippocratic dictum "first do no harm," it is important for health care providers to also consider other nonpharmaceutical interventions with fewer medical risks. This is especially important given that patients in a primary care setting often do not adhere to antidepressant medications due to side effects, lack of improvement in symptoms, or because they actually feel worse (Haslam, Brown, Atkinson, & Haslam, 2004).

Whether one takes a "do no harm" or a cost-benefit approach to treatment, it is impossible to ignore the fact that antidepressants are not medically benign treatments. The short-term side effects of SSRIs are well-established and commonly include agitation, sleep disruption, gastrointestinal problems, and sexual dysfunction (Antonuccio et al., 1999). Side effects and medical risks (including risk of dying) increase when SSRIs are combined with other medications (Dalfen & Stewart, 2001), as is often the case (Antonuccio et al., 1999). In addition, the withdrawal symptoms of SSRIs are substantial for many, if not most, patients (Coupland, Bell, & Potokar, 1996; Fava, 2002; Rosenbaum, Fava, Hood, Ashcroft, & Krebs, 1998). Although the data are mixed and somewhat controversial, other potential risks that warrant further investigation include the association (although not an established causal relationship) of SSRIs with breast cancer (e.g., Cotterchio, Kreiger, Darlington, & Steingart, 2000), acts of deliberate self-harm (e.g., Donovan et al., 2000; Healy, 2002), manic episodes (e.g., Preda, MacLean, Mazure, & Bowers, 2001), and the possibility of irreversible biochemical changes predisposing some susceptible patients to chronic depression (e.g., Baldessarini, 1995; Fava, 1995, 2002). When medical cost offset (Hunsley, in press), relapse, and side effects are considered in a cost-benefit analysis, psychological interventions can be very cost-effective, particularly in a psychoeducational (e.g., therapist-assisted bibliotherapy) or group format (Antonuccio, Thomas, & Danton, 1997). Dr. Ruthven makes the case that such interventions for depression should be tried first.

Our cultural preference for medication interventions creates a need to encourage health care providers and patients to consider psychological interventions instead of medication prescriptions as a first-line treatment for depression because (1) psychotherapy (particularly cognitive therapy, behavioral activation, and interpersonal therapy) compares favorably with medications in the short term, even when the depression is severe (e.g., DeRubeis, Gelfand, Tang, & Simons, 1999), (2) psychotherapy appears superior to medications when long term follow-up is considered (Antonuccio, Danton, & DeNelsky, 1995; Hollon, Shelton, & Loosen, 1991), and (3) there are no apparent medical side effects. Several meta-analyses, reported in both psychiatry and psychology journals covering multiple studies with thousands of patients, are remarkably consistent in support of the perspective that psychological interventions are at least as effective as medication in the treatment of depression (e.g., Conte et al, 1986; DeRubeis et al., 1999; Dobson et al., 1989; Hollon et al, 1991; Robinson et al., 1990; Steinbrueck et al., 1983; Wexler & Ciccheti, 1992).

It is impractical for health care providers in a primary care setting to deliver effective psychotherapy for depression; however, it is reasonable to assume that they may be able to practically deliver components of empirically validated psychotherapies in the form of what I call brief "behavioral prescriptions". For example, one such empirically validated treatment is bibliotherapy for depression (Ackerson, Scogin, McKendree-Smith & Lyman, 1998; Cuijpers, 1997; Jamison & Scogin, 1995; Gould & Clum, 1993; Pantalon, Lubetkin & Fishman, 1995; Scogin, Jamison & Davis, 1990; Scogin, Jamison, Floyd, and Chaplin, 1998; Smith, Floyd, Scogin, & Jamison, 1997). Cuipers' (1997) meta-analysis of bibliotherapy and depression examining six studies yielded an impressive mean effect size of 0.82 (with a 95% confidence interval of 0.50 --1.15). Behavioral prescriptions can be adaptations of treatments that have already been empirically validated. The Feeling Good book (Scogin et al. 1989; Scogin et al., 1990; Scogin et al., 1998; Smith et al.,1997), behavioral activation (Hopko et al. 2003), aerobic exercise (Babyak et al. 2000; Blumenthal et al., 1999), relaxation training (McLean & Hakstian 1979, 1990), and social skills/assertiveness training (McLean & Hakstian 1979, 1990) already have established efficacy in the treatment of depression.

In accepting that psychological interventions have efficacy comparable with that of antidepressants, it is not necessary to give up the biological model completely, because there is evidence of metabolic changes associated with improvement in psychotherapy that are similar to those seen with antidepressants (Brody et al., 2001; Martin, Martin, Rai, Richardson, & Royall, 2001). In fact, distinct metabolic (Mayberg et al., 2002) and electroencephalogram changes (Leuchter, Cook, Witte, Morgan, & Abrams, 2002) have also been documented in patients who respond to placebo.

There is no doubt that depression is a costly condition. An estimated 60% of office visits do not result in an official biological diagnosis (Cummings, Pallik, Dorken & Hinke, 2000). It's likely that many of these patients are reporting somatic complaints, including sleep, appetite, and concentration problems that are related to depression. Among individuals diagnosed with major depression, research has supported a link between the presence of chronic psychological conditions and emergency room visits. One of ten episodes of treatment involve an emergency room visit and can lead to a higher usage of inpatient services, costing at least $2500 per individual diagnosed with major depression (Cucciare & O'Donohue, 2003). A number of recent studies (Guthrie et al, 1999; Simon et al., 2001;McLeod, Budd, & McClelland, 1997) focus on the reduction of health care utilization cost via the development of psychosocial intervention programs including bibliotherapy for a variety of psychological conditions such as depression. In the era of managed care, it is not enough to be effective; treatments must be cost-effective. Cost-benefit analysis demonstrates that CBT interventions are at least as cost-effective as antidepressant prescriptions. For example, one analysis (Antonuccio, Thomas, & Danton (1997) showed that over a 2-year period, fluoxetine alone may result in 33% higher expected costs than individual CBT treatment for depression and the combination treatment may result in 23% higher costs than CBT alone. Integrating such psychological treatment into primary care settings results in a medical-cost offset or reduction in overall costs (Cummings et al., 2000).

Some might suggest that because there appears to be a small advantage over placebo, antidepressants should still be considered a first line treatment for depression. However, there may be several reasons why nondrug alternatives ought to be considered before medication is used. First, most of the drug conditions in studies of antidepressants use supportive weekly visits adjunctively (e.g., Elkin et al., 1989) and do not adequately evaluate the efficacy of medication alone. The resultant therapeutic alliance (e.g., Blatt, Sanislow, Zuroff, Pilkonis, 1996) may enhance the efficacy of the medication and give an inaccurate picture of the effectiveness of these medications in a typical managed care environment where antidepressants are often delivered in conjunction with infrequent visits to a mental health professional.

Some might argue that antidepressants are important to stave off suicide in very depressed patients. However, there is no evidence that antidepressants reduce the risk of suicide or suicide attempts in comparison with a placebo in randomized controlled trials (Khan et al., 2000; Storosum, van Zwieten, van den Brink, Gersons, & Broekmans, 2001). Finally, most patients seem to prefer a psychotherapeutic intervention when given the choice (Chilvers et al., 2001; Hall & Robertson, 1998; Jorm, 2000; Paykel, Hart, & Priest, 1998; Priest, Vize, Roberts, Roberts, & Tylee, 1996). Despite this repeated finding, it is often concluded that consumers just need more "education" about the benefits and safety of antidepressants to bring their preferences in line with accepted practice (e.g., Paykel et al., 1998; Priest et al., 1996).

As detailed by Dr. Ruthven, the analyses of the FDA antidepressant database (Kirsch et al., 2002) have convincingly demonstrated, using pharmaceutical industry data, that the image of antidepressants as powerfully more effective than placebo is not supported by the data. The small advantage over inert placebo credited to antidepressants is quite possibly a methodological artifact (Moncrieff, 2002). It could be argued that the patients randomly assigned to placebo are the lucky ones, because they derive a benefit virtually comparable with the medication condition without the associated medical risks. We are left with the current paradox regarding the use of antidepressants in children, i.e., there is enough evidence of harm to warrant a black box warning but there is not enough evidence of benefit to be able to say these medications are more effective than placebo.

The silver lining in these results for health care providers is that the health care provider, or at least something about the therapeutic relationship, and not the pill, appears to facilitate improvement in depression. Figuring out ways to enhance the therapeutic alliance, originally pioneered but recently marginalized by organized psychiatry, may prove more fruitful than modifying the selectivity of antidepressants. There is no doubt that antidepressants have a biochemical impact on the brain, but the valence of that impact is open for considerable debate, and whether it corrects a chemical imbalance is in grave doubt. Recent events have caused Americans to become more skeptical of the pharmaceutical industry as a source of information about pharmaceuticals in the same way that most Americans are reluctant to rely solely on the manufacturer for information when buying a car. When the logical arguments and the advertising blitz fail to discredit the evidence of minimal benefit and when we begin to fully appreciate the cost of side effects and long-term health risks associated with antidepressants, American medicine's preference for these medications as the primary treatment for depression may change. Other popular medical practices have certainly proven ineffective or too risky over time. One day we may look back and marvel at the stroke of marketing genius that led to calling these medications antidepressants in the first place. As the FDA analysis shows, just because a pill is called an antidepressant, it doesn't necessarily make it so.

This book helps to explain some of the events that led up to this state of affairs. Dr. Ruthven takes the position that (1) depression does not necessarily result from a chemical imbalance, (2) extensive industry influences have resulted in a biological bias in depression research, (3) much of the antidepressant research is fatally flawed, (4) the practice of relying on antidepressants in combination with other psychotropic medications may actually be driving up risk and mental health costs, (5) evidence of harm in children from antidepressants far outweighs evidence of benefit, and (6) patients report high satisfaction with psychological interventions alone. The case examples and transcripts in the patients' own words are particularly revealing. It is wonderful to see a managed care administrator thinking "outside the box" when it comes to safe, effective treatment for depression. In the end, the patients will reap the benefits.

INTRODUCTION

In 2003, Americans spent thirteen billion dollars on antidepressant drugs, most of which were prescribed by the family physician. Most of these dollars were spent on the newer variety antidepressants, the Selective Serotonin Reuptake Inhibitor and related drugs (SSRIs) such as Prozac, Paxil, Zoloft and approximately a dozen others. These drugs are typically the most frequently prescribed drugs in any pharmacy benefit plan and compete in cost with the class of drugs to treat cardiovascular diseases.

Currently about one million children a year are taking antidepressant drugs. During 2003 seventeen million antidepressant prescriptions were written for children. In 2002, children received about 7% of the total number of antidepressant prescriptions. The youngest children using antidepressants were about one month old.

Dr. Gianna Rigoni has estimated that there are over 157 million prescriptions annually for SSRI and atypical antidepressants dispensed for all ages in 2002. Sertraline (Zoloft) was the most prescribed drug of the ten products at over 31 million prescriptions, followed closely by paroxetine (Paxil) with 30.5 million.

Meanwhile, the problem of depression in the United States today and the cost of treating it is a staggering burden to society and our health care system. About 17.5 million of us have a diagnosable depression at any one time and 20% of the adult population will have at least one diagnosable episode during their lifetime. Add to this the 25% or so with a diagnosable anxiety disorder, which is now also treated by SSRI antidepressants. The market potential for these drugs—and the financial cost to society—is indeed mind-boggling.

In 1999, 3 of the top 10 best-selling drugs were the SSRIs Prozac, Paxil, and Zoloft, which had combined revenues of $6.7 billion (Louie, 2001). Revenues for SSRI drugs are increasing by about 25% each year (Kroenke, K., et al., 2001). One in eight adult Americans has taken an antidepressant in the past ten years, and 3.5 billion doses of SSRIs were consumed in 1999 alone (Langer, 2000). Of those polled, 60% had taken antidepressant drugs for more than 3 months, whereas 46% had been taking them for a year or more.

The "Proponents"

The marketers of these drugs from the above sales figures have done extremely well for themselves; rightly or wrongly they have sold people on a panacea. The drug company manufacturers may feel assured that their future prospects are bright, but they do face some challenges for continued growth:

- the difficulty of keeping many patients on these drugs,
- the high relapse rate when drugs are discontinued,
- a wide variety of adverse drug side effects,
- rising and persistent questions about their safety,
- mention in the media from time to time on research reports that question their effectiveness, and
- a few mental health professionals, like myself, who question the very foundation from which this industry has risen—that depression is a biological or brain disease and drugs are its primary treatment.

Fortunately for the marketers, the drug companies have some powerful forces in society on their side to assist in the expansion of drug treatment of these problems. All in all, the future looks very bright indeed for the drug companies and their antidepressant wares. The forces assisting the drug makers include some major players: the profession of psychiatry as a whole, the medical establishment, the National Institute for Mental Health (NIMH), the Food and Drug Administration (FDA), antidepressant drug psychiatrist-researchers (with few exceptions), patient advocacy groups such as the Alliance of the Mentally Ill and others, the mass media by and large, many state and national politicians who have become handmaidens for the industry, and even a sizable number of trained psychologists who have accepted the conventional wisdom that drugs combined with psychotherapy are better than therapy alone.

The Questions

Some who are not yet caught up in the antidepressant mainstream ask some questions that seem (to the marketers) to hang around annoyingly:

- What research evidence do we have to support the chemical imbalance theory of depression?

- How do we know that depression is a *biological* disease? Does this mean that it necessitates *biological* treatments?
- Are there any alternative theories about depression and its treatment? How do these stack up with the chemical imbalance theory?
- What about side effects of these drugs? Some say they can cause suicide or homicide? Is there anything to that?
- If these drugs cure or alleviate depression, how do they work?
- If depression and anxiety are mental health problems, is having non-psychiatric physicians prescribe most of these drugs a good idea? Is this good treatment and does it save money?
- Can depression be caused by non-biological factors in a person's life?
- Some depressed people *seem* to have problems in their life that *might* bring about depression. Can a drug treat the problem without attention *to* the problem?
- How much better is drug treatment of depression for a depressed person than no treatment at all? Or how much better is an antidepressant drug in treating depression than a sugar pill?
- Are we getting good value for this part of the health care dollar?
- Do we need to put *more* people on these drugs or *fewer* people?

The above seem to be fairly reasonable questions that one might legitimately ask about antidepressant drugs and of those who champion their use. I hope to answer these and many other questions regarding all of these issues.

Open Mind Needed

If you believe in the power of antidepressant drugs to cure depression and subscribe to the notion that depression is a biological disease, I would like you, as you read these pages, to keep an open mind and to suspend judgment until all of the evidence has been examined.

If, as a primary care physician, psychiatrist, psychologist, psychiatrist drug researcher, media person, a supporter of patient advocacy or other, you endorse the drug model of treating depression, do not discount my thesis out of hand but let's look at the scientific evidence and try to separate scientific truth from any marketing hype that might exist within the industry.

Rationale

I have spent my whole career diagnosing and treating a full range of mental disorders with patients of all ages, including the vast majority of those who present with primary stress and mood problems, including diagnosable depression and anxiety. However, I would hesitate to write such a book based upon my clinical experience alone since anecdotal reports of successful therapy — as indeed reports of successful drug therapy — are no measure of scientific proof.

I must admit that six years ago I started this enterprise in somewhat of a defensive posture. Eighteen years ago I founded what has become a medium sized, national managed behavioral health organization (MBHO), Preferred Mental Health Management, Inc. (PMHM) of Wichita, Kansas. In the early years I found that my ideas about depression and anxiety and their treatment were almost diametrically opposed to the MBHO industry as a whole, perhaps because the industry has largely been a creation of the field of *psychiatry* rather than psychology. As a practicing psychologist I had never found the need to add drugs to my behavioral treatment of either anxiety and/or depression. Moreover, in the founding of PMHM, I saw no need to substitute or add drugs to therapy for those calling PMHM for services to arrange treatment for depression and anxiety.

Mine, however, is not the model in the MBHO industry as a whole. In my industry, antidepressant drugs rather than behavioral interventions drive the treatment.

Even though at PMHM we have an exceptional national panel of providers with the highest credentials, I was somewhat shocked to find that a number of our own panel psychologists and clinical social workers seemed to favor *combined* treatment over therapy alone. This, as you could imagine, would and did bring about problems for PMHM in arranging and managing care. Since the *drugs* first philosophy in treating depression is so endemic in society today, not only did we have to educate our *callers* with depressed mood to accept a *therapy* first approach to their problems, but some of our *providers* needed education as well.

Moreover, since the conventional wisdom about depression and its treatment is so prevalent in society today, including human resources/health benefit managers, I thought PMHM might be at a competitive disadvantage in the market. I needed some way to address this issue when it arose. For example, many MBHOs do not reimburse for psychotherapy for depression unless the therapy is *combined* with drug treatment. I really did not want to hide the fact the PMHM endorses the behavioral or non-drug model of treating both depression and anxiety, yet I knew some benefits' managers who hire MBHOs are advocates for drug therapy.

About six years or so ago I did not think I could marshal a cogent argument of a *behavioral* model based upon my clinical experience alone. Therefore, I began to examine the research literature on drug and non-drug treatment of both depression and anxiety. I focused on *scientific* studies. I looked at FDA antidepressant clinical trials using placebo controls for comparison purposes, and other controlled research regarding outcome of drug and behavioral treatment, including research comparing combined treatment versus drugs or therapy alone.

When I started this review of the research literature I was open to the possibility that combined treatment *might* be advantageous in *some* depressions. I did not think that most depression treatment required drugs. Although I knew the SSRIs had adverse side effects, I did not believe these side effects included suicide and homicide even though these events had been reported from time to time for some of those on the newer antidepressants.

I wanted to have the best evidence available to answer these questions and this very long process has culminated in this book. I looked at the research and drew conclusions based upon my unbiased examination of the data. From the outset, I determined not to look at the research simply to support my position. Ph.D. psychologists have an advantage over all other mental health professionals since we alone are trained to design and conduct controlled research and to review and examine the research of others. From my examination of the relevant research and my clinical experience I came to the following conclusion: I do not endorse the current, popular, biologically based theory of depression and its treatment. Alternative, non-chemical imbalance explanations of the facts are much more plausible and the reader is invited to test his or her views of depression against the scientific evidence.

This book is meant for a wide audience, including PMHM's employer clients who have retained PMHM to manage their Employee Assistance Program/Mental Health Benefit.

I don't doubt that many bright and educated readers in contemporary society will have a very strong commitment to the conventional theory about depression and its treatment. The drug treatment theory of depression is very prevalent and embedded in the popular culture of today and many mental health professionals espouse its tenants on television and in newspaper articles. We have been conditioned to believe that a very complex mental disorder can be treated effectively with a little pill prescribed by the family doctor. What a marketer's dream! If you have bought this prevailing theory about depression you should not feel badly about it — you are in some very good company. Still, I ask you to look at the following evidence impartially and then test your beliefs against the additional evidence.

Comments on My Use of Certain Terms in This Book

(1) **Current generation antidepressant drugs (SSRIs)**: these have a specific focus on various neurotransmitter systems of the brain such as the serotonin system. Drugs that principally focus on the serotonin system are called Selective Serotonin Reuptake Inhibitor Antidepressants (or SSRI drugs for short and include the big three, Prozac, Paxil and Zoloft). These drugs keep serotonin more available at the synapses between brain cells, which may aid in firing the next neuron (brain cell) in the chain. Some drugs also impact the norepinephrine system, (e.q., Effexor).

(2) **Chemical Imbalance**: The theory that mood (depression, anxiety and OCD) is caused by an imbalance of serotonin or norepinephrine in the brain.

(3) **Tricyclic Antidepressants**: These were the earlier or first generation antidepressants such as Elavil, which are still in current use today but these drugs are overshadowed by the current generation drugs such as Prozac, Zoloft, and Paxil.

(4) **"Believers"**: those lay people who have a strong commitment to the use of antidepressant drugs in the treatment of depression and anxiety or both. These people endorse the commonly accepted idea that depression is a disease, a

chemical imbalance in the brain, which is effectively treated by an antidepressant drug alone.

(5) **"Proponents"**: those who have a vested interest with an extremely strong commitment to these drugs for monetary, professional turf, or public "welfare" reasons. All "proponents" and most "believers" are strongly committed to the notion that depression is basically a *biological* disease and any approach to treating it behaviorally or non-biologically is doomed to be inadequate.

(6) **Cognitive Behavioral Therapy (CBT)**: one of several types of psychotherapy for treating both depression and anxiety. It came out of the work of Aaron Beck, M.D., a psychiatrist, and many psychologists. Their theory is that it is not so much what happens to us to make us depressed; rather, it is what we *tell ourselves* about what happens to us that makes us depressed. A significant part of the therapy is to help the patient to become aware of their erroneous thoughts that makes them and keeps them depressed.

(7) **Schizophrenia**: A psychotic disorder characterized in the active phase by hallucinations, delusions, disorganized thoughts-speech, disorganized or catatonic behavior and apathy.

(8) **Bipolar 1 and 2 Disorder**: Bipolar 1 is a *psychotic* disorder characterized by one or more manic episodes. It is a new term for the older Manic-Depressive Psychosis. Bipolar 2 is used when the patient has *not* had the history of a manic (psychotic) episode, but seemingly shares other characteristics with bipolar 1 patients.

(9) **Anxiety Disorders** include Panic Attacks, Agoraphobia (avoidance of places or situations in which help may not be available during a panic attack), Specific Phobias (e.g., riding an escalator), Social Phobia, Acute Stress Disorder, Posttraumatic Stress Disorder, Obsessive-Compulsive Disorder (OCD), Generalized Anxiety Disorder (GAD), Anxiety Due to a General Medical Condition, Substance-Induced Anxiety Disorder, and Anxiety Disorder Not Otherwise Stated.

(10) **Anxiolytic drugs or Anxiolytics**: A drug class to treat anxiety, many of which are benzodiazepenies such as the earlier Valium and currently Xanax. These drugs are addictive and should only be used for short-term use. These drugs are

habituating in that dosage increases are required to maintain the same effect. Withdrawal from these drugs usually requires detoxification in a hospital.

(11) **Rebound phenomena**: The tendency for the fear reaction (e.g., panic attack) to increase in frequency and intensity over its pre-treatment level when the anxiolytic drug is stopped.

(12) **Atypical Antipsychotic Drugs or Atypicals**: Newer drugs for Schizophrenia or Bipolar Disorder. The atypicals are much more expensive than the earlier generation drugs such as Haldol, which are still in use to some extent.

(13) **Organic Disease**: A disease attended with morbid (serious, progressive) changes in the *structure* of the organs of the body or in the compositions of its fluids; as opposed to "functional" disease.

(14) **Antidepressant Drug Clinical Trial, Double-blind, Placebo-Controlled Study**: The depression and anxiety clinical trials of a new drug to obtain approval by the FDA are conducted by psychiatrist-researchers and largely paid for by the sponsoring drug company. Subjects, once selected for the study, are randomly assigned to the drug condition or an inert placebo-controlled condition. These studies are referred to as "double-blind," meaning neither the subject nor the prescriber-rater knows whether the subject is on the drug or placebo

(15) **Effect Size**: A statistical operation that gives the power of a drug or a procedure (e.g., a program of exercise or a program of remedial tutoring) on the *dependent* variable (such as reduction of depression or weight loss). A strong Effect Size is 1.00 or above (standard deviations). A weaker Effect Size are those less than 1.00.

(16) **Personality Disorders**: These are enduring, life-time patterns of maladaptive behavior that deviate markedly from the expectations of the person's culture, is pervasive and inflexible and has an onset in adolescence or early adulthood. The specific disorders are called Paranoid, Schizoid, Schizotypical, Antisocial, Borderline, Histrionic, Narcissistic, Avoidant, Dependent, Obsessive-Compulsive, and Personality Disorder Not Otherwise Specified. These are *incurable* disorders and most competent therapists *manage* rather than *treat* these disorders since the name "treatment" implies a possible cure.

CHAPTER I

DEPRESSION: IT'S NOT AS SIMPLE AS THEY THINK

"If you've seen one depression, you've seen one depression"

Two of our major public health problems in the United States today are stress and mood problems, and their diagnosable counterparts – clinical depression and the anxiety disorders. These symptom problems – and the inappropriate *medical* treatment of these problems – is a major cause of our escalating health care costs and increasingly poor health care. Most Americans seem to like everything about their health care except its cost. However, in addition to the cost problems, there are many quality care problems. One of these major quality health care problems is the inappropriate medical (drug) treatment of psychological problems.

Cost of Depression and Anxiety

Depression and anxiety, even excluding the normal stress and mood problems to which all of us are subjected, have an enormous economic burden on all of society. Untreated depression costs American business as much as 43 billion dollars annually in medical treatment, the number of sick days, loss of productivity, disability, and employee turnover (Boyd, J. H., 1982).

It has been estimated that 17.5 million Americans have some form of depression at any one time, and that 9.2 million have major depression, the most serious form (Boyd, 1982). Depression typically shows up with "physical" symptoms and when it is not diagnosed and competently treated, these patients are notoriously high users of both inpatient and outpatient general medical services. There is a very high incidence of depression (perhaps 50%) in those who are hospitalized for conditions *other* than depression – diabetes, asthma, gastrointestinal problems, and others. Often it does not seem to be the *primary* disease that necessitates the hospitalization; *mental health* problems aggravate the primary disease and make the hospital care necessary.

Cost of Psychiatrist Treatment of Depression

In the conventional wisdom on depression and its treatment, one reason given to justify drugs over psychotherapy in treatment of depression is the costs. How much does pharmacotherapy of depression cost as delivered by a psychiatrist, for example?

Terry (Terry, Christine, et al., 1998) examined the cost of drug treatment of major depression by psychiatrists in one large managed care plan. In this study 4,250 depressed patients were followed for twelve months and the average cost per Patient Treatment Episode (PTE) was $2,287.

In this cost of drug treatment ($2,287) per case, are we getting a good return on money spent? We know depressed patients as a group have a high utilization of physician and medical services. Such depression treatment with drugs *may* be reasonable *if* the treatment improves general health, reduces future depressive episodes, and lowers general medical costs of these patients. Because of the almost exponential increase in the use of these drugs since the SSRIs first appeared on the market in 1987, we must ask if drug treatment of depression – by either psychiatrists or primary care physicians (PCP) – is indeed an appropriate and effective treatment of these health problems?

The Chemical Imbalance Theory

Ten to twelve years ago my psychiatric colleagues were telling me that depression was not only a disease but also a disease of the serotonin system. The "reasoning" went something like this: an SSRI inhibits the reuptake of serotonin in brain synapses, that is, it keeps more serotonin around in the synapse. The additional serotonin allows the one brain cell to fire the next one in the chain more easily, allowing increased behavioral output. Thus, the SSRI cures the depressive episode. Therefore, depression is a disease of the serotonin system!

When Prozac, a drug that worked principally on the serotonin system came out in the late 1980s, it was a drug in search of a disease, a disease that became known as a "chemical imbalance." Since the medical community prefers to think in terms of *diseases* rather than behavior, it has become popular to speak of depression, anxiety, OCD and other mental health diagnoses as diseases of the serotonin or other neurotransmitter systems.

It is true there is no *proof* of serotonin depletion in the depressed patient, or if there was, that the "depression" was *caused* by the serotonin depletion; nevertheless, psychiatrists were quick to say depression was a biological disease. Psychiatrists were pleased because they could now treat patients in just the same way as their medical colleagues — make a diagnosis of organic disease and treat it with drugs.

Even if it were shown that there were some brain change or brain "abnormality" associated with depression, there remains the question of whether this change is a *cause* or an effect of the "depression." At least one brain-scan study found that simply asking normal people to *imagine* or recall a negative situation would make them feel sad and resulted in significant changes in blood flow in the brain (Pardo, Jose V. et al., 1993).

The Biological Marker Hope

Psychiatry's hopes were temporarily raised fifteen or so years ago when a lab test seemingly identified a *biological* marker for depression. Prior to that supposed marker all mental disorders were diagnosed through the patient's behavior, whether schizophrenia, depression, dependent personality, or others.

Psychiatrists believed that with this *biological* marker they now had a lab test to diagnose depression, a test that supposedly picked up an excessive amount of a stress hormone (cortisol) in the blood. The test is called the Dexamethasone-Suppression Test or DST; although once very popular, the DST is no longer in use except for a few psychiatrists who refuse to compromise their belief in the biology of depression. However, the theory behind this test and the claims of its usefulness were found to be mistaken since "so many patients with well-defined depressive illness have normal DSTs" (Anderson, Nancy, 1984). Similarly, in an Archives of Internal Medicine article, three physicians concluded: "Data from studies currently available do not support the use of the Dexamethasone Suppression Test" (Shapiro, M., et. al., 1983).

I suppose the thought was to diagnose *sub-clinical* depressions and treat these patients with antidepressants *before* a full-blown depression emerged. Perhaps the marker would also confirm the clinical diagnosis of depression, which might help to convince the patient to take *and stay on* antidepressant medication.

Everyday Mood Problems? A Slippery Slope

Both the psychiatrist and the non-psychiatric physician believe that, if there could be a pharmaceutical solution for (well-diagnosed) clinical depression, why not the *same* solution for everyday mood problems that all of us are subjected to, mood problems that do not reach the level of diagnosable depression? That is, if depression *is* a chemical imbalance in the brain (the drug treatment view) then why *couldn't* the everyday mood problems be *minor* chemical imbalances that might also be subject to the same pharmaceutical solution (i.e., an SSRI antidepressant)? The answer of course is it *could be* and on such a hope we have seen a large industry grow into what might be described as the "medicalization" of almost all psychological problems. Now probably 60 to 70% of patients on antidepressants do *not* have a diagnosable depression—and these drugs do not have FDA approval for such populations. There is no scientific evidence to justify the use of these drugs in this way. It is true there is a *theory*, but a theory is not evidence.

Thus far there have been *no* antidepressant drug clinical trials submitted to the FDA for patients with stress and mood problems that fall short of *diagnosable* depression or anxiety. Despite this lack of evidence these drugs *are routinely prescribed* to such persons. Presently physicians prescribe these drugs for minor stress and mood problems under off-label use.

Defining Clinical Depression

I am limiting the discussion of depression to *unipolar* depression because of its prevalence. In the Diagnostic and Statistical Manual of Mental Health Disorders (DSM-IV™) the depressive disorders are divided into Major Depressive Disorder, Dysthymic Disorder and Depressive Disorder Not Otherwise Specified. The latter two are differentiated from Major Depression (which is one of the psychotic disorders) on severity, chronicity, and persistence. I will focus on Major Depressive Disorder (MDD). In MDD, unlike the temporarily down moods of most of us, the depressed mood must be present for most of the day, nearly every day, for a period of *at least two weeks*. I mention the duration of the mood disturbance because all antidepressant trials require the patient meet these and other diagnostic criteria.

Despite the fact that all depression is self-limiting (i.e. it goes away in time), depression is one of the most important health problems we have today. It is destructive of what is most human about us, our health and well-being, our ability to be productive and creative, innovative, to laugh, to feel optimistic, to enjoy a full range of pleasure and enjoyment in our relationships with others. First, depression is *real* and devastating to the individual, those around the depressed person, and society as a whole. Clinical depression – the failure to diagnose it and the failure to treat it effectively – is one of the major causes of our high and escalating health care costs. It is a very serious health care problem, and it is, perhaps, second to stress in its impact on society.

<u>MDD Symptoms</u>

To be diagnosed MDD according to the DSM-IV™, the patient must have *five* or more of the following (Diagnostic and Statistical Manual of Mental Disorders, 4th edition, 1994):

(1) depressed mood most of the day, every day,

(2) diminished interest or pleasure in all, or almost all activities most of the day,

(3) significant weight loss when not dieting or weight gain (a change of more than 5% of body weight in a month),

(4) insomnia or increased sleep nearly every day,

(5) agitation or slowing of thinking/behavior nearly every day,

(6) fatigue nearly every day,

(7) feelings of worthlessness or excessive or inappropriate guilt nearly every day,

(8) impaired ability to think or concentrate, or difficulty making decisions nearly every day, and

(9) recurrent thoughts of death or recurrent suicidal thoughts.

At least *one* of the five symptoms the MDD patient has must include either (1) depressed mood or (2) loss of interest or pleasure.

As one can see from the above symptoms, depression affects almost all areas of the patient's life and the patient's ability to master the demands of everyday living. From reading the above, one might think that the diagnosis of depression is a fairly simple task, but it is not. PCPs fail to diagnose 50% of their patients with depression, and the same physicians frequently diagnose depression when it is *not* present. A number of hysterics unconsciously *play* a depressed *role* rather than *being* depressed and others may be consciously assuming the role of a depressed person for financial or other secondary gain. Psychiatrists, unlike psychologists, are generally limited to the interview, clinical history or consultation with family members to make a diagnosis. The diagnosis is made from the patient's behavior (self-reported behavior and the reports of others at times) and nothing but the patient's behavior.

Life and Psychological Tests Correlate

Psychologists have an advantage over psychiatrists in diagnosis because we can observe the patient's behavior not only in daily life but also their behavior on standardized psychological tests. If the patient *were* depressed in daily life (or behavior), the patient would also be expected to behave "depressed" on relevant psychological tests. If a patient *were* schizophrenic in everyday life, the patient would be expected to behave "schizophrenic" on certain psychological tests. In both cases we would not anticipate an exact parallel between behavior and life and behavior on tests, since the latter is only a *sampling* of behavior and the psychological test is probably less demanding than real life.

If there is evidence (self-report or observation) of fatigue, low energy, slowness in thinking, etc. in the person's *behavior* in real life, then these same symptoms would be anticipated in the depressed person's *behavior* on psychological tests. Let's take the Rorschach or inkblot test as an example. Patient A and patient B during interview and clinical history may both be diagnosable as MDD, but let's look at their differential responses (percepts) on the same inkblot. Let's also say A and B are similar in intelligence (since IQ is correlated with many aspects of Rorschach behavior). Patient A, on one card/blot, gives a "bat," and, after encouragement by the examiner, gives "an empty glass." Patient B, who seems equally depressed in his *behavior*, gives four responses including "circus bears performing tricks" and a "Matisse nude in a colorful boudoir."

Patient A's Rorschach responses are *consistent* with a diagnosis of unipolar depression, but patient B's Rorschach responses are simply incompatible with unipolar depression. We would have to look elsewhere than depression to account for patient

B's "depressive" behavior during the interview and his *non-depressed* behavior in his response to the Rorschach. Why? There might have been poverty of thought in patient B's interview behavior clinically, but there was certainly no lessening of patient B's richness of thought on the test.

Self-Limiting Depression and Victimhood Treatment

All depression is self-limiting, that is, assuming the depressed person does not commit suicide, depression goes away in time whether or not the patient receives any treatment. When you hear that person A has been continuously depressed for twenty years, you know that factors *other* than depression are operating in the patient. If it is a *primary* depression, it goes away without treatment, and if the patient receives *effective* treatment, recovery occurs sooner rather than later and future depressive episodes are reduced. It is probably much more difficult for depressed patients to get over their depression when they are exposed to poor or inadequate drug or psychological treatment or both than if the depressed patient were left alone and not exposed to treatment of any kind.

Psychiatric or psychological approaches that support "victimhood" make it difficult for the depressed patient to get over depression. Telling someone he or she has a chemical imbalance is underwriting victimhood as much as telling them their depression was caused by bad mothering or by being sexually molested as a child.

Poor Diagnostic Understanding, Poor Treatment

The following examples demonstrate that a diagnosis of depression is not as simple as it might appear despite what general physicians seem to say.

Manipulative Depression

There is a sizeable group of persons who show up to their physician, psychiatrist, or psychologist offices with what "appears" to be a depression, but the "depression" is not a "real" depression. It takes good clinical skill to be able to make a correct diagnosis in these cases, and with a correct diagnosis, both drugs and cognitive therapy with these patients are doomed from the start. These people *are* unhappy and wear their "depression" as a badge, but the "depression" is designed primarily to make significant others meet their needs. The "depression" may represent the message: "You are not doing right by me, you are not taking care of me, and I want you to." The "message" will vary in each person, but all *pseudodepressions* must be recognized if there is to be any hope of providing effective treatment for these persons. Psychologists have to be very alert to pseudodepressions to make the difficult, but important diagnosis. Although conscientious, hyperresponsible persons are more subject to depression than others, in this pseudodepressive group we hear too much *other* blaming for it to be a "real" depression.

Deliberately Falsifying

In my work of reviewing mental health care, I have occasionally been asked by an employer client to look into a long-term disability case to give some possible direction to be considered in the disabled employee's recovery. Based upon my experience in these cases, which were obviously selected for my advice rather than strictly *random* cases, there is a very high incidence of malingering.

Playing a Role - John

John was a patient who had been on disability for six years for a so-called major depression. From a close reading of his psychiatric history (a schoolteacher with a history of an alcohol problem), I believed there was some kind of a personality disorder involved. This was not just a failure to respond to treatment, and this was not a primary depression. John had been on a variety of antidepressant medications without positive benefit. He had been on lithium (just in case he was bipolar), several antipsychotic medications (there was no history of psychosis), several antianxiety drugs, etc., all without any improvement.

On a note to the disability insurance carrier, the psychiatrist said that this was one of the *worst* cases of depression he had ever seen and that John's only hope was that the pharmaceutical industry would one day develop a new antidepressant drug that would effectively treat his patient's depression! This psychiatrist, although very intelligent and of sound mind, had bought the biologically based view of depression so much that he failed to look at his patient. He was blind to the inconsistencies in the patient's history and current behavior that were *not* compatible with a clinical depression.

I later found John was consciously *playing a role* of a depressed patient. He was no more depressed than the psychiatrist. John had a pretty good life. He was receiving disability payments he didn't deserve. He no longer had to deal with authority figures in his daily life. He had a good rationalization for his failures in life. He had a great deal of sympathy from his psychiatrist on a continuing basis.

Next to lower back pain, chronic depression is the *second* leading cause of vocational disability. I fail to understand why a physician would *ever* tell even a genuinely depressed patient not to work. What can make one more depressed than staying home everyday and not being productive, not working? One must keep the depressed patient as active and productive as he or she can be within the limits of the severity of the depression at the moment.

The Taj Mahal

In Karl's case, I reviewed treatment notes on a worker's compensation case with a diagnosis of chronic depression following a job injury (Karl fell from a scaffold and hit his head). Both a psychiatrist (with drugs) and a psychologist with what the psychologist described as "cognitive behavioral therapy" (CBT) were treating the patient. My diagnostic antenna was out because the patient had been off work for two years. He was, if anything, getting worse rather than better, and all things being equal as a depressed person he *should* be getting better. He described typical and continuing depressive symptoms such as low energy, impaired concentration, insomnia, and severe fatigue, etc. In reading the treatment notes I discovered that in the midst of his chronic depression Karl, a concrete finisher, was building and had completed a miniature Taj Mahal out of concrete, a creative pursuit that was completely incompatible with the impairments that arises from clinical depression.

A severe depression is simply *not* compatible with having the mental energy, self-confidence, concentration and creativity to carry out such a project even if the physical work had been done by others. Depression erodes all of one's independent and creative powers. When depressed it is difficult to rise above one's self-doubt and indecision to carry out even everyday life demands and a creative challenge that requires innovative and imaginative thinking such as this "depressed" patient demonstrated is incompatible with depression.

Because of this incompatibility, I drew a conclusion of conscious malingering or deliberate falsifying of a depression for disability payments. When I confronted the psychologist and psychiatrist with my doubts about the genuineness of Karl's depression, both professionals defended their diagnosis and rationalized Karl's seeming energy by saying he had gotten the neighbors to do the actual physical work. It is hard to believe that these professionals could have been so clinically naïve and to have been so taken in by their patient.

Impaired Individuals Need Their Mental Powers

Stress and mood problems, including full-blown anxiety and depression often occur with any serious injury to a breadwinner. The stress or anxiety associated with the injury has powerful adverse effects on the recovery process. Impaired individuals attempting to cope with the fear over their bodily injury and altered physical and social status need all of their remaining mental powers to meet adaptive challenges. Therefore, mental health drugs should be avoided because of the cognitive impairing side effects of these drugs.

Behavioral therapy already has effective *behavioral* treatments for the problems of anxiety and depression whether or not the patient has a physical injury. These techniques and treatments are and should be rendered *without* accompanying drug impairment of brain tissue for the patient recovering from the injury/disability. Behavioral interventions by a trained professional (a psychologist) is needed to help impaired workers learn to manage their stress (fear) and mood problems and promote a return to a productive life.

There is a large group of very poorly treated work injury patients. The treatment is poor because general physicians in their desire to help their patient deal with the stress and mood problems secondary to an injury overuse these medications. I would estimate that more than one-half of workers' compensation patients are prescribed psychotropic drugs despite the lack of any evidence that these drugs assist the recovery process. These drugs are being given off-label since most workers' compensation cases would not meet diagnostic criteria for either depression or an anxiety disorder.

In worker's compensation injuries, quality *medical* treatment of the tissue damage is mandatory. Unfortunately, rather than physicians rendering circumscribed care, we have a "medicalization" of the total rehabilitative and recovery process, which often compounds the major cost and quality problem in many worker's compensation cases.

There are important personality, psychological, and family factors that are critical in the patient's rehabilitation. Often, there is no attempt to address these factors directly except through general medical care and drug treatment. The problems that disabled workers have when they are injured – fear, the loss or jeopardy of a major life role and changed relationships – are complex and multidimensional and the thought that a pill would cure these problems is at best naïve.

Depression as Learned Helplessness

This theory of depression as learned helplessness (Seligman, M, 1992) came about in the late 1960s and 1970s through the animal research of the psychologist, Martin Seligman, and colleagues (Seligman, 1968). Learned helplessness may be defined as a *learned* state produced by exposure to noxious, unpleasant situations in which there is no possibility of escape or avoidance. In the original studies rats (and in later studies other animals and then humans) were traumatized by being placed in a noxious situation in which there was no escape. In the rat studies the rats received a shock no matter what the animal did or did not do. Normal, non-traumatized rats in such situations learn to *avoid* the shock by jumping over a barrier when a signal appears (a light, for example). At least 1/3 of traumatized rats, those that had no control over the noxious stimulus, failed to learn an avoidance response (jumping over a barrier) to the signal *even when conditions changed* and they could escape by jumping the barrier in response to the signal and thus avoid the punishment. The *learned helplessness* rats continued to do nothing (they seemingly gave up) and continued to receive the punishing electric shock.

The *learned helplessness* model of depression has much merit. Mood and depressive problems tend to have snowballing effects. The mood problem and its associated thoughts or affects (despair, pessimism) result in *decreased* activity. When activity is curtailed we are removed from pleasurable activities (called competence-engendering) that give a feeling of confidence and self-esteem. When we are cut off from what psychologists refer to as "self-reinforcing" behaviors, despair and discouragement increases, activity further declines and the depression is deepened.

Removing Learned Helplessness

Depressed people stop responding and therefore remove themselves from any positive reinforcement or possibility of solving their problems. Even before the advent of cognitive therapy, the whole key to treating the depressed person successfully was to help the depressed person to become more active, to find more positive reinforcement in their daily life. Telling a seriously depressed person to just "get with it" or to just "do something about it" will not work because the patient will only have a greater sense of failure and a greater sense of helplessness will evolve.

As in cognitive therapy, also an ahistorical approach (we did not take the depressed patient back to their childhood), the patient is given gradual reintroduction of positively reinforcing behaviors that are doable for the patient given the current state of the patient's depression. The patient contracts with the therapist to do some things before the next session (e.g., write a brief note to a friend). However, the demand (request) must be neither too much, in which case the patient would fail and get more depressed, or too little, which would not be sufficiently positively reinforcing. The therapist must request behavior or activity that would be emotionally gratifying or pleasurable to the patient given the *patient's* level of depression.

Prior Behavior Important

To find out what behavior to induce, we must look to the patient's adjustment and behavior *prior* to his/her depression to find out what behaviors to re-institute in the patient's life. In the hands of a skilled clinician this was and is a very effective way of treating depression, although in retrospect the relapse rate was probably somewhat high because the patient's tools were very limited in preventing the return of another episode. Cognitive therapy, unlike this earlier treatment approach, challenges or modifies, when applicable, the patient's maladaptive beliefs and attitudes in a systematic way, which gives the patient tools to resist future bouts of depression.

The learned helplessness model shows why a therapy such as emotional support would be ineffective at best and counterproductive at worst. In my behavioral management experience I have seen many treatable depressed patients stay the same or get worse on a combination of pharmacotherapy and supportive therapy. At the very least the patient needs encouragement for engaging in *productive* pleasurable activities once again. Sympathy alone only reinforces helplessness.

<u>Bonnie</u>

For instance, Bonnie had weekly medication visits with a psychiatrist for six years and weekly "therapy" sessions with a clinical social worker with no improvement over the six years. Listening to her phone call, I learned that her engineer husband of many years had a habit of ridiculing her when the couple was in social situations. This was a key item of information that gave me an insight into the patient's personality and her maladaptive way of relating to others. Her core problem was *not* a chemical imbalance; it was her passive submissive approaches in response to her husband's actions. Trying to change people's disrespectful conduct toward her by being nice and doing for others was not working for Bonnie. She continued to be depressed.

I gave Bonnie feedback about what I believed to be her core problem, not asserting her right to be treated with respect. I referred her to a social worker for reinforcement of the knowledge that she had rights equal to others and to teach her how to be normally assertive toward her husband. Bonnie's previous treatment reinforced her passive, helpless, victim role. What she needed was the encouragement to take charge of her life and her behavior. Her assumption of an active role worked against her depression and was the cure for *her* depression.

<u>Why?</u>

It was not enough to know that Bonnie *was* depressed. The diagnosis itself does not tell us what we should or could do for her or for any depressed person for that matter. We needed to know why *she* was depressed and when we knew the answer to that we had a rational treatment plan. We need to know why *this* woman is depressed and we need to know what core difficulty is feeding the depression. We need to have a *definitive* understanding of this person's depression, which requires the services of a *trained* expert in human behavior and mental disorder.

Phyllis

For example, to say that Phyllis is depressed because her husband of twenty-five years, Marty, died a year ago is no explanation. To find out why Phyllis is depressed we are going to have to get to know her, her mental make-up, her history, her relationship with Marty, her current life, her needs and fears. This can often be done in one or two sessions. Let us look at some plausible explanations that *might* account for Phyllis's depression.

1. Phyllis had been totally dependent on Marty and now it is as if she is adrift at sea. She needs help to learn ways to manage her life more independently, perhaps learning to drive, paying the bills, starting a social life, etc. As she acquires these skills she will become less depressed, or
2. Marty's death was difficult for Phyllis not so much for the loss (she responded with normal grief), but because through it she was smacked in the face by her *own* mortality. She had never before dealt with this in herself, and she is at a loss to deal with her own mortality, or
3. Phyllis is depressed by Marty's death because, after a twenty-five year relationship with him, she does not have a genuine feeling of loss and this scares her and she wonders what kind of person she is, or
4. Phyllis is depressed by Marty's death whom she loved because at a life choice point she married rather than pursuing a career in advertising. Since Marty's death she no longer has responsibility for another person and she is completely free to follow her own needs and wants. This complete freedom scares her and she is depressed.

Endogenous Depressions

Some psychiatrists in reading the above would argue my point and say, "What about endogenous depressions?" Depressions have been grouped into *reactive depressions*, i.e., those that arise as a consequence for an adverse life event or events (perhaps the death of a spouse, e.g.) and so called *endogenous* depressions that do not seem to be triggered by *any* external event. Psychiatrists love the term endogenous depression, which seems to support their belief that depression is a *biological* disease and must be treated with drugs. Many psychiatrists say that some *reactive* depressions *can* be effectively treated with psychotherapy alone but an endogenous depression requires drug treatment.

The latter belief is very much alive in psychiatry today. However, there is simply no substance to this myth since cognitive therapy is effective whether the depression is "reactive" or "endogenous." The term itself may be invalid because most "endogenous" depressions are a result of triggering events when one is sufficiently clinically skillful to discover it. Moreover, in some of these so-called endogenous depressions, the patient's dysfunctional patterns of thinking are fueling the depression and should be the primary focus in CBT rather than the patient's environment or relationships.

Content-Free Depression

For a number of years many mental health care professionals used the term "content-free depression." A patient was obviously depressed, but questioning could not elicit any current or past thoughts of a depressing nature. The content free depressed person did not report any ongoing depressive thoughts such as suicidal ideation, guilt, etc. The patients would report a feeling of physical malaise (low energy, impaired sleep and the like) but they would deny any *mental* content of a depressive quality. No doubt some of these endogenous depressions are similar to this content free group.

I tend to see these content-free depressed patients as having, in addition to a depression, a hysterical personality make-up. Hysterics are characterized by an over reliance on repression and denial in relating to conflict and dealing with their social world. The hysteric's ability to dissociate emotion from the corresponding mental content is a process that could be operating in some of these content-free depressions; some of these "depressions" may be "real" and others not. Some hysterics *can* become depressed.

Complexity of Diagnosis – Understanding the Patient Sets the Course

Even though there are *symptoms* of depression that are common to all depressed persons, before we can begin to treat it, we need to determine how and why depression arises in *this* particular person. What is it about *this* person, his or her history, personality make-up, patterns of thinking and current life difficulties/stress that give rise to *this* depression. Seeing depression in this way says it is something *more* than a biological disease and implies that *psychosocial* factors are critical in both the understanding and treatment of depression. Therefore, I recommend intervention by a well trained specialist.

<u>Jeopardy</u>

When I was on call one night a thirty-year-old male from Detroit wanted to be hospitalized for depression secondary to girlfriend and on-the-job problems. The day of Philip's call his supervisor had been very critical of his work performance. He described a litany of symptoms often characterized as depression, but in the midst of reporting these depressive symptoms, he announced: "And I used to be a whiz at the TV game show Jeopardy, but now I can't do it anymore."

This last observation, and the way he reported it, did not fit a depression, so I asked, "Have you ever had a head injury?" It was not that he could not *enjoy* watching the TV show anymore; what he was implying was that he no longer had enough "smarts" to handle the cognitive demands of the game show. In response to my question about a head injury, he said he had been knocked out in an automobile accident eight months ago, but he was told his brain was all right. He had been given a CT Scan in the hospital to rule out any bleeding in the brain— but this test does not pick up the microscopic brain lesions that occur in the vast majority of traumatic brain injuries and Philip demonstrated consequences of a brain trauma.

Philip was experiencing cognitive deficits from his head injury, probably in the more executive functions such as organization, planning, judgment and flexibility of thinking. I deduced the latter was true because he was reporting difficulty in both his job and in his relationship with his fiancée, both of which require complex problem solving skills. He probably was diagnosable as clinically depressed, but neither drugs nor cognitive therapy would be appropriate for his "depression." I explained to him what I suspected was going on in his depression and adjustment difficulties and referred him to a clinical neuropsychologist for diagnosis and help in mastering work and relationship demands.

Gerrie Had Lost Eight Pounds in the Past Six Months Unrelated to Diet.

Gerrie, with a husband of six years and two small children, called with concern over unhappiness and an unwanted and unexplained eight-pound weight loss over the past six months. She was employed and felt overwhelmed by her job and household and mothering duties. Her physician had put her on Prozac a few months ago with no apparent effect. It was possible that she was diagnosable as clinically depressed, especially in view of the eight-pound weight loss. She was concerned that she might have some *physical* problems to account for the weight loss.

As she talked about her life, it became apparent that her depression was reactive to problems in her marriage. Her husband was mentally abusive on the weekends when he was drinking (he used to drink beer nightly but went to only drinking beer on weekends on his wife's insistence) and he claimed loss of memory for his periods of mental abuse. To her credit Gerrie did not let him touch her sexually when he was drinking. I thought it was positive that she could set and enforce some limits on her husband's drinking behavior.

During the first of our two telephone consultations she said that her husband had not been *physically* abusive toward her. I concluded from her reports that her husband's behavior manifested a diagnosis as an alcoholic, which was a surprise to Gerrie. Beyond this he had character shortcomings that would make it difficult for him to participate in a mature, equal, and mutually give and take relationship. The patient and not the "therapist" has to be responsible for all the important decisions in the patient's life, because the patient and not the *professional* will experience the *consequences* of those life decisions. However, at the same time the professional has a duty to give informed opinions on matters of concern to the patient *on the basis of current but often far from complete information on the issue in question.* Gerrie's husband did not show a favorable prognosis. There was a likelihood the alcoholic husband would react physically and abusively if she placed reasonable demands on him. I suggested she receive counseling for herself and gave her a referral to a psychologist whose practice included work with alcoholics and families of alcoholics.

Gerrie called me again a week later and informed me that her husband *had* been physically abusive to her on a recent occasion. Her husband had implied that *she* was largely to blame for the abusive episode. Fortunately, the husband's attempt to place the blame on his wife for the abuse did not work. Gerrie had him remove himself from the home.

Does Gerrie Have a Disease?

According to the biologically-based theory of depression, Gerrie not only has a disease, but she also has a chronically relapsing disease (even though this is her first and only episode of depression thus far). In looking at Gerrie, a psychologist must decide if Gerrie is an emotionally normal person with serious depressive symptomology or a woman caught up in a bad marital situation with an alcoholic. Does this woman need information and guidance or does she need treatment? Certainly it is very normal for a person like Gerrie caught up in such a distressing situation to react with such distressing symptoms. Does she need to get out of such an unhappy situation to be free of symptoms, or does she have to learn ways to better cope with her life without depressive symptoms, or does her head (better yet her thinking and attitudes) need to be examined—by a cognitive therapist? There is a tendency for lay persons (and unfortunately many mental health professionals) to over-pathologize normal behavior, that is, to see something about a person as representing something *pathological* rather than something that *may* be a part of normal behavior.

Many people, seeing Gerrie and her situation, might think she was masochistic in the Freudian sense and would need therapy to resolve this before she could function in a "normal" marital relationship. Many women get caught in these unfulfilling marital relationships, but is this due to their inherent pathology? Or does this reflect an outcome derived from the "normal" rearing of many females in our culture? I am not sure in Gerrie's case (this is one reason why I referred her to a psychologist), but I believe her need is for *counseling* to deal with a bad situation rather than "therapy" to correct intrapsychic problems. Counseling rather than therapy may be needed because she took charge of her life previously when she refused her husband sexually when he was drinking and, when he physically abused her, she ordered him from the house. With Gerrie and others this is an important distinction to make between behavior that is pathological or "normal." All too often many people (including many mental health professionals) err on the side of overestimating a pathological origin to a part of what may be normal behavior.

If we are treating non-existent pathology we are doing just that, treating something that isn't there. Of course we can also err on the other side, that is, seeing something as "normal" when indeed it is not. My point is that many things are not as simple as they often appear and persons making these clinical judgments about people should be very thoroughly and broadly trained *behavioral health* professionals.

<u>Do We Need to Know What Depression is to Treat it?</u>

We certainly do not have to know the cause of a variety of health conditions to be able to treat them competently. Often effective treatment of a condition, disease or other is established empirically, that is, we have found a treatment works, although we are not sure *why* it works. Even though we certainly do not know everything about depression that we would like to know, we do know enough to know how to treat it. The *indiscriminate* use of cognitive therapy is not the answer for all depressions, since cognitive therapy is not appropriate treatment for *some* depressions. As we have seen, the diagnosis of depression is not sufficient in itself to determine what treatment is appropriate for *this* depressed person. We need to understand why depression has come about in *this* depressed person, how does the depression fit in with the person's personality structure, history, current life situation and the conflicts-demands he or she is facing? We try to find out the *crux* of the problem and have our treatment address it.

The Confusion between Unhappiness and Depression

People tend to confuse unhappiness with depression. Not all unhappy people are depressed, but perhaps it is safe to say that depressed people are unhappy. Unhappiness is a broader term and, conceivably, an acute bout of unhappiness (e.g., failure to get a desired promotion) *could* work its way to a full depression in *certain* people but not others. Often people become unhappy when they do not get something that they want, especially if they feel as if they *deserve* or are entitled to have what they want. When their response is anger or other-blaming rather than self-blaming, these people are not likely to be on the road to depression. The difference has most to do with the mental make-up of the person — those who are over-conscientious, hyperresponsible, and have a tendency to blame themselves are at greater risk for developing depression. For instance, I think the school shooters are much more other-blaming than self-blaming, although these shooters are often incorrectly considered to be depressed.

Husband Murders Ex-Wife, Children, Then Commits Suicide.

Unfortunately the above headline is not a rare event in American society today. Most people think the husband and father in the above case must have committed such acts in the throes of a severe depression. Not so. Here is a case of confusing *unhappiness* with *depression*. We had an unhappy and angry man but not a *depressed* man. If we had gotten him on Prozac, or cognitive therapy, before the act, it would have made no difference. But one might say: "But what about his suicide, didn't that prove he was depressed?" No, not in the least! It is true the risk of suicide is substantially higher in depressed people, but all suicides do *not* arise from depression, this example being a case in point. By killing himself the husband-killer avoids going through the consequences of his acts, that is, a life of imprisonment, which is not very compatible with anyone with an inner feeling of entitlement. The murderous acts may have been precipitated by a loss of control initiated by his wife's leaving him, but in his last moments his murderous acts, including the murder of himself, restores his complete dominance over his world. A depressed person does not feel in control of his world.

A corollary of the biologically-based belief is that depression is not only simple to treat (an appropriate pill), but it is also very easy to diagnose by any physician. This belief exists although we'll find that general physicians continue to fail to diagnose it 50% of the time. Rather than a chemical imbalance, clinical depression differs only in *degree* and not *kind* from the more minor mood problems of everyday life. Depression does not resemble the pathophysiological characteristics of a disease. To try to make it into a brain disease is reductionist at best. It does a disservice to the complexity of depression as a *biopsychosocial* disorder to think that it is a simple disorder that can be treated effectively with a drug alone.

CHAPTER II

STRESS/ANXIETY: ONE ROAD OR TWO?

"I always thought I was just a worrier. I'd feel keyed up and unable to relax. At times it would come and go, and at times it would be constant. It could go on for days. I'd worry about what I was going to fix for a dinner party, or what would be a great present for somebody. I just couldn't let something go."

"I'd have terrible sleeping problems. There were times I'd wake up wired in the morning or in the middle of the night. I had trouble concentrating, even reading the newspaper or a novel. Sometimes I'd feel a little lightheaded. My heart would race or pound. And that would make me worry more."

Depression gets the majority of media attention, but problems of stress/anxiety are more prevalent in society today, touch more people in their daily lives, and probably have a much greater devastating effect on health status than problems of mood/depression. Again, by using the designation of stress/anxiety as with mood/depression in Chapter I, I am saying that there is *one* continuum in each disorder. The diagnosable anxiety disorders differ in *degree* but not in *kind* from the stress to which all humans are subject.

There is more than a moot difference between viewing anxiety disorders as *diseases* versus extremes of what is found in normal human behavior. We have in the latter a *continuum* and in the former, the view of anxiety as a disease, a *discontinuum* that appears when the anxiety reaches diagnosable proportions à la the DSM-IV™ (*The Diagnostic and Statistical Manual of Mental Disorders, 1994*).

Fear and Anxiety—Normal

Physiologically, when we know what fear is, we know what anxiety is. Fear is anxiety and anxiety is fear when it comes to bodily reactions. We do not have to go to college to know fear (anxiety). It is a part of being human and since we have survived these 100 thousand years with fear, we know that fear *must* be adaptive. It is true most of us do not like it, it is very unpleasant, but we simply cannot get along without it. It is a signal for danger and our body prepares itself to deal with the danger.

When is it "Irrational"?

Those who want to make anxiety into a disease will quickly point out that there *is* a big difference between a normal fear reaction (a bear about to attack us) and the Obsessive Compulsive shaking with an irrational fear of being contaminated with germs as he thinks of grasping a doorknob. The former is rational ("It makes sense to be afraid when we see a bear about to attack us.") and the latter "irrational." However, does the *irrationality* make the fear of contamination into a disease?

The "proponent" of anxiety as a disease says, of course, "Yes, it is a disease if we fear that we will be contaminated by touching a door knob." However, such reasoning implies that normal people do *not* engage in irrational thinking or irrational behavior, and I think it would be very difficult for our psychiatric brethren to convince us that normal people do not engage in irrational thinking or irrational behavior. Moreover, what is so irrational about the obsessive-compulsive's fear of touching a doorknob? Actually he or she is right; there *are* germs on doorknobs and we can and *do* get the flu and other diseases from them.

I am no more obsessive-compulsive than most people are (actually, anyone who gets through graduate school has to be obsessive-compulsive to some degree). I am a little skittish about touching the inside doorknob of a public rest room door and will make as little contact with the door handle as possible. Does this mean I have a disease? Or even that my behavior is irrational? My caution with public rest room door handles does not interfere with my life in any way. Even if fears *do* interfere with a person's life to a restricting or disabling degree, does their condition imply that they have a disease? The anxiety may be so disabling or so restricting in the person's life that he or she may and should do something about the fear; in the same way if we broke our leg, we would want it fixed.

Genetic and Constitutional Factors

We know that there are important genetic and constitutional factors involved in how individuals deal with risk and pending danger in their lives. Others might consider some "fearless," but this is not because these people are oblivious to the danger or to their fearful response. These persons have a high tolerance for risk compared to shy or timid individuals who withdraw at even the slightest surge of adrenaline. There is no doubt that these two hypothetical persons are genetically opposed in make-up and will behave quite differently in their lives despite whatever environmental or rearing factors they were exposed to in their development.

Psychiatry stresses these genetic factors more than psychologists, and psychologists put more stress on the environmental and rearing factors involved in fear behavior. Psychology, however, is a biological *and* a social science, and to understand most complex human behavior requires an understanding of both dimensions. Certainly fear is one such complex human behavior.

Psychologists, not discounting the importance of biology in fear, realize that learning plays a vital role not only in how we respond to fear-engendering situations but in how we respond to novel situations of any kind. Our internal wiring is not the only thing that makes us respond fearfully; there are also powerful environmental, rearing, cultural and gender factors that operate in fearful behaviors. These factors provide powerful effects on how we respond to fear-provoking situations. Early fearful trauma, irrespective of how the person is programmed, sensitizes the individual in later fear or anxiety-provoking situations.

Some children are very timid in novel situations while others respond more boldly to them, and psychologists attribute such individual differences to both *nature* and *nurture*. Much of this type of emotional learning, psychologists believe, occurs on the basis of *modeling* others in our environment. Lori as a child was told by her mother never to run with a lollipop in her mouth because if she fell she could be hurt. I was never told this as a child and, in fact, I did disobey the "rule" but never came to harm. Lori, a psychologist, is very good at treating anxious patients, perhaps partly as a result of her *empathetic* ability with these patients, her ability to understand their struggles against their fearfulness.

There are probably male-female differences in how we respond to novel and fear-arousing situations. However, environment is important. Remember that, except perhaps for recent years, females more than males have been reared in more protective environments that stressed safety and less risk taking. Perhaps because of this differential gender rearing, women are more likely to be diagnosed with an anxiety disorder than men. Since this is the case, would our psychiatrist colleagues tell us that women have the *disease* more often than men? I do not think the concept of anxiety as a disease is either useful or supported by the facts.

If we can explain the known facts quite well without the disease concept, that there is only *one* dimension of anxiety and the diagnosable kind of anxiety differs in degree and not kind from the milder forms, there is no need to bring in the concept of disease to separate the severe form from normal fear-anxiety. The simple fact that psychiatrists treat anxiety with drugs does not make anxiety a disease. Psychologists (and the anxiety outcome literature as a whole) seem to do quite well in treating anxiety behaviorally and without drugs. Drugs *do* provide temporary relief; they mask and lower sympathetic nervous system arousal. However, drugs certainly do *not* address the *causes* of anxiety. As with depression, anxiety is caused by *biopsychosocial* factors and the cure comes from emotional re-learning or re-education.

When we speak of irrational anxiety there are always stimulus-response connections that were acquired and, once learned, these cues or stimuli trigger the anxiety. Moreover, these connections are never unlearned by themselves. Although the person may spend a life-time avoiding whatever it is that makes him or her anxious (e.g., getting on an elevator), the anxiety will return as strongly as ever if the person is again placed in the feared stimulus situation.

<u>Only Way</u>

The only way for the unlearning of the anxiety to occur is for the person to allow himself to be placed in or confronted with the feared stimulus and learn a *new* response (e.g., relaxation) to the anxiety-arousing stimulus situation. This process of emotional relearning is referred to in anxiety treatment as counterconditioning. A simple example is Pavlov's dog who learned to salivate at the sound of a bell (the conditioned stimulus); after the bell had been paired with the appearance of food (the unconditioned stimulus), a dog salivates automatically (the conditional response) when the bell is presented. After the conditioned response became quite strong, the food was no longer paired with the bell and the conditioned response (salivating at the sound of the bell) would finally extinguish. A stimulus-response connection had been formed and the connection was unlearned through the process of *extinction*.

In treating anxiety it is helpful when we know the cues eliciting anxiety (touching a doorknob, not checking four times that the stove has been turned off). Still, even when cues are *not* readily apparent, such as in Generalized Anxiety

Disorder (GAD), we can treat it with the same techniques as those used when stimulus-response anxiety connections are known or suspected.

Fear has a gradient; as we get closer to the feared object, the level of anxiety increases, and conversely the anxiety *declines* in intensity as we put distance between the feared object and ourselves. Our desire to avoid increases in intensity as we come closer to the feared object, and avoidance declines with distance from the feared stimulus. If there are positive as well as negative aspects of the feared stimulus (going on an airplane to enjoy a trip in Hawaii), the individual is caught up in a normal approach-avoidance conflict. As long as avoidance rules the day the anxiety is never mastered and the fear never abates.

Fear restricts our mobility. When mobility is severely compromised, *mood* can be affected, which is one reason why anxiety often accompanies depression. This relationship can also occur the other way; anxiety can arise secondary to the consequences of a mood problem. In such cases the clinician's task is to determine which is the more fundamental problem, anxiety or depression, and direct treatment to the more fundamental disorder.

Autonomic Nervous System

The key to understanding stress and anxiety is to have some appreciation of the structure and function of the *autonomic* nervous system, the part of the nervous and hormonal system that is involved in emotion.

The autonomic nervous system is divided into two main divisions. The *parasympathetic* system is associated with the more *pleasant* emotional and bodily feeling states. The *sympathetic* division is the division under the control of the hormone adrenaline, which is activated automatically when the individual perceives that he/she is under attack. We might say the parasympathetic system is active under the more *positive* emotions and the more *negative* or unpleasant emotions arise from activation of the sympathetic system.

Antagonistic Systems

What is important for later discussion is that these two systems are *antagonistic*. When we are under attack, the sympathetic system holds sway and predominates, which is of course adaptive for survival. When we are relaxed the parasympathetic system dominates. For example, listening to a Beethoven symphony at night in our living room is certainly a very emotionally pleasant experience and our body responds accordingly. Our heart rate decreases, blood is withdrawn from the head and brain and large muscles of the body, blood goes to the gastrointestinal system (which aids digestion), our hands and extremities become warmer, sweating and respiration decrease, our senses become less acute, and the body's physiology reflects a very pleasant and enjoyable emotional state, a feeling of well-being and safety. This emotional state is more than pleasurable and it too has survival benefits; it strengthens our immune system to assist healing and to ward off present and future threats to our health.

Emotions Affect Physical Health

The emotions—positive and negative—have very powerful effects on both our general health and how we cope with disease. In one study of hospitalized patients, one group could see trees from their hospital window and the other group could only see bricks and mortar. The patients who could see trees and vegetation from their windows recovered faster and left the hospital sooner than their counterparts who were not visually exposed to nature during their hospital stay.

Being hospitalized is a major stress for most of us and, even under these stressful conditions, the opportunity for pleasant emotional experience aids healing. This is true whether we are in reasonably good health or are dealing with any of a variety of diseases. Cancer patients, everything else being equal, who are able to cope effectively with the stress of cancer, do better, live longer, and even have lower health care costs than their counterparts who have not been able to master the stress of their disease.

Rorschach and Cancer

The Rorschach (the ink blot personality test) expert, Bruno Klopfer, reviewed blind Rorschach response data (blind in the sense that someone else had gathered the data). Knowing only age, gender, and education (and nothing about each patient's cancer), he was said to be able to accurately separate those patients whose cancer would be *rapidly* progressive versus those cancers which would be more *slowly* progressive. He was able to determine cancer prognosis on the basis of personality/emotional differences among these cancer patients as reflected in their responses to the inkblot test.

One might argue that the very progressive cancers produced the dyphoria/hopelessness picture in these patients' Rorschach responses. From what we know about the effects of anxiety and depression, the reverse appears to be true. The patients' *positive or negative* emotional attitude on health was the *causative* factor of rapid progression rather than the reverse.

The body's sympathetic nervous system response to attack (threat) is *adaptive* because it enables the individual to deal more effectively with the threat in terms of the well-known fight or flight response. It is important to know that this sympathetic body response to physical threat differs only in *intensity* but not in kind from non-physical (or psychological) threat. One might think that psychological threats (e.g., I am a complete failure unless I get an A on this calculus test) are less devastating to the individual than physical threat of attack, but that would be wrong.

The *intensity* of the sympathetic body response is certainly stronger under *physical* attack than when under some forms of *psychological* attack, but with some exceptions (e.g., prolonged battlefield combat) physical threat is typically an acute rather than a more prolonged situation. Recovery, in the sense of the body returning to normal or to a non-stressed state, is quicker under an acute threat of physical harm than when one is under *continuing* psychological harm.

Trauma

Certainly there are major and persistent mental health consequences that can and do arise following certain trauma (e.g., sexual assault, physical assault with bodily injury), and these health consequences may be diagnosable as a post-traumatic stress disorder (PTSD), which requires professional treatment. Some resilient individuals are able to get through seemingly severe trauma fairly unscathed emotionally while others are emotionally devastated by what seems to outsiders to be "milder" trauma. The former recover quickly in the absence of treatment, return to a normal life and a normal emotional state more quickly, and the latter even with treatment often experience the emotional effects of the trauma for longer periods of time.

Fortunately, most of us are spared such severe trauma, but none of us is spared psychological threat or the normal stresses of everyday life. The concept of "normal stress of everyday life" covers a very wide territory and includes relationship problems (e.g., divorce), job stress, a child not doing well in school, a spouse with health problems, the death of a good friend, a downturn in finances or the stock market, even such "positive" changes in our life such as a job promotion. These normal life events are stressors, cause worry, and are adaptive challenges, and our body is literally wired to defend itself against these attacks.

Causes of Fear-Anxiety

Individuals who seem to have been overprotected during their development tend to be more fearful than others are and also have less environmental and social mobility. The overprotectiveness in itself instills in the child fear of the environment and since the child is exposed to fewer risks these children have fewer opportunities to learn how to deal with challenging or "high risk" situations.

I have seen the consequences of this past overprotectiveness in many women now in their sixties, women who would not be diagnosable as having an anxiety disorder. Twenty-five years ago my wife, who was then in her forties, took several long cross country automobile trips with our children when I could not get away from my practice. Many women who knew her, many non-patients as well as patients (my wife is also a psychologist), were amazed that she would have the guts to drive alone cross country with her children and face the possible dangers alone of such a trip. Many commented that they would never even contemplate taking such a trip without their husbands, and some had never taken even a short trip by themselves outside of their home community.

These women all had scary thoughts about the dangers that could happen. The women could not even imagine how they would go about contending with various threats (e.g., if they had a blowout). Fear-anxiety is quite endemic in our society. It is self-limiting to most of us but disabling to some of us.

Panic Attack a Disease?

The ex-football coach, John Madden, is afraid of flying and will not get on an airplane. I understand he is driven to his television appearances as a football commentator in a motor home. Does John Madden have a disease? If you could get him on an airplane, he would have as strong an anxiety attack as anyone with diagnosable panic attacks, but should we speak of the one with panic attacks as having a disease, and not John Madden, or do they both have a disease? It's true the one with panic attacks is much more emotionally *impaired* than John Madden. Of course, John Madden can "work around" his fear much more capably than his counterpart, but an anxiety attack is an anxiety attack despite how often or infrequently it occurs.

The language of disease applied to either the whole spectrum of anxiety or restricted to the diagnosable anxiety disorders adds nothing to our understanding of fear and anxiety. Environmental, non-biological factors form and shape anxious behavior and to think that anxiety arises as a disease of the brain seems reductionistic as best.

Anxiety, like depression, is a *biopsychosocial* disorder and each is so much like the stress and mood problems of all of us that we gain nothing when we bring in the concept of (brain) disease to describe the more disabling forms at the extreme.

The Stigma of Anxiety

Some advocates for labeling anxiety as a disease believe that it decreases the stigma of this problem. We are told persons with anxiety or depression would be much more likely to seek help for their problem if it were viewed as a disease. The disease model of anxiety and depression puts people more in the light of having a problem just like any other *medical* problem such as in heart disease or diabetes, etc. Anxiety is then a problem that is not of the person's making and one which the person has no control over. The biologically-based theory and treatment says to the person with the problem (and to the family of the patient), you are not accountable for the problem because the anxiety or depression is due to a chemical imbalance in your brain.

This belief *does* harm – it encourages patients with anxiety and depression to look for a *chemical* answer, and later we will see some of the harmful effects of such a conception. Certainly, all of us want to *reduce* the stigma for persons to encourage them to get professional help with these problems. Moreover, I think the supposed "cure" of the stigma problem is more likely to *raise* than *lower* the stigma of those with the problem. The disease model *removes* these people (with the so-called chemical imbalance) from the rest of us. Actually, the *continuum* view of anxiety and depression is *less* rather than *more* stigmatizing than the disease model because it views the diagnosable forms in terms of *severity* rather than a difference in kind from what *all* of us experience in everyday life.

The disease model takes the solution to the problem out of people's hands – they are passively in need of a pill to correct their chemical imbalance. As mentioned with depression, the disease model also encourages victimhood. "I am a victim of this chemical imbalance; I didn't deserve it," and "it must have come from my parents," and "will I pass it on to my children?" and "woe is me." Nothing is gained for those who suffer diagnosable anxiety or depression when describing these disorders as *diseases* of the brain.

Many of the above groups who espouse the *disease* view of anxiety and depression also use the same simplistic logic in speaking of schizophrenia and bipolar disorder as *diseases* of the brain as if the environment plays little or no role in how these disorders are expressed in patients with these disorders.

These psychotic disorders are *not* diagnosed through brain imaging but through a very comprehensive assessment of the patient's *behavior*. This is *not* to say that there are not very important *biological* factors operating in these psychotic disorders — and that appropriate medication is not crucial in the effective treatment of these disorders — but if we *only* look at the patient's biology, and if our treatment addresses only so called *biological* factors, we have less than quality treatment. We know that the culture, the subculture, personality characteristics, life and family have *enormous* influences on our behavior whether we do or do not have schizophrenia or bipolar disorder. Our failure in meeting the needs of the mentally ill are due not to lack of money but to a very narrow view of these disorders that stresses *medication* and neglects important *psychosocial* factors of the mentally ill among us.

"Examples of Normal Stress"

The following are some case examples of persons experiencing a variety of stress who called my company and talked to me or other PMHM psychologists for help with those problems. About 90% of these callers had one twenty to thirty minute telephone counseling session, which often was sufficient for the person to achieve adequate resolution without a second call or the need for face-to-face therapy.

These callers, as a group, were encountering significant emotional stress in their lives, which often affected their mood as well. Although many would not have met criteria for a diagnosis of depression or an anxiety disorder, their distress was sufficient to impair their health, their sleep, their productivity, and certainly their general happiness. If these distressed callers had seen their primary care physicians first, these callers would have been offered either an SSRI antidepressant or an anxiolytic, or both.

The Harried Department Manager

Julie called from work with a sharp edge in her voice and a headache that had lasted for a week. She had been trying to meet an important work deadline for a project two weeks from her call and aspirin and other pain relievers had not helped. She was about to go to her physician for something to ease the pain, but she thought she would first use the Employee Assistance Program, hence her call to me.

I did a quick assessment of her and her situation. I found out that she had not been having any nausea or vomiting (which are often associated with headaches from a brain tumor). I asked her to close her office door, and I would give her ten minutes of relaxation training to decrease or possibly eliminate her chronic headache. She was a little skeptical but, knowing how people are when in pain, I knew I would gain her full cooperation, which I did.

I had her turn the office lights off, close her eyes, get comfortable in her chair with her feet flat on the floor, and turn her attention to her breathing and my voice. I had her breathe deeply and slowly from her abdomen, rather than her upper chest. Upper chest breathing is characteristic of those, like Julie, who are in heightened emotional stress. When pain accompanies stress (such as a headache or lower back pain), the pain *automatically* increases the stress. For example, the headache is an additional threat to the person, which again activates the body to defend itself against the new threat, which intensifies the stress response in a vicious circle.

Julie's whole body was wound tight like a drum to prepare to defend itself from the threat, but she was warding off a *psychological* rather than physical attack. What I was doing was to help her to take herself in the other (relaxation) direction by controlling her breathing and attention. Again, we have a case of thoughts controlling emotion or in this case the stress response.

I was not doing hypnosis (although some of the techniques are similar, e.g., helping the person to narrow their attention), but I was getting her to actively lower her stress reaction by directing her attention to the relaxation response. When we are undergoing stress we can feel *out of control* and the *first* step to manage stress is to get *personal* control over it. Here the physician and the psychologist are at odds.

Relaxation and tension (stress) are antagonistic and I was helping Julie to re-program her thoughts to shape bodily relaxation. Within five minutes the headache was gone, even when I had her open her eyes. I took another five minutes to explain how she had come to have the headache, how she had turned her body around to get rid of it, and how she would have to modify her work behavior and attitudes to see that this type of thing did not happen again. In addition to learning a stress reduction technique, I told her she would have to learn how to take care of herself at work and not to try to do more than she could. When she did this, she would find herself to be *more* rather than *less* productive at work.

Julie learned something very important about herself in those few minutes that she will be able to use all of her life to improve her emotional well being and her health. She will enjoy improved health as a result, and being better educated about herself, will be a more informed health care consumer in the future. Yes, pain is very motivating and we can see how emotionally normal people when confronted with pain are very open to learning maladaptive or adaptive ways to find relief.

A Mother Who Can't Let Go

Margaret, mother of a grown son in the military called in distress over a daughter-in-law's possessive manipulation of her husband. Margaret's son was assuming almost total care and responsibility for the couple's child. The unemployed daughter-in-law left most of the household and caretaking duties to her husband, who seemed to accept a situation that most of us would consider unfair.

Margaret was also distressed because of her problem in gaining non-interrupted access to the grandson on visits. Margaret had given the son good advice on several occasions about his relationship with his wife. Margaret told him his wife *should* assume more responsibility for the child and the marriage, but the "counseling" was to no avail. It was possible that Margaret's son would be transferred to another installation (the wife and child would remain behind), and the caller was concerned about possible neglect or abuse of the grandson by the daughter-in-law after her son was transferred.

I came to the conclusion that the daughter-in-law was likely to have some sort of a personality disorder and was not depressed as Margaret thought or hoped. Margaret was in a no-win situation in trying to get her son to initiate changes in his marriage. I added the fact that the relationship was apparently meeting her son's needs. It would be best for Margaret's own well-being to *accept* the situation as it was and cease efforts to "make it right or better". To do otherwise would be to risk alienating her son and jeopardize her contact with the grandchild.

I realize many people would say that the daughter-in-law was wrong, that she *should* be a better mother and that she *should* consider that other people had rights equal to her own, etc. These may well be true, and it would be nice if Margaret *were* facing a different situation, but Margaret has no direct control over her daughter-in-law and her behavior. Margaret had no parenting relationship with her, and no direct control over her son for that matter.

Rather than continuing to fight a losing battle, it would be best for Margaret to accept the situation as it is, stop trying to change it, and deal with it as best she could. Her goal should be to maintain a good relationship and access to her son and grandson and to have a "good" relationship with her daughter-in-law as a way to achieve the caller's primary goals.

I addressed the caller's fears about the safety and well being of her grandson when her son is transferred, especially since her son had been the principal caregiver. I advised Margaret to monitor the situation. She should call Child Protective Services if she saw signs of abuse or neglect. I told her the daughter-in-law would most likely provide child care when she was forced to and the child would not be in harm's way. Probably the grandson would not receive the *best* of care from his mother, but fortunately many people do well in life even though they received less than the best of care during their rearing.

Let It Alone or Leave

Mary called my company for help with her marriage of eight years. The couple, who was childless, had known each other for twelve years and had difficulty in the past year, ostensibly since the husband, Steve, became aware of his wife's previous brief sexual infidelity some years in the past.

Steve continued to bring up the incident and caused much distress for them both. Steve and Mary worked different shifts and had limited time together. Nevertheless, when their schedules were compatible, Steve would often reject his wife's wishes to be together and have an outing with friends.

I advised Mary to stop being a victim of her husband's abuse, to refuse to discuss or listen to the topic of her past infidelity and not to organize her life around his, since he obviously did not organize *his* life around hers. I suggested she invite him to do something with her at their next available opportunity, but if he would not commit, she should make her own plans without him and hold to them, even if he *changed* his mind and wanted to be with her. For her own well being, she had to become less vulnerable, refuse to be abused and less dependent. I offered to have a telephone counseling session with Steve and to make a referral to a therapist.

I talked to Steve a few days later and he came across as an injured party, although I pointed out the "injury" was four or five years ago. Rather than responding sympathetically, I told him he was being abusive to his wife and that he had to either divorce her or stop bringing up the infidelity. He must put it out of his mind and become a loving husband once again or leave.

I told him it was not his wife's problem, although I had advised her in ways to protect herself from his abuse. If he wanted a marriage, he *had* to stop his abusive behavior. This was not a case for marriage counseling, which I felt would only be another stage for Steve to abuse his wife.

He went to see a therapist on my referral, but Mary later told me he quoted the therapist as attributing his abusive behavior toward his wife to "his mother's desertion of him when he was a child." The latter may have given him some comfort, but the most important thing for him to do was to *stop* his abusive behavior and for Mary to *not* allow herself to be abused. The competent therapist must focus on the here and now, i.e., the patient's *abusive behavior* and not past history, which may or may not have been true or contributory.

Abusiveness is a pattern of behavior under *voluntary* control. As with all voluntary behavior, it can be stopped. The immature personality *wants* to believe that his behavior is involuntary, or that the person deserves his wrath or that he is helpless to control it. In a situation like this, the therapist has a very difficult job because he must help the husband to take personal responsibility for the behavior, to change it, and to avoid a premature termination on the patient's part. Mary appeared determined to no longer take her husband's abuse, which indicated a good prognosis for her emotional well-being, if not the marriage. She had learned to see her husband's behavior as what it was – abusive meanness. There could now be a good outcome – whether a better marital relationship or a divorce.

Mother's Concern About a Grown Daughter

Mrs. Quinn called with a concern about her 24-year-old single daughter who has a BA in psychology from a large university in her hometown. Sue didn't have a career in mind, but she had a job offer at a child development center. In listening to Mrs. Quinn, I noted Sue seemed to have social service interests and she liked to write (her father is a technical writer). A BA in psychology does not prepare one for any specific career, but it would be useful in a child development center. I suggested Sue take the job, but also take the Strong Vocational Inventory at her university counseling center as a part of career counseling. Interest and aptitude tests would give her useful information to help in her career decision-making. Mrs. Quinn was pleased with the advice and direction for Sue to consider. Some problems of stress can be resolved with good information and advice on which an action can be taken.

Mother's Concern About an Introverted Son

Lay people and many inadequately trained mental health professionals often confuse and attribute *emotional* pathology to what is many times normal human behavior. Mrs. Greene's call about a shy, introverted 10-year-old son was a good case in point. Justin did very well in school. He played baseball and had several friends. He was, however, fearful of new situations and he did not talk much and spent much more time in solitary pursuits than her other children.

I explained to Mrs. Greene that shyness is a normal trait and introversion is a normal trait also. I said society seems to idealize the emotionally outgoing extrovert, and these people have fewer problems adapting to the social environment, but those who are high on introversion are among many of our future scientists, engineers, writers, artists, and other groups.

Mrs. Greene did say her child seemed interested in science and spent long hours with a chemistry set. He would doubtless manage on his own to adapt to his social world, but his mother needed to accept him as he is, an introverted person whose inner world takes precedence over his social world. She accepted this interpretation of her son's behavior, and I may have helped her to see her son as *different* but not as impaired or ill. Stress prompted this call — the mother's fear that her son might be mentally ill — and the information offered seemed to reduce the mother's stress and perhaps as consequence her son's as well.

A Frantic Caller

I took the call at night from Tina, a divorced 32-year-old female who was in crisis over several recent stressors in her life. She had been beaten by her ex-husband and was recently involved in a near fatal gas oven explosion at her house. Following this, she was diagnosed as having Post-Traumatic Stress Disorder (PTSD) by her family doctor. There was a history of being a victim of a sexual assault, she was involved in a child custody battle with her ex-husband, was getting ready to remarry, and claimed no memory of striking her fiancé during a recent argument.

She called in a state of panic and demonstrated what is known as pressured speech in reporting the above. She verbally expressed a feeling of having an absence of any inner controls or any ability to modify her heightened emotional state.

Tina is a good case that demonstrates my point that one should be very well trained before offering oneself to the public as a therapist for mental health problems. This patient is one that a therapist could cause great harm.

We can see from Tina's adjustment that she *already* has a low anxiety threshold and we certainly don't need to give her anything else (drugs or the wrong kind of behavioral therapy) that will add to her problems and maladjustment.

We have many marriage and family therapists and other licensed counselors who render mental health services to the general public today as well as to patients such as Tina. Like most psychologists, I have strong reservations about whether the training these persons receive is sufficient to treat the Tinas of the world or many other patients as well.

Tina is the type of patient who can be easily harmed in treatment, and she is not an easy patient for a therapist to really help. With some patients, if the therapist does something wrong, the patient will not return to therapy and this is good because such a patient might get to a more effective therapist later. However, with Tina, the therapist can do many *wrong* things and she will *still* return. She will not make any progress or get better, but she will be back on the therapist's doorstep weekly, twice weekly or more often if the therapist or managed care company allows. I am not sure any therapist would be comfortable with a Tina, but the thought of a therapist trying to treat Tina with less than the full training and experience of a psychologist is extremely scary.

Each Individual Must Be Treated Individually

When symptom disorders (depression or anxiety) arise secondary to adverse life events, the therapist must concentrate on working with the adverse life event rather than with drugs or cognitive therapy. However, action in the individual case requires clinical judgment based on broad training and experience. If the focus is on the adverse events in Tina's life, as many limited or poorly trained therapists might do, at least six major adverse events or areas in her life would have to be addressed. That approach would have her in therapy for twenty years, and at the end of twenty years we would be no closer to helping her. As a psychologist I had to identify her "core" problem, the problem that was most disabling to her adjustment and, in this brief telephone assessment, I formulated the following treatment plan.

The place to start with Tina was her sense of emotional vulnerability, her experience of herself as being unable to control her panic and chaotic emotional life. After identifying this core problem to Tina, I told her our starting point was to help her to learn to control her emotions, not to address the problems in her life. The key to controlling emotions is to first control one's thoughts, which is the defining approach in cognitive therapy. I gave her a start on controlling her emotions through a brief course of progressive relaxation over the telephone. However, the job could not be completed in one telephone call and I referred her to a psychologist in her community to finish the job. Getting control over her emotions was the initial task, a task that had to be completed *before* she would be able to resolve other problems in her life. Actually, a good cognitive therapist would never get around to Tina's adverse life events because Tina's major therapeutic need was to gain control over her emotional life.

Tina might well have met criteria of PTSD, and she was certainly in a high state of anxiety, but unlike "medical" illnesses with mental health problems, it is not enough to know the diagnosis – we have to know the person. This is especially true when the patient is presenting symptoms of anxiety or depression. Moreover, Tina was considerably more anxious and dysfunctional than many of the above cases. Nevertheless, the therapeutic approach is much the same no matter where the patient is on the stress-anxiety dimension, reduce disabling anxiety by giving the person control over their own anxiety.

Borderline Personality Disorder

In talking with Tina about her chaotic life, I suspected that her distressing symptoms and maladjustment were arising from a more fundamental *borderline personality* disorder. There are a variety of personality disorders, but all of these have in common that they are fixed, permanent, life-long patterns of maladjustment that are essentially unmodifiable. Moreover, many of the behavioral expressions of these disorders are said to be experienced by the person as "ego-syntonic," a fancy word meaning that these behavioral expressions, far from being considered "wrong" by the individual, are considered acceptable and even worthy.

On the other hand, an "ego-dystonic" behavior or trait is one that the person finds wrong, objectionable, and wants to change. Depression, for example, is ego-dystonic for the individual. It is unpleasant, and the depressed individual is motivated to get rid of it – not so for *ego-syntonic* behaviors, thoughts, self-appraisals, or maladaptive ways of relating to others. The narcissistic personality disorder believes, and accepts, that they are *inherently* superior to others and their second belief is their *entitlement* – that people *should* admire and envy them because of their superiority – is completely acceptable to the self and certainly *not* in need of change (from the narcissist's point of view).

We have, then, personality disorders that are not only fixed, life-long patterns of maladaptive behavior, but the core disorders are not seen by the patient as undesirable or in need of change.

Persons with personality disorders are likely to encounter serious mental health problems, e.g., they are very subject to stress and poor mood. Their mental health problems arise in their relationship with people because of their maladaptive ways of perceiving and relating to others.

Cure or Management?

The mental health world is divided into two broad camps on what is considered to be appropriate treatment for these personality disorder patients. One group seems to have come from the ideas of Sigmund Freud and the psychoanalytic tradition and the attempt is to *cure* the disorder through long-term analysis or psychotherapy. Others, like myself, see from the nature of the disorder that cure is impossible, and that these patients do better with a *management* approach. A management approach helps these patients to cope more effectively with distressing situations and relationships and to improve their ability to get along with others. Unfortunately, many psychiatrists in my professional experience seem bent on trying to cure these personality disorders with drugs, a futile task to my point of view.

Drugs for Stress/Anxiety?

In the above, and especially in the case examples, I have tried to show that all of us are subject to stress and that all of us are susceptible to experiencing the unpleasant bodily effects of stress. I have taken the position that stress and diagnosable anxiety (such as panic attacks) differ only in degree but not kind from one end of the spectrum to the other. Moreover, the callers who were encountering normal stress in their lives have solutions to their problems that are really quite similar to the solutions for those with the more severe and diagnosable anxiety disorders.

Those reacting with stress or anxiety need information about what they are experiencing and the tools or skills to control the extent of their emotional reactivity. Perhaps the distressed person needs an altered *perception* of a situation or a new cognitive interpretation of the stress-inducing situation. Managing stress or treating a diagnosable anxiety disorder requires behavior change and changes in the pattern or content of our thinking, that is, what we are telling ourselves about what we are experiencing. Drugs for stress/anxiety only mask the *physiological* expressions of the bodily distress and do not address the *causes* of the various threats we encounter in our daily lives.

I hope the reader will also see that in order to understand and treat the person's stress or anxiety disorder — much as in the case of clinical depression — the therapist needs to know something about the person in order to plan appropriate treatment.

The Stress-Anxiety Continuum

Earlier in this chapter, I advocated for a stress-anxiety continuum in contrast to the politically correct discontinuity model, which says that anxiety is a disease that differs in kind and not just degree from those stress causing situations emotionally normal people experience.

In the continuum the treatment at both ends of the spectrum was seen as essentially similar and examples were offered showing the need for information, behavior change, changing the patient's perception of a stress inducing situation, providing tools for self-mastery or perhaps helping the patient to change their cognition (thoughts) of themselves or some situation confronting them.

Here I would like to demonstrate the stress-anxiety continuum by discussing an example of an anxiety disorder, namely, panic attacks.

Panic Attacks

A *panic attack* is a discrete period in which the person is seemingly in the grip of a powerful fear, apprehension, or terror, often associated with feelings of impending doom. Panic attacks often include symptoms such as shortness of breath, palpitations, chest pain or discomfort, choking or smothering sensations, and often include fear of "going crazy" or losing control.

Needless to say such an event must be a very frightening experience for the person and we might characterize the panic attack as a fear of fear. Sometimes these attacks are triggered by external cues or events (the person attempting to get on an escalator, e.g.) or they seem to just come out of the blue as if from nowhere.

DSM-IV™ describes the Features of a Panic Attack and for discussion purposes I would like to offer the features of a panic attack here.

> Because Panic Attacks occur in the context of several different Anxiety Disorders, the text and criteria set for a Panic Attack are provided separately in this section. The essential feature of a Panic Attack is a discrete period of intense fear or discomfort that is accompanied by at least 4 of 13 somatic or cognitive symptoms. The attack has a sudden onset and builds to a peak rapidly (usually in 10 minutes or less) and is often accompanied by a sense of imminent danger or impending doom and an urge to escape. The 13 somatic or

cognitive symptoms are palpitations, sweating, trembling or shaking, sensations of shortness of breath or smothering, feeling of choking, chest pain or discomfort, nausea or abdominal distress, dizziness or lightheadedness, derealization or depersonalization, fear of losing control or 'going crazy,' fear of dying, paresthesias, and chills or hot flushes. Attacks that meet all other criteria but that have fewer than 4 somatic or cognitive symptoms are referred to as limited-symptom attacks.

Individuals seeking care for unexpected Panic Attacks will usually describe the fear as intense and report that they thought they were about to die, lose control, have a heart attack or stroke, or 'go crazy'. They also usually report an urgent desire to flee from wherever the attack is occurring. With recurrent attacks, some of the intense fearfulness may wane. Shortness of breath is a common symptom in Panic Attacks associated with Panic Disorder with and without Agoraphobia. Blushing is common in situationally bound Panic Attacks related to social or performance anxiety. The anxiety that is characteristic of a Panic Attack can be differentiated from generalized anxiety by its intermittent, almost paroxysmal nature and its typically greater severity.

Panic Attacks can occur in a variety of Anxiety Disorders (e.g., Panic Disorder, Social Phobia, Specific Phobia, Posttraumatic Stress Disorder, Acute Stress Disorder). In determining the differential diagnostic significance of a Panic Attack, it is important to consider the context in which the Panic Attack occurs. There are three characteristic types of Panic Attacks with different relationships between the onset of the attack and the presence or absence of situational triggers: **unexpected (uncued) Panic Attacks,** in which the onset of the Panic Attack is not associated with a situational trigger (i.e., occurring spontaneously 'out of the blue'); **situationally bound (cued) Panic Attacks,** in which the Panic Attack almost invariably occurs immediately on exposure to, or in anticipation of, the situational cue or trigger (e.g., seeing a snake or dog always triggers an immediate Panic Attack); and **situationally predisposed Panic Attacks,** which are more likely to occur on exposure to the situational cue or trigger, but are not invariably associated with the cue and do not necessarily occur

> immediately after the exposure (e.g., attacks are more likely to occur while driving, but there are times when the individual drives and does not have a Panic Attack or times when the Panic Attack occurs after driving for a half hour).
>
> The occurrence of unexpected Panic Attacks is required for a diagnosis of Panic Disorder (with or without Agoraphobia). Situationally bound Panic Attacks are most characteristic of Social and Specific Phobias. Situationally predisposed Panic Attacks are especially frequent in Panic Disorder but may at times occur in Specific Phobia or Social Phobia. The differential diagnosis of Panic Attacks is complicated by the fact that an exclusive relationship does not always exist between the diagnosis and the type of Panic Attack. For instance, although Panic Disorder definitionally requires that at least some of the Panic Attacks be unexpected, individuals with Panic Disorder frequently report having situationally bound attacks, particularly later in the course of the disorder. The diagnostic issues for boundary cases are discussed in the 'Differential Diagnosis' sections of the texts for the disorders in which Panic Attacks may appear. (DSM-IV, 1994)
>
>

Certainly the above describes a very severe attack of anxiety, but severity, in and of itself, does not mean that we are dealing with something that differs *in kind* from the more milder forms of stress-anxiety. Certainly the more severe forms of anxiety such as in a panic attack are much more disabling to the individual's social and emotional adjustment than the milder forms. In science, if two theories explain all facts equally the simpler of two theories is considered correct. If we bring in the concept of a brain disease to account for some or all of the diagnosable anxiety disorders, to contrast these with the milder stress reactions of everyday life, the onus is on "proponents" of such a belief to show us some proof. Don't just *tell* us about your theory, "Show us the *Beef*."

<u>Too Loose with Language</u>

I am not arguing that people with diagnosable anxiety disorders are not different in many ways from the rest of us who only experience "normal" stresses of everyday life, but we are playing too loose with language when we think of anxiety disorders as either "illnesses" or "diseases".

Biopsychoeducational Process

Behavioral intervention throughout the whole stress-anxiety spectrum is essentially a bio-psychoeducational process. First, the person is given a detailed description about the biopsychological processes involved in stress/anxiety. When we have knowledge of something, the knowledge itself makes it less scary, and when something is less scary it is more manageable.

The bodily physiological reactions occurring under the impact of stress/anxiety (increased heart rate, increased breathing and the like) are described to the patient as essentially "normal" reactions. The person is responding quite normally (if the anxiety is severe enough) to a *perceived* external threat. This knowledge very adaptively prepares the person to deal with the threat (the well known fight or flight response).

The reactions themselves are taken as normal, that is, they are quite appropriate and adaptive *when we are indeed under actual physical attack.* The abnormal part is our misperception of the threat, usually our substitution of a *physical* threat to our safety or integrity for a *psychological* threat.

In the above we are beginning here a *cognitive* process with the patient to determine what external or internal *psychological* threats are giving rise to the anxiety. Are there resolvable adverse life situations or conflicts triggering the stress/anxiety? If so these need to be the primary focus — rather than the anxiety itself — and the anxiety should give way with more effective problem resolution. At other times personal attitudes and unrealistic self-appraisals trigger the anxiety response. These self-defeating thoughts need to be modified by the therapeutic process. There is both a science and an art to treating the full range of anxiety and there is no substitute for expert clinical judgment.

Loss of Control

Anyone experiencing severe stress or anxiety is very likely to be experiencing a sense of loss of power in connection with the anxiety. The most frightening aspect of anxiety is our fear that we are completely vulnerable to it and cannot control it. We need to teach the patient not only what is happening to them (e.g., they may fear that they might become crazy but they will not go crazy) but also how to manage the anxiety. I have talked to many persons over the telephone who were experiencing a full-blown anxiety attack, the caller hyperventilating, feeling dizzy and expressing a litany of environmental stressors or problems.

If a patient shows up at their physician's office in such a state the patient is given Xanax and perhaps an SSRI antidepressant as well. Of course with such an approach the message to the patient is, "There is nothing *you* can do about your anxiety and problems, so I will give you something to control what *you* do not have the power to control yourself."

The Key to Control

At the psychologist's office — even *before* taking a history — the patient is given the knowledge and opportunity to gain some *immediate* control over their anxiety. In just a few minutes, we can give the anxious patient tools and have the patient practice retraining their own anxiety. Listening to their problems and stressors at this point would *only* increase their anxiety when in such a state; teaching *self-mastery* is the first order of business. Teaching the patient to govern their anxiety is an important approach that is common throughout the full range of treating stress-anxiety problems.

To the general physician or a lay person, a patient in a severe anxiety state can be overwhelming. Not knowing what to do, he/she places reliance on a drug to calm the person down as the *only* alternative. The patient in a severe anxiety state is in a highly *motivated* state to do something about the anxiety, and he or she is very receptive to offers of help, unlike some other kinds of mental disorders.

Behavioral treatment of anxiety does not preclude the use of drugs, especially in the acute stages if the anxiety is overwhelming, but if drugs can be avoided in the acute stage so much the better. If the highly anxious patient can attend to the therapist and follow directions, the patient in the hands of a skilled therapist has an excellent opportunity to experience the benefits of self-mastery of the anxiety. The drug provides only temporary relief. It does not address the sources of distress nor the *solutions* to the problem.

Anxiety Not Self-Limiting

If we want good health, we *have* to be able to manage our stress. If we have a diagnosable anxiety disorder we need effective treatment, which includes the learning of tools to manage our problems in the future. Anxiety, unlike depression, does not go away by itself. If it is a specific fear (e.g., fear of closed spaces), the fear will be of a permanent nature unless we are taught techniques to resolve the specific fear.

Drug Not a Cure

A drug addresses only the *biological* symptoms operating in anxiety and not the causes or psychosocial factors. Unless the latter are treated, the drug has only provided relief, not a cure. A drug only approach ensures that the psychological issues giving rise to the anxiety will continue to feed it but in attenuated form due to the drug. In treating diagnosable anxiety — as in treating diagnosable depression — the standard should be a complete *remission* of symptoms — not temporary *relief*. Unlike drug therapy to *reduce* symptoms for both anxiety and depression, our goal should be complete and permanent *remission*, that is, cure.

Some people who seem more genetically constitutionally disposed than others to respond anxiously will, unless environmental circumstances were very favorable, develop a diagnosable anxiety disorder at sometime in their life. Although with some cases a successfully treated patient in a very stressful situation may need to return for one or more "booster" sessions with the cognitive therapist; the prognosis with cognitive treatment of the anxiety is very good for a return to a more normal *stressful*, but less disabling life.

Stress is a normal part of everyday life and the key is not to get rid of it – the only way we can do that is to die – but to *manage* it or cope more adaptively with the stress we encounter in our lives. *Managing* stress is not the same thing as *reducing* the physiological effects of stress – having one or two martinis or a Valium from our doctor will do this quite nicely and we will feel better temporarily. In using alcohol or Valium (SSRI antidepressants as well) we are *masking* the effects of stress but we are not coping adaptively with the psychological threats in our lives.

CHAPTER III

THE BIOLOGIZING OF MENTAL HEALTH PROBLEMS: A HISTORY

The biological bias that underlies the drug treatment theory affects the way clinical trials and outcome studies are run and how these clinical trials are interpreted. To understand how this bias could happen, let's look at the background of the training of physicians and psychiatrists. What is the need behind the "biologizing" of mental health problems? What is the history? Let's look at some of the reasoning in physician endorsement of the disease model of depression and anxiety.

The Real and the Unreal

Most physicians tend to see organic disease as *real* and all other health problems, including all *mental* health problems and behavior in general, as unreal. In their minds, the former belongs to the "hard" sciences, which are tough-minded, the latter to the "soft" sciences and the tender-minded. The "real" health problem must show up in lab work or a scan of some kind, and the real health problem must be treated with medicine, surgery, or, in a few cases, nothing. If the condition *only* shows up in the patient's behavior, as in all mental disorders despite propaganda to the contrary, it is *not* seen as "real" and does not belong in *real* medicine. It took me some time, but I finally discovered that most physicians do not see behavior as real. This last point requires some explanation. If I were to confront a physician about this I am sure the physician would not deny the reality or "realness" of human behavior, but when engaging in professional practice the physician *acts* as if behavior is not real.

Physicians have tended to see mental health treatment as arising from the so-called soft sciences as mentioned above such as psychology rather than the "hard" sciences such as biochemistry and neurophysiology. For this reason, most physicians are more comfortable with the idea that depression is a *disease* affecting the serotonin system. Needing a pill to correct the imbalance fits their frame of reference much more readily than psychology's approach which says that a depressed person can gain and maintain a more normal mood by learning to modify the patient's own negative attitudes and inappropriate thinking.

Most physicians, brought up on anatomy and biochemistry as they are, see the latter as mumbo-jumbo. There is nothing in a psychosocial model for physicians to relate to in their own training or in the way physicians practice medicine. However, when a psychiatric colleague talks to them about dopamine receptors and corticotrophin-releasing factory, or CRF, psychiatry is seemingly back in the medical fold and treatment of mental disorder is now back within medicine.

Since 1987, with the introduction of Prozac, general physicians began (with the help of the pharmaceutical industry, modern psychiatry, the National Institutes of Mental Health, and other groups) to believe that they were now in possession of a drug for effectively treating the vast majority of patient ills. This included the vast majority of patients showing up in various states of physical distress arising from everyday stress and mood problems.

No longer was referral to a highly trained specialist needed, especially to a specialist surrounded by the stigma of mental illness. No longer was it necessary to confront the primary care patient with the *non-biological* origin of what ails him or her. No longer was it necessary to *remove* the patient and his or her problems from the real world of medicine to what most physicians see as hocus–pocus, the world of *mental disorder* for its treatment. There *are* important biological and genetic factors involved in those who are susceptible to developing depression, but these factors do *not* represent a disease nor do these biological factors dictate the type of treatment.

For several years, psychiatrists got lab work on many of their patients. As I mentioned earlier, psychiatrists thought that they had found the depression marker, but the only result was a waste of money and professional and patient time. For awhile the lab test *did* make the psychiatrist *appear* to be closer to his medical colleagues in his or her everyday practice.

Psychiatry

Almost from the start of the profession, psychiatry has been divided between those in the profession who look for organic, biological causes versus those who look for psychological or non-organic causes. The difference in conceptualization is important because it directs treatment.

Sigmund Freud is perhaps the most important name of those who espoused a *psychological* view of mental disorder and "behavioral" or non-organic forms of treatment. Sigmund Freud was not a psychiatrist (he was trained in neurology), and although his work was in the field of psychology (he was not *trained* in psychology) he and his followers had a tremendous impact on the field of psychiatry and the conception and treatment of mental disorder.

The German psychiatrist, Kretschmer, postulated that there were three basic body types (ectomorphs, lean and thin; endomorphs, round in the middle; mesomorphs, triangular with broad shoulders). He found that endomorphs, as a group, were more predisposed to depression than ectomorphs, who were predisposed to schizophrenia, and mesomorphs, who were disproportionately associated with what is now called sociopathic personality. Spurred on by these findings, psychiatry has been looking almost exclusively at the *biological* side of depression and other mental disorders and investigating a variety of *somatic* treatments, not just drugs but insulin shock therapy, electroconvulsive therapy, hydrotherapy, lobotomies, and dozens of other physical treatment over the years.

From time to time one side would dominate and then would lose power. A noticeable shift in power toward the *organic* side was occurring in the 1980s and the advent of the SSRI Prozac in 1987 was a harbinger of things to come. With Prozac the organic view became ascendant and captured the field of psychiatry with very few exceptions. Residency training in psychiatry shifted to a drug and organic model and psychiatry hit upon a great funding source for psychiatric research, the pharmaceutical industry. Meanwhile, the National Institutes of Mental Health was moving in the same direction as biological psychiatry and research money for non-organic factors in mental disorder were becoming less available

The movement of the 1980s and 1990s to make all mental health problems biologically-based was founded on the work of the 1950s and 1960s. In the 1950s and 1960s biological psychiatry made major strides because of the introduction of drugs for the effective treatment of the *psychotic* disorders, schizophrenia and manic-depressive psychosis. Then the introduction of Prozac, which was seen by psychiatry as holding the promise of the more effective treatment of clinical depression than the earlier tricyclic antidepressants such as Elavil, psychiatry, now married to neuroscience, saw a new age of drugs to target brain neurotransmitters. Psychiatry pointed to the fact that the manipulation of the dopamine system had resulted in more effective drug treatment of schizophrenia and asked why couldn't the same be accomplished with improved drugs to treat depression and the anxiety disorders? In anticipation of this great future, psychiatry began to re-conceptualize depression as a biological disease, a disease affecting the serotonin system and perhaps other neurotransmitters. Depression, despite any other non-organic etiological factors that might be involved, represented a chemical imbalance in the brain and Prozac and other drugs in the pipeline would correct these chemical imbalances. The depression would be relieved and in many cases cured.

Modern psychiatrists are now no longer trained in non-drug forms of treatment. After an article of mine, "A Politically Incorrect View of Depression," appeared in print, I received a call from a psychiatrist at a medical school with many years of experience who was teaching psychiatric residents. At first, I thought he was a psychologist because he thanked me for what I had written. Then he mentioned the frustration that he and others of his peers encounter in trying to get the field of psychiatry to look at more than drug treatment.

Psychiatry's status, through its disease-drug treatment model of mental disorders, has now been seemingly raised to the same level as its non-psychiatric medical colleagues. The fact that the model is based on public relations and is much closer to propaganda than science makes no difference. It is a message that medicine and psychiatry *want* to hear. The belief in the disease model has no scientific basis but it has a very compelling *emotional* appeal. That is, if a drug can cure anxiety and depression then drug treatment would bring these health problems back into medicine.

Psychiatry Residents in Treatment Prefer Psychotherapy to Medication

Even though psychiatry has been promoting drug-treatment for treating depression and anxiety in the public arena, there seems to be some lingering interest among psychiatric residents at least in old-fashioned psychotherapy. A psychiatric residency as with any residency is a time of challenge and stress. To what do psychiatric residents turn to in addressing their mental health needs? In one large psychiatric residency program (Psychiatric News, 2004), about two-thirds were in individual psychotherapy only, 17% received psychotherapy *and* psychiatric medications and less than 1% received medication only. This certainly does not sound like a strong endorsement of drugs to me.

Since the 1950s, psychiatry and psychology have been in a battle over what psychiatry sees as its turf – the diagnosis and treatment of mental disorder. The profession of clinical psychology emerged after World War II when the Veterans Administration contracted with doctoral programs at universities to train psychologists to diagnose and treat returning WWII veterans with mental health problems. These veterans were entering the VA hospitals and outpatient VA clinics across the country. The university psychology programs provided the core training of psychology students during the academic year and the VA provided summer clerkships and one-year clinical internships under psychology departments at VA hospitals across the country.

Psychiatry has been attempting to dissociate itself from the rest of the mental health field, especially psychologists. The means of doing this has come through defining drugs as the primary treatment for all mental disorders. In doing so psychiatrists are emulating their non-psychiatric medical colleagues who look to drugs to treat diseases. Over the years, psychiatry has painted itself into a box; a box that many of us believe has only one tool, drugs. Psychologists have the best and most comprehensive training in the diagnosis and behavioral treatment of mental disorder and with prescribing privileges and the additional training in psychopharmacology, where is the need for psychiatry?

Currently, psychiatry is alive and well and basically does drug treatment in hospitals and outpatient care. In addition to treating schizophrenia and bipolar disorder with drugs, psychiatrists are now using drugs alone to treat stress/anxiety and mood/depression problems.

Medical Psychotherapy?

The "biologizing" by psychiatry of mental health problems continued unabated in several directions. About twenty years ago, psychiatrists, in filling out patient insurance claims, began to use the term *medical* psychotherapy rather than the procedure code psychotherapy, as if psychotherapy delivered by a psychiatrist is different from psychotherapy delivered by a psychologist or other non-psychiatric mental health professional. The term "medical" psychotherapy has no meaning but it enjoys widespread current use. There have been, and are, procedure codes that psychiatrists and other physicians use for medication management. However, the use of "medical" psychotherapy is another example of psychiatry's continuing attempt to "medicalize" the field of mental health, to try to separate what it does from what is practiced by non-medical behavioral health professionals.

A second and final example of the "medicalization" of mental health by psychiatry is the arbitrary division of mental health problems into *biologically* and *non-biologically* determined mental illnesses. As my wife says, "When correctly viewed everything is lewd." Psychiatry—without any scientific justification at all—has determined which mental health problems are *biologically* and which are *non-biologically* based. The reader can decide whether psychiatry has been conservative or liberal in distinguishing one from the other. It appears that psychiatry has decided that any diagnosis for which there is a drug is a *biologically* based illness. One might expect the usual psychiatry suspects such as schizophrenia, bipolar disorder, depression, the full range of anxiety disorders, anorexia and a host of others. This exercise for psychiatry is more than mental masturbation because it has effects in the real world, in third-party and government reimbursement for mental health services.

Especially in the past fifteen years, psychiatry has been moving more toward the drug treatment of *all* mental disorders and away from psychotherapy and behavioral treatment.

Since all human health and mental health problems have *biological* and *psychosocial underpinnings*, it makes no sense to make such a distinction. However, psychiatry has thus far been successful in making this "distinction" in the legislatures in about fifteen states.

Licensing

In the 1950s, states began to license and regulate the practice of psychology, and general medicine and psychiatry opposed these proposed state laws. Psychologists, of course, promoted them. I was in Kansas during the successful licensing attempt, and the legislature heard from psychiatry that if this bill went through and psychologists practiced independently, psychologists would be unable to diagnose the organic diseases of their patients and many patients of psychologists would commit suicide. Apparently, the legislature did not listen to this slippery slope rhetoric and the bill was passed.

In the late 1960s, I was legislative chairman for the state association lobbying for third-party insurance reimbursement for psychologists. At that time, only psychiatrists or other physicians could bill insurance companies directly for psychiatric and psychological services, the latter supposedly under the direct supervision of the physician. This system kept psychologists under the economic servitude of physicians, since psychologists would need insurance reimbursement to establish the independence of their profession.

Again, the legislature heard that if the law was adopted, independently practicing psychologists would fail to diagnose organic diseases that were giving rise to their patients' mental symptoms, and patients of psychologists would be committing suicide in record numbers. Again, the legislature turned a deaf ear to psychiatry's rhetoric and the law passed in the early 1970s, the year after the chiropractic insurance reimbursement bill went through the Kansas Legislature.

Psychiatry is still trying to protect its turf vis-à-vis psychology. One major issue is related to prescription privileges for psychologists who have appropriate extra training for prescribing classes of drugs to treat various mental disorders. The Air Force has trained dozens of psychologists to prescribe these drugs, and these drug prescribing psychologists are currently doing this independently with military personnel and dependants. New Mexico has become the first state to extend psychotropic prescribing privileges to psychologists meeting additional training. In 2004, Louisiana became the second state to grant prescribing privileges to psychologists with prescriber training. How do you think American psychiatry will respond to prescription privileges for psychologists? Just take a look at this recent press release form the American Psychiatric Association on the New Mexico psychologist prescribing law.

APA Press Release, January 6, 2004

> ARLINGTON, Va., Jan. 6 – Today the American Psychiatric Association (APA) reiterated its opposition to New Mexico's psychologist-prescribing law, which will take effect tomorrow, January 7, after a long and controversial process to develop regulations for it. The law originally passed in 2002 and would grant psychologists – who are not physicians and who lack sufficient medical training – the right to prescribe psychotropic medications. In recent months there has been rumor of an effort to expand the scope of the dangerous law and

weaken the educational criteria through legislation expected in the upcoming session of the state legislature.

> "We believe the current law is a threat to public health and safety in New Mexico," wrote APA Medical Director James H. Scully Jr., M.D., in a letter to New Mexico Gov. Bill Richardson. "We are particularly disturbed by ongoing reports that legislation will be introduced in the pending session of the legislature to both broaden the reach of the current law and weaken the educational standards established under current law even before the current law, as inadequate as it may be, is in place and any psychologists have gone through the conditional supervised program. ...Weakening the standards or broadening the scope in this precipitous manner is folly. On behalf of our patients, we respectfully urge you to strongly oppose any such legislation."

Parity

In the past five years or so, mental health parity laws correcting the traditional *lower* level of insurance reimbursement for mental health versus "medical" problems have been introduced or enacted on both a federal and state level.

Twelve or thirteen states have enacted such laws to end such discrimination. There has been much opposition to this legislation by insurance companies, employers, and Chambers of Commerce, the fear being that enactment of parity would *raise* health care costs.

Psychiatry and supporters of psychiatry such as the drug companies stepped in and said, "How about parity for the *biologically*-based mental illnesses and the traditional *lower* reimbursement for the *non-biologically* based illnesses?" Say, what a great *self-serving* solution to the problem, one which would save money on the non-biologically based problems—perhaps problems treated by non-medical behavioral health professionals? Would it then become a *crime* for a non-physician to treat a *biologically*- based illness? Have any psychiatrists thought of that?

This legislative issue varies from state to state, but "biologically" based mental illnesses usually are defined legislatively to include schizophrenia, bipolar disorder, depression, anorexia nervosa, bulimia, obsessive compulsive disorder, attention deficit disorder, and all of the anxiety disorders. All other disorders are referred to as non-biologically based and – what is important – are reimbursed at a *lower* rate than the biologically-based disorders.

With these parity laws enacted, providers (psychiatrists, psychologists or others) will want their patient's mental health services to be reimbursed at the highest rate possible. Of course, *everything* coming to the doorstep of a psychiatrist will be diagnosed as a *biologically*-based illness and, of course, psychologists will make the same diagnosis. Remember when correctly viewed everything is a *biologically*-based mental illness. Psychiatry feels it has an advantage in these parity laws with their concept of biologically-based mental illness. Since this concept of mental illness appeals to the undiscerning mind of some laypersons (at least ten or twelve state legislatures bought this), why not a State or Federal Law that a biologically-based mental illness *must* be treated by a drug? Such a law would have great appeal to many groups and the drug companies would be glad to lend their financial support to the lobbying effort in support of psychiatry.

Psychiatry has indeed made major strides with such legislation despite the ludicrousness of such a theory. It is certainly an *empty* theory, but as marketers say "it *does* have legs."

There *should* be parity of reimbursement in insurance from the medical plan to the mental health part of the plan, but there is no real parity when some forms of mental disorder are reimbursed at a lower rate than other mental or indeed "medical" problems. Some "minor" medical problems are not reimbursed at a *lower* rate than more "major" medical problems, such as cancer or heart disease. True parity requires equal treatment on *both* sides of the plan. Besides, such differential reimbursement on the mental health side will "eliminate" treatment of the non-biologically based mental disorders. These disorders will no longer be diagnosed because of the higher co-payment to the patient and the reduced reimbursement to the provider. What will happen is that *all* patients receiving mental health reimbursement will be diagnosed with a so-called *biologically*-based illness in order to give the mental health patient maximum coverage.

This is not to say that genetic and constitutional factors do not play important roles in both "medical" and "mental health" problems, but believing in a *biological* origin for all health problems strains and violates both logic and common sense.

First of all, it is as illogical to conceive of a *biologically* based mental illness as it is to think of a *biologically* based "medical" illness. Perhaps a bacterial or virus infection might be considered biological illnesses if we forget that stress compromises the immune system. However, 98% of what physicians treat could *never* be legitimately considered a *biological* illness. Most diseases that physicians treat (e.g., type II diabetes, heart disease and others) are *lifestyle* caused, and *lifestyle change* rather than drugs is the most effective treatment.

Politics of Anxiety and Depression as a Disease

The view of anxiety or depression as a disease is a belief (not supported by any scientific facts) that serves the needs of those who subscribe to the belief. Despite the absence of scientific facts to support it, a disease model is the current politically accepted view of depression and anxiety.

The belief is endorsed and supported by many groups:

- the National Institute of Mental Health,
- mental health patient advocacy groups, such as the National Alliance for the Mentally Ill,
- organized medicine,
- psychiatric and non-psychiatric physicians with a few exceptions,
- non-psychiatric prescribers of drugs (physicians' assistants and nurse practitioners),
- the pharmaceutical industry,
- large segments of the media,
- and many patients who are users of antidepressant and antianxiety drugs.

These diverse groups rally around the disease model for different reasons, not always monetary.

Mental Health Advocacy Groups

The National Alliance for the Mentally Ill (NAMI) and other advocacy groups have bought into and promote the disease model of mental disorders and have found a home in modern psychiatry. NAMI accepts this oversimplified thinking about the complex mental disorders such as schizophrenia, bipolar disorder, or depression because the belief that these disorders result from a brain disease, which will remove or decrease the stigma of getting mental health treatment. The party line, however, promotes a drug approach. Despite the necessity of drug treatment for most cases of schizophrenia (not all schizophrenics need drugs) and bipolar disorder, much more than drug treatment is needed. I strongly support the search for new and better drugs for these disorders, especially drugs of equal or greater benefit but with fewer side effects that would help patients who needed these drugs to stay on these drugs.

I am certainly not attacking the mental health advocacy groups, since these lay groups play a very important role in getting society to pay attention to the mentally ill and their rights. However, their *brain disease* focus works against more effective solutions with more comprehensive treatment that would address the *psychosocial* needs of these patients in addition to their medication needs.

Current treatment of chronic schizophrenics is largely drugs by psychiatrists and inadequately trained case managers or lesser-trained "therapists" in the public sector to deal with the patient's psychosocial needs. At a recent conference, a national director of a mental health advocacy group gave the usual brain disease argument at the beginning of her talk. However, in addressing the *treatment* needs of the mentally ill, she brought up environmental, non-drug changes – better living situations, vocational skill training, job placement, improved recreational-social and leisure time pursuits, and other opportunities for skill development and social learning. It is obvious even to the biologically-biased that drugs alone are not the answer for those with persistent mental illness. If improved treatment is to be provided for the mentally ill, society must address the psychosocial needs of these patients.

The National Alliance for the Mentally Ill And The Pharmaceutical Companies

NAMI and the pharmaceutical companies are in bed together; there is no other way to put it. The pharmaceutical companies could have written NAMI's script: all mental illnesses are *biologically* based and *drugs* are the primary treatment. According to one investigation (O'Meara, K.P., 2000), NAMI has received an enormous amount of funding from drug companies. Eli Lilly and Company donated nearly three million dollars to NAMI between 1996 and 1999. According to Ken Silverstein (Silverstein, 1999), NAMI took in more than eleven million dollars from eighteen drug companies for the same period. Eli Lilly and Company loaned one of their executives to NAMI for "strategic planning" purposes. The facts suggest that NAMI is basically a marketing arm of the drug companies since they seem to share much the same goals, that is, selling more psychotropic medication. According to NAMI's 2002 Annual Report, seventeen drug companies and related businesses were corporate sponsors. These included two large *behavioral health management firms*, PacifiCare Behavioral Health, Inc. and Magellan Health Services.

The National Institute for Mental Health (NIMH)

NIMH has had and continues to have a strong drug bias in treating mental disorders, including depression and anxiety. NIMH knows the antidepressant drug outcome research but it still maintains the belief that antidepressant drugs should provide the core treatment for moderate to severe depression despite the absence of any evidence to support this position.

For the past twenty years, NIMH has been funding demonstration projects to teach primary care physicians (PCP) to treat depression with drugs alone and to have two drug failures before referring the patient to a mental health specialist. What is the reasoning behind this?

Twenty years ago PCPs failed to diagnose 75% of their patients with depression. After NIMH spent hundreds of millions of dollars teaching PCPs to diagnose and treat depression with drugs, these physicians now fail to diagnose only 50% of their patients with depression! What an improvement!

Not only does the NIMH model represent psychiatry's drug bias, but there is no strong internal voice within NIMH for behavioral or psychosocial interventions in mental health delivery. There are psychologists at NIMH, but they also seem to go along with the drug treatment bias. If I were a psychologist at NIMH, I would probably last ten minutes before I was terminated.

I think we need an institution such as NIMH, but we need to try to build something that is based on science rather than hype or getting into bed with the drug companies or being a captive of psychiatry.

Federal Drug Administration (FDA)

The major problem with the FDA is that the bar for efficacy in drugs to treat depression and anxiety is far too low. The FDA's concern for safety of drugs is admirable, but drugs to treat diseases or health conditions must be more than safe – *drugs must be effective as well.* They must work! They must be effective! We have to define effective. Should drugs be approved if they work *just a little bit better than no treatment or a little better than a placebo*? I think not.

I learned recently that the FDA receives on average $500,000 from the drug companies for each drug it approves. Since the FDA is regulating the industry, it should remain completely independent and objective. I am afraid the FDA does not maintain its independence from the industry it regulates. I would like to see more proactive regulation.

For drugs to treat depression and anxiety, we must raise the *standard of efficacy*. If we raised the standard of efficacy to one not influenced by vested interests, we would probably do without 70% of current prescription drugs on the market today. Moreover, if we did this, the country would enjoy an immediate and substantial improvement in the overall health of its citizenry. In accepting this physician model of health care, the exclusive use of pharmaceuticals or surgery to treat *symptoms* of disease, the FDA ignores the *efficacy* problem in a wide variety of drug treatment.

The Pharmaceutical Industry

All of us, entrepreneurs and non-entrepreneurs alike, should have our behavior modified by the greater good. Self-interest *should* be guided by ethics.

However, the pharmaceutical industry appears incapable of making any changes from within. It will only change when it is forced to change from without. I see an analogy between the pharmaceutical industry and the illegal drug industry. Right now, despite our efforts, we cannot stop the flow of illegal or legal drugs. To get the flow under control we have to stop the end users (the patient and the drug pusher, and in many cases the patient and his physician). We will have to intervene in this dyad if we are *ever* able to achieve affordable health care. The intervention must not only be with the prescribing behavior itself but also with *payment* for the behavior. We must have mechanisms that will only pay for *appropriate* health care and appropriate prescription drug use.

The drug companies, seeing higher profits in antidepressant versus non-antidepressant drugs, have been getting into the fray by proposing "depression disease management" programs, which is the exact *opposite* of what PMHM is doing in its own drug management program. Depression disease management programs, often a joint drug company-HMO or MBHO (managed behavioral health organization) enterprise, is designed not for *appropriate* treatment, but to get more people on antidepressants and *to keep these patients on antidepressants for as long as possible.* The drug companies found out they were leaving money on the table because *large numbers* of antidepressant users were *discontinuing* drugs either the first month because of side effects or ineffectiveness or before the recommended six to nine months for drug treatment. I am sure many drug companies give these depression disease management programs away "free," but there are big dollars to be had in keeping these patients on drugs.

I am sure the drug companies justify these programs, and the expense to the payer of these programs, by saying: "Depression is a chronic, relapsing disease and because of the relapse rate after acute treatment, 35% of depressed patients will require life-time drug treatment." Could this philosophy be called self-serving? The drug company's philosophy is built on the fact that drugs have little more than placebo value. Why shouldn't we expect high relapse with placebo cures? Just throwing more drugs at the problem will not solve it.

Managed Care

Managed care has saved a few health care dollars but by and large, it has been a big disappointment. After a few years of level costs, healthcare costs are now rising again. The great hope of managed care for some of us was not only to *lower* costs but also to deliver *better* care. Managed care *can* lower costs and raise the quality of care, but only if done correctly. The reason it has failed is that it has the same *biological model of care as the health providers* it attempts to manage.

We have a health delivery system centered on *symptom* reduction with drugs and surgery for patients with modifiable diseases such as type II diabetes, cardiovascular and other diseases. Prevention and changing patients' behavior to promote health is ignored. An overweight patient who eats three double cheeseburgers a day is prescribed a cholesterol reducing drug and also an antihypertensive. That is a pattern of care that is approved by the managed care company because it and the provider share the same model. Giving drugs to reduce symptoms (high blood pressure and high cholesterol) only *lowers* the patient's motivation to changing behavior to lose weight, get on a program of exercise, and have a nutritious (lower fat) diet.

The patient may have high blood sugar, high cholesterol, and high blood pressure secondary to obesity, high fat diet, and lack of exercise, all of which may be completely or partially controllable with weight loss and exercise. The physician knows that without the modification in life style, drugs to reduce the *symptoms* may not *appreciably* reduce the risk of heart attack in his patient. The physician does not recommend lifestyle change because the physician does not expect his patient to change, but if the patient refuses lifestyle changes, the physician will prescribe a drug regime. The patient is happier, but he or she receives poorer care, and the physician lowers his liability risk.

The physician can tell the patient that because of a sedentary life style and thirty excess pounds, the patient is at a high risk for a heart attack *without these lifestyle changes*, and drugs alone may not reduce the risk appreciably. However, the patient may opt for drugs. In such a case, the physician is a "winner," i.e., the physician gains financially from prescribing and monitoring the drugs and enjoys decreased liability if the patient has a heart attack. The patient, however, is a loser because of inappropriate health care. The other loser is the payer (society in general) because the payer is reimbursing for inappropriate and ineffective health care.

Until we stop giving drugs to patients who won't modify their health risk behaviors, we will continue to have both poor and unaffordable health care.

Type II diabetes is an excellent example of rewarding irresponsible health risk behavior. Physicians tell us most type II diabetes is due to obesity and lack of exercise. Most type II diabetes is preventable and largely reversible with lifestyle changes. Because type II diabetes raises the risk of heart attack, physicians are treating the cardiac risk of type II diabetes much more *aggressively* than previously. Physicians now want their type II diabetes patients' LDL cholesterol under 100, and diastolic blood pressure below 80. Many type II diabetic patients are put on three or more medications in an attempt to reduce heart attack risk *even if the patient does not make healthful lifestyle changes.* Should society pay for pharmaceuticals for symptom reduction when the treatment does not address the *causes* of disease? Obviously, I do *not* think we should pay for inappropriate medical care that only rewards irresponsible health risk behavior, but all of us continue to pay for inappropriate health care.

The discussion of type II diabetes leads us directly to healthcare's Quality Assurance Industry.

Will NCQA/HEDIS Take Health Care to the Promised Land?

A Standard of Care Is Needed

In recent years, there has been a great deal of discussion in HEDIS and elsewhere on implementing standards of care as a way of improving health care and lowering costs. There is a push to follow *treatment standards*. There is still too little discussion about what standards are right and what standards are wrong. I think most of us – health care professionals or not – can agree on the rightness of many standards such as childhood vaccination, but many other treatment standards, such as treatment reduction of high blood pressure through medication alone, are either questionable or wrong. Moreover, providers are often forced to follow a standard of care even when the provider knows the standard of care to be wrong.

At a health care conference NCQA had a vendor's booth and I talked with the exhibitor in charge about the dearth of preventive standards in the NCQA treatment standard. I was surprised that this NCQA representative agreed with me. He said originally the standards incorporated preventive lifestyle changes but these proved unpopular with physicians and were dropped from the final treatment standards.

For example, in the mental health area, some managed behavioral health care organizations will not reimburse psychotherapy for depression *unless the patient is receiving antidepressant drug therapy* as well. Behind this policy is the assumption that psychotherapy for depression combined with drugs is better and more effective than psychotherapy alone. That is simply wrong.

A couple of years ago I was asked by a local Mental Health Association to be on a professional task force for improving child mental health services in the community and to secure increased funding for treating emotionally disturbed youth. Others on the committee saw drugs as the primary treatment, not just the psychiatrists but other mental health professionals.

The other non-psychiatrist mental health professionals saw their roles as *adjunctive* to the drug treatment and they seemed quite satisfied with the status quo.

The problem with the belief that drugs are the most effective treatment for depression is that there is simply no scientific support for it. The scientific literature as a whole favors psychotherapy over drugs for depression, even when psychotherapy is combined with drugs. Often the practitioner who is not a "believer" in the drug treatment model will still follow unsupported and unproven treatment standards because of patient expectations or legal liability. The patient may expect to be given the standard of care, drugs, and even if the practitioner *knows* the standard of care is wrong the practitioner may comply with the wishes of his or her coercive patient.

The United States has been dealing with a prescription drug problem under the Medicare Program. There is no rational way for society to be able to afford to pay for these drugs if the status quo continues.

I once reviewed a hospital psychiatric case of an 11-year-old sociopathic child and the psychiatrist wanted to keep the child in the hospital a few more days to see if Klonopin would help the child's impulsiveness, an off-label use of this medication. I told the psychiatrist I could not allow reimbursement for an extended stay because we had no evidence drugs could address the problem of a deficient conscience. If the psychiatrist *believed* that Klonopin was a cure for lack of conscience development, then he should conduct a controlled scientific research project to study the effects of Klonopin on sociopathic children.

Such a position is not only unacceptable to physicians (how can a non-physician tell a physician what or what not to do), but also to many other people, I am sure. At the very least, non-physicians and physicians acting on the best science must control *reimbursement* of all prescription drugs. When this control occurs, we will be able to have reasonable prescription drug costs and we will also enjoy improved health care. Much of our poor health care today is due to the misuse, overuse, and inappropriate use of prescription drugs. We will have better health care when the misuse is eliminated or reduced. As long as healthcare is driven by a *symptom* reduction as opposed to a *prevention* model we are destined to have unaffordable healthcare and poor quality healthcare. One must grant that the disease model is expensive. For better physical health and mental health care, we have to move from the present "drug medicated symptom reduction model" to treating *causes* of our physical health and psychological problems.

The NIMH—Its Biological Bias

When one goes to NIMH's web site on depression, its biological bias becomes clear. In its treatment recommendations for depression, antidepressant drugs are stressed. It says, " these drugs are widely used, effective treatments for depression."

The second paragraph discusses several types of psychotherapy, including CBT and IPT (Interpersonal Therapy) that are referred to as being "helpful." So would a cruise to Bermuda be helpful for a depressed patient.

NIMH is ignoring its own sponsored research evidence as well as the preponderance of the scientific literature to promote its *biological* model of mental disorder. Yes, body-mind dualism is unfortunately still very much alive in health care today. Any illness involves the *whole* person and the division of what is "mental" and what is "physical" is completely arbitrary and without substance. We have to treat the *whole* person with a health care problem. Unless we do effective treatment of the person as a whole, health care outcome is compromised and the cost is horrendous as we are seeing.

Mental Health Advocacy Groups

One can see how all of the above entities endorse without question the politically correct view of anxiety and depression, that these conditions are brain diseases and that drugs are necessary if not sufficient in their effective treatment.

I don't think one has to be a trained psychologist to predict how the FDA (or NIMH or patient advocacy groups) will respond in the future to the accumulating scientific evidence of the dangerousness and ineffectiveness of antidepressants. These groups are committed to the belief that drugs are the key to the safe and effective treatment of depression (not necessarily these drugs but future drugs), and it will take more than science to change the FDA's thinking or behavior about antidepressant drugs.

Not all Psychiatrists are Fooled by the Drug Companies

An FDA staff psychiatrist on September 13, 2004, testified before a select House Committee on oversight looking into the dangerousness of antidepressant drugs for treating depressed children. His FDA superiors asked him to examine the FDA submitted clinical trials for the efficacy and dangerousness of these drugs with children. His report (which was at first suppressed) came up with conclusions that his superiors did not want to hear. His conclusions that these drugs are dangerous and have limited or no efficacy with depressed children were unacceptable to promoters of these drugs within the FDA. This psychiatrist had a greater allegiance to scientific truth than to his economic self-interest, and for this we have to respect and admire him for his courage to stick to the truth.

CHAPTER IV

THE BENEFITS OF ANTIDEPRESSANTS: REAL AND PERCEIVED

Drugs are evaluated in terms of a benefits/risk ratio. If the benefits outweigh the risks, society accepts that we have come up with a good or useful drug. Any drug that is likely to have any benefit will undoubtedly have some risk associated with its use. The risks always have to be evaluated not in themselves but against the *benefits* of a particular drug, and against the disease, disorder, or condition the drug is treating.

A drug or medical procedure may have a risk of brain damage in 5% of the cases, which would not in itself preclude the appropriate use of the drug when all circumstances are considered. However, if the drug were designed to treat a hangnail, for example, the risks (causing 5% brain damage) would not justify the use of the drug. For one thing, a hangnail is not a life-threatening ailment; for another, there are a number of drug and non-drug means of treating the problem quite well. Many cancer drugs *do* have a high risk of causing significant brain damage, but they have (and should have) FDA approval because these drugs are treating a life-threatening disease in which there may not be any alternatives with lower risk. The decision on the use of any drug comes down to a matter of judgment based on an evaluation of the patient's condition and the drug's benefit/risk ratio.

Another consideration has become added to the equation, one that historically physicians have not considered, and this added consideration is the *cost* of the drug. With escalating health care costs, which presently account for over 14% of the Gross National Product, we can no longer afford to ignore the *cost* of a drug or medical procedure. We *have* to bring cost into the equation along with the benefit/risk ratio to evaluate a drug's utility.

Data compiled by PMHM suggests that antidepressant and related drugs represent over 20% of total pharmacy costs in some benefit plans. In one analyzed plan, 22% of the covered lives annually received one or more prescriptions for either an antidepressant, an antianxiety drug or both. Moreover, the patients on these drugs accounted for 45% of the plan's *total* pharmacy costs.

How Do We Assess a Drug's Benefit?

First, a drug approved by the FDA must be one that treats a specific disease, disorder or condition that is recognized in a generally accepted medical classification system. A drug cannot (and should not) gain FDA approval because it makes the person feel better. It must be a drug that treats a specific *disease.* If the drug treats a specific disease and the drug treated person feels better, that is just fine. For example, the FDA has approved an antibiotic drug because it has been judged safe and, in two double-blind, placebo-controlled trials, it proved that it was more effective in treating infection than placebo. When our infection is treated successfully we often *feel better* as a result, but the drug is not approved because it makes us *feel* better.

Measure of Improvement and the Placebo

The efficacy of a drug simply cannot be established except by comparison with a placebo-control group of patients with the same disease, disorder or condition.

The drug-treated and placebo-treated patients are compared on a pre-selected measure of improvement, in the case of an antibiotic a reduction in infection. This design with the placebo-control group attempts to isolate the effectiveness of the drug itself from other non-drug factors that might have an influence on improvement. For example, some infections are time-limited, that is, the infection gets better without treatment. Without a placebo comparison one would not be able to attribute the observed improvement to the drug rather to other non-drug factors. In these drug-placebo comparisons on differential improvement, we look for *statistically* significant differences. A difference, even a seemingly large difference, can be the result of chance factors rather than properties of the drug itself. Statistical analysis is used to assure we will be able to detect a *true* difference between drug and placebo when it in fact *does* exist with a definite level of confidence.

Placebo Effects

The placebo (the sugar pill, meaning a pill with an inert substance) has been called the most powerful drug because of its widespread effects on both physical and mental status. Of course the power of the placebo is not in the placebo *but in what it means* to the person taking the placebo. The *message* it communicates from the physician to the patient is, "This will help you." To assess drug effectiveness on any disease we have to separate *drug* effects from *placebo* effects. This can *only* be accomplished through scientifically controlled, double-blind, placebo-controlled studies. There is simply no other way other to assess the effectiveness of any drug, including antidepressants and anxiolytic drugs.

Double-blind

By double-blind we mean neither the patient *nor* the physician prescriber knows if the patient is in the drug or the placebo (treatment) condition. The outcome could be compromised if *either* the patient or prescriber becomes aware that the patient is taking the drug or the placebo. In such a situation one or both have penetrated the "blind" and the results would be contaminated.

The Problem with Inert Placebos

Unfortunately all of the antidepressant drug clinical trials and many, if not most, of the other double-blind, placebo-controlled drug outcome studies have serious experimental design flaws that make it difficult to assess whether there is a significant *drug effect* beyond a *placebo effect* in treating diagnosed depression. The antidepressant drug clinical trials employ *inert* placebos. The blind is more difficult to maintain for both patient and prescriber because the inert placebo, unlike the antidepressant drug, has absolutely *no physiological* effect on the patient. Thus, the patient and the prescriber are much more likely to know that the patient is receiving placebo and not the drug, which can affect outcome.

In antidepressant drug clinical trials the prescriber not only dispenses the drug or placebo but in most trials also *rates* the patient on the improvement instrument, usually the Hamilton Depression Rating Scale (HAM-D), and prescriber knowledge of the patient's experimental condition (drug or placebo) *can* influence the patient and the prescriber's rating of the patient on improvement.

The Active Placebo

Psychologist researchers recommend the use of an *active* placebo, which decreases the possibility that either the patient or the prescriber will penetrate the blind. With the active non-antidepressant drug, the patient has physiological effects (often side effects similar to antidepressant drug side effects) and may report these side effects to the prescriber. Both patient and prescriber are more in the dark about whether the patient is on the antidepressant drug or on the active "placebo," which makes for more accurate assessment of improvement. By maintaining a stronger blind than the use of an inactive placebo one can better assess the true *drug effect* of the antidepressant if there is indeed a drug effect.

In these antidepressant drug clinical trials we want to determine if there is a *drug effect* beyond a *placebo* effect. If improvement in the condition reflects only a placebo effect we have an ineffective drug. In so called open-label studies in which both the patient and prescriber know that the patient is taking the real drug, improvement *cannot* be attributed to the drug because of uncontrolled placebo effects. These *open-label* studies are comparable to what is called anecdotal evidence, which is really not evidence at all. Of course, drug companies like to sponsor these antidepressant open-label studies because they *appear* to be science.

Feel Good Drugs

Dr. Jones may give his depressed patient, Christa, an antidepressant drug and Christa, according to Dr. Jones, gets less depressed, which is all that can be said. We cannot take the next step and say the drug was effective in treating Christa's depression because there has been no control for placebo effects or recent environmental factors (e.g., Christa's husband just returned from the war) that might have influenced Christa's depression. Christa may also report that she feels better on the drug, and feels worse when she stops the drug, and doesn't this prove that the drug is a good drug? Even if we accept Christa's "good feeling" as an effect of the drug, remember a drug must treat some *disease* or *disorder* to be approved by the FDA. If Christa "feels good" secondary to the effects of a drug on treating a disease, that is one thing. If Christa is looking for a drug to make her feel good she should not be looking for a pharmaceutical licensed by the FDA.

An antidepressant should be a drug to treat *depression*. If depression is treated effectively by the drug, improvement of mood is an expected consequence. "I just feel better when I am taking my Prozac" is not justification for the use of the drug. Illegal drugs or tonics might give some of the same effects, but certainly their use would not be justified even though there may be many happy users. Most of those illegal drugs are harmful and should not be used despite the high rates of satisfaction from their users. We have to be much more careful about *licensed* drugs when these drugs are not only treating a disease but also having an effect on mood or well being.

The SSRI antidepressants have been called by some people "mood brighteners." This term is not only used with depressed people but with "normals" as well. If their use is as a mood brightener rather than a treatment for depression we have a use that is more analogous to the use of an illegal drug. In such a use the prescriber becomes more of a pusher than a healer despite his or her protestations to the contrary.

We have a similar situation with the anxiolytic drugs, especially the benzodiazepines such as Valium and Xanax. There are legitimate *medical* uses for these drugs, for example, to bring someone out of having a brain seizure through the drug's ability to raise seizure threshold. These drugs are, however, one of the "feel good" drugs. As with the antidepressants, we have to be extra careful that these drugs are being used to treat legitimate mental or other disorders and are not used just for their "feel good" effect. In general I would have to say that both classes of drugs — SSRI and related antidepressants and anxiolytic drugs — have and are being used more for this "feel good" effect rather than for legitimate medical or mental health purposes.

The benefits of antidepressant and to a lesser extent anxiolytic drugs must be restricted to how well these drugs treat the respective "diseases" or disorders for which they have gained approval by the FDA.

I know this definition will not be acceptable to a few users, such as Sally, who wants to believe that her Valium twice a day has been a lifesaver to her over the past five years or Jane who swears by her Zoloft that makes her feel good. However, there is simply no other acceptable standard to determine whether or how much a drug is effective in treating a disorder than from *scientific* double-blind, placebo-controlled outcome studies.

Popularity of the drug, testimonials of satisfied users and prescribers, are simply no measure of proof, even though the antidepressant industry has flourished more on the basis of advertising and testimonials than on the scientific evidence. With this foundation, let's turn to assessing the benefits of these drugs by looking at the scientific evidence.

Reviewing the Literature

Before turning to the outcome studies, I would like to say something about my ability to objectively review this literature in a fair and unbiased manner. Any review of such a vast literature is selective at best, and this review is no different from others, but I have tried to come up with as unbiased a sample as I possibly can. I began the review about six years ago to answer some of my own questions about antidepressant and anxiolytic drugs. Actually the review changed some of my own thinking.

Although I had never had to use these drugs in my own practice for treating depression and anxiety, my experience did not *prove* these drugs were not useful. I had referred schizophrenic patients to psychiatrists for medication, but I did not find the need to refer patients with primary depression or anxiety to psychiatrists. I shared the conventional point of view at the time that for *some* depressions perhaps *combined* treatment (psychotherapy *and* drugs) might be more effective than either one alone.

Initial Classification of Tricyclics and SSRIs

Before looking at the scientific literature with respect to the benefits, some initial classification would seem to be in order. Tricyclic antidepressants (e.g., Elavil) were the first generation antidepressants and many of the depression outcome studies came from evaluation of the tricyclic antidepressants. Aside from the antidepressant drug clinical trials submitted to the FDA for approval, perhaps 60% of the outcome studies involved *tricyclic* antidepressants rather than the current generation SSRI drugs such as Prozac, Paxil, Zoloft, Effexor or others. However, all studies comparing current generation antidepressants against tricyclic antidepressants find that *neither antidepressant* drug class is superior (*or inferior*) to the other (AHCPR, 2002).

FDA Standards

In order for an antidepressant drug to gain FDA approval, the drug company must submit to the FDA two double-blind, placebo-controlled trials in which the antidepressant was found to be superior to an (inert) placebo in treating well-diagnosed cases of depression to a statistically significant degree.

The FDA does not set a standard such as an *amount* of difference between drug and placebo improvement, only that there proves to be a *statistically* significant difference between improvement on the drug versus improvement on placebo.

Improvement might be defined in the clinical trial as a reduction in scores on the Hamilton Depression Rating Scale (HAM-D) at the fourth, sixth, or eighth week of antidepressant (or placebo) treatment. Lower scores defined by averaging the improvement scores for both groups at each rating or assessment period would reflect improvement or a reduction of depressive symptoms for the antidepressant and placebo groups. A *statistically* significant difference in favor of the drug might be defined as one that could have been observed due to chance alone (and not due to a real treatment effect) in less than 5 times in 100 such experiments.

<u>Meta-analysis</u>

In the following you will see the term "*meta-analysis*." This statistical technique allows a researcher or a reviewer to combine a group of independent research studies on the same topic in order to come up with *stronger* data than by analyzing each individual study alone. Not all studies in a particular area are selected for inclusion in the meta-analysis. The researcher or research team will come up with specific *selection* criteria for inclusion or exclusion. The team might remove any studies without a placebo-control group, studies with insufficient or questionable measures of improvement and the like. The meta-analysis is not without its critics, but in general, it is an accepted method of combining research studies to make more powerful inferences than one could make from the data in each study taken separately.

Obstacles to the Scientific Trial

A statistically significant difference is no guarantee that the drug trial was carried out in a scientifically controlled and unbiased manner. Drug companies rarely do their own clinical trial research. The drug companies farm this out, in the case of mental health drugs to Psychiatric Research Centers that typically conduct only drug studies for drug companies.

<u>Funding Dependence</u>

These research centers are almost exclusively financially dependent on drug companies for their revenues and they must deal with the problems of maintaining their scientific objectivity versus being influenced by economic motivations. We will see later that some researchers not being paid by the drug companies believe that these drug clinical trials are not unbiased and favor the drug treatment outcome. These possible clinical trial biases will be looked at later.

<u>Other Funding</u>

The federal government through the National Institute of Mental Health funds some of the antidepressant outcome studies submitted by psychologist or psychiatrist researchers on topics of interest and concern to NIMH. Universities may fund antidepressant outcome studies using money from a variety of sources including the drug companies. Some drug companies fund independent researchers to conduct specific research on topics of interest to the drug company and the independent researcher as well.

It is a good idea in reviewing an antidepressant outcome study (or any study for that matter) to look at the credentials of the researcher and the funding source. Most of these outcome studies appear in scientific or professional journals, which are juried, that is, "independent" experts review the experimental design, results and statistical treatment of the data before the research is selected for publication in the journal. The expert reviewer typically has excellent research credentials in the same area as the researcher who is submitting his/her study for publication. However, even in jury reviewed drug research we often have the case of a *psychiatrist-reviewer* with income from the drug companies reviewing the work of a fellow psychiatrist researcher who received drug company money to conduct the study. If you believe this arrangement can be somewhat incestuous you are right, much as is the common practice of drug company hiring former FDA officials.

How Do We Measure Depression for Antidepressant Outcome Studies?

There is a saying in science that if something exists we should be able to measure it because if we cannot measure it, we cannot set up an experiment to examine it. If depression exists, and I think all of us agree that it does, we should be able to measure it. In the physical sciences we can measure things very exactly such as the pressure of a gas, for example. However, in the non-physical sources we do not need such a degree of exactness in measurement to have a useful and accurate measuring tool. In depression treatment outcome studies the most widely used tool is the HAM-D, which appears below in its entirety.

THE HAMILTON RATING SCALE FOR DEPRESSION

(to be administered by a health care professional)

Patient's Name

____

Date of Assessment

____

To rate the severity of depression in patients who are already diagnosed as depressed, administer this questionnaire. The higher the score, the more severe the depression.

For each item, write the correct number on the line next to the item. (Only one response per item)

---

1. DEPRESSED MOOD (Sadness, hopeless, helpless, worthless)

______ **0** = Absent

1 = These feeling states indicated only on questioning

2 = These feeling states spontaneously reported verbally

3 = Communicates feeling states non-verbally—i.e., through facial expression, posture, voice, and tendency to weep

4 = Patient reports VIRTUALLY ONLY these feeling states in his spontaneous verbal and non-verbal communication

2. FEELINGS OF GUILT

______ **0** = Absent

1 = Self reproach, feels he has let people down

2 = Ideas of guilt or rumination over past errors or sinful deeds

3 = Present illness is a punishment. Delusions of guilt

4 = Hears accusatory or denunciatory voices and/or experiences threatening visual hallucinations

3. **SUICIDE**

______ **0** = Absent

1 = Feels life is not worth living

2 = Wishes he were dead or any thoughts of possible death to self

3 = Suicidal ideas or gesture

4 = Attempts at suicide (any serious attempt rates 4)

4. **INSOMNIA EARLY**

______ **0** = No difficulty falling asleep

1 = Complains of occasional difficulty falling asleep—i.e., more than ½ hour

2 = Complains of nightly difficulty falling asleep.

5. **INSOMNIA MIDDLE**

______ **0** = No difficulty

1 = Patient complains of being restless and disturbed during the night

2 = Waking during the night—any getting out of bed rates 2 (except for purposes of voiding)

6. **INSOMNIA LATE**

______ **0** = No difficulty

1 = Waking in early hours of the morning but goes back to sleep

2 = Unable to fall asleep again if he gets out of bed

7. **WORK AND ACTIVITIES**

______ **0** = No difficulty

1 = Thoughts and feelings of incapacity, fatigue or weakness related to activities; work or hobbies

2 = Loss of interest in activity; hobbies or work—either directly reported by patient, or indirect in listlessness, indecision and vacillation (feels he has to push self to work or activities)

3 = Decrease in actual time spent in activities or decrease in productivity
4 = Stopped working because of present illness

8. RETARDATION: PSYCHOMOTOR (Slowness of thought and speech; impaired ability to concentrate; decreased motor activity)

______ **0** = Normal speech and thought
1 = Slight retardation at interview
2 = Obvious retardation at interview
3 = Interview difficult
4 = Complete stupor

9. AGITATION

______ **0** = None
1 = Fidgetiness
2 = Playing with hands, hair, etc.
3 = Moving about, can't sit still
4 = Hand wringing, nail biting, hair-pulling, biting of lips

10. ANXIETY (PSYCHOLOGICAL)

______ **0** = No difficulty
1 = Subjective tension and irritability
2 = Worrying about minor matters
3 = Apprehensive attitude apparent in face or speech
4 = Fears expressed without questioning

11. ANXIETY SOMATIC: Physiological concomitants of anxiety, (i.e., effects of autonomic overactivity, "butterflies," indigestion, stomach cramps, belching, diarrhea, palpitations, hyperventilation, paraesthesia, sweating, flushing, tremor, headache, urinary frequency). Avoid asking about possible medication side effects (i.e., dry mouth, constipation)

______ **0** = Absent

1 = Mild
2 = Moderate
3 = Severe
4 = Incapacitating

12. SOMATIC SYMPTOMS (GASTROINTESTINAL)

______ **0** = None

1 = Loss of appetite but eating without encouragement from others. Food intake about normal

2 = Difficulty eating without urging from others. Marked reduction of appetite and food intake

13. SOMATIC SYMPTOMS GENERAL

______ **0** = None

1 = Heaviness in limbs, back or head. Backaches, headache, muscle aches. Loss of energy and fatigability

2 = Any clear-cut symptom rates 2

14. GENITAL SYMPTOMS (Symptoms such as: loss of libido; impaired sexual performance; menstrual disturbances)

______ **0** = Absent

1 = Mild

2 = Severe

15. HYPOCHONDRIASIS

______ **0** = Not present

1 = Self-absorption (bodily)

2 = Preoccupation with health

3 = Frequent complaints, requests for help, etc.

4 = Hypochondriacal delusions

16. LOSS OF WEIGHT

______ **A.** When rating by history:

0 = No weight loss

1 = Probably weight loss associated with present illness

2 = Definite (according to patient) weight loss

3 = Not assessed

17. INSIGHT

______ **0** = Acknowledges being depressed and ill

1 = Acknowledges illness but attributes cause to bad food, climate, overwork, virus, need for rest, etc.

2 = Denies being ill at all

18. DIURNAL VARIATION

______ **A.** Note whether symptoms are worse in morning or evening. If NO diurnal variation, mark none

0 = No variation

1 = Worse in A.M.

2 = Worse in P.M.

B. When present, mark the severity of the variation. Mark "None" if NO Variation

0 = none

1 = Mild

2 = Severe

19. DEPERSONALIZATION AND DEREALIZATION (Such as: Feelings of unreality; Nihilistic ideas)

______ **0** = Absent

1 = Mild

2 = Moderate

3 = Severe

4 = Incapacitating

20. PARANOID SYMPTOMS

______ **0** = None

1 = Suspicious

2 = Ideas of reference

3 = Delusions of reference and persecution

21. OBSESSIONAL AND COMPULSIVE SYMPTOMS

______ **0** = Absent

1 = Mild

2 = Severe

Total Score________

Adapted from Hedlung and Vieweg, The Hamilton rating scale for depression, *Journal of Operational Psychiatry,* 1979; 10(2): 149-165

Scores

In the Hamilton Rating Scale for Depression (HAM-D) scores can vary from 0 to 68. The higher the score the more depressed is the person. Scores in the 60s, however, are rarely encountered in these studies, especially if the outcome study is being conducted on outpatients. A score from 10-13 is considered mild depression; 14-17 mild to moderate and greater than 17 moderate to severe depression. A score of 7 or below (sometimes 5 and below) represents *remission* (recovery) or not depressed.

Seven Areas

The instrument is considered both reliable (repeat scores are roughly comparable given stable mood) and valid, that is, the scale *does* seem to measure depression. Physicians, psychologists and psychiatrists can be trained to obtain the ratings reliably (two or more raters would obtain approximately the same score on the same individual) and the instrument takes about fifteen minutes to administer. The instrument assesses the individual in seven symptom areas: Somatic Symptoms, Insomnia, Working Capacity and Interest, Mood, Guilt, Psychomotor Retardation, Agitation, Anxiety and Insight. You will notice that a number of items refer to what we might think to be "mental" content of depression (e.g., feel sad), and others refer to what might be called a general feeling of bodily malaise.

Administration of the HAM-D

The instrument, in the research study, is given several times during the course of the study by the prescriber (of antidepressant or placebo), e.g., as a baseline *before* the study for selection purposes. Next, all subjects are given a five-to-ten day placebo washout period and subjects who improve by 20% or more on the placebo are *removed* from the study. Following this, depressed subjects are *randomly* assigned to the drug or placebo condition. Placebo and drug subjects are then rated at weeks four, six, and eight, and again in some studies at one or more follow-up periods after the drug/placebo has been discontinued. In any research of this type one is bound to lose some of the subjects before the end of the study. Researchers hate to throw away data when a drug or placebo patient drops out, say at the four-week assessment period. When this happens, researchers carry forward the last obtained measure (LMCF) and by doing this the researchers *assume* that the subject would not have gotten worse if he or she had completed the study. Many of us consider this assumption to be a weakness of these drug trials and believe the *best* measure involves all subjects who *complete* the study.

Differences in Improvement

Researchers also look at differential improvement on the HAM-D of the drug and placebo patients, that is, all of those completing the study. Typically improvement (the responders) in the drug and placebo subjects is defined as a reduction in depressive symptoms by 50% or more. Remember that *response* is not the same as *remission* or *recovery*. Remission is a higher standard and may be defined by the researcher as a HAM-D score of less than 7 or less than 5. The "responders" in both the antidepressant and placebo groups usually end up at termination with a HAM-D score representing *mild* depression, much improved but still mildly depressed.

In looking at the results of double-blind, placebo-controlled studies we have to keep in mind that all depression is self-limiting. If one were to select depressed patients using the HAM-D and were to reassess them with the same instrument on a schedule comparable to that used in depression treatment outcome studies, the patients as a group *would get better over time* without drug or placebo or treatment of any kind. We are really interested in knowing not just how much more powerful an antidepressant is over an inert or active placebo, but we also want to know *how much more powerful the drug is over doing nothing.*

For example, one meta-analytic study (Dobson, K.S., 1989) compared psychotherapy and wait-list controls in nineteen separate studies on improvement. The control subjects, after identification and inclusion in the study, received *no* treatment during an interim period or the treatment period for psychotherapy treated subjects. Psychotherapy groups had mean effect sizes of 0.62 to 2.87 and wait-list controls in these nineteen studies had mean effect sizes of -.28 to 1.00. In one study, the wait-list subjects got worse (-.28) as a group, but most no treatment controls got better, but the improvement was far less than the psychotherapy treated subjects.

The psychotherapy groups had a mean, or average, effect size of 1.60 (standard deviations) versus 0.37 for wait-list or no treatment controls.

Psychotherapy from this data is over *four* times more effective than no or wait-list "treatment," but more importantly at this point of the discussion is that people with mental health problems as a group get better. They get better with no treatment or on a wait-list or on an *antidepressant* drug for that matter.

To be considered clinically effective, the antidepressant not only must be more *effective* than placebo, but it must also be more effective than the expected improvement that occurs with *no* treatment.

The FDA standard for drug approval is a two trial *statistically significant* drug-inert placebo differences in favor of the drug but beyond this the FDA *requires no standard effect size of the drug over placebo to grant drug approval.*

Summary of Findings from Antidepressant Outcome Studies

One Third of all Antidepressant/Depression Outcome Studies Found No Difference in Improvement Between Drug and Placebo (Steinbrueck, S.M., et al., 1983).

We know immediately from the above that antidepressants have *very limited* effectiveness in treating depression. Compare this with antibiotic drugs in treating various infections. If antibiotic drugs were no more powerful in treating infection than antidepressants were in treating depression, would we even have a class of drugs such as antibiotics?

We also know that antidepressant trials with *positive* results are more likely to be published than similar trials with *negative* results, i.e., results that did not show superiority of the drug over placebo. When this "file drawer" phenomena is factored into the above, the "superiority" of the antidepressant over the placebo in the FDA clinical trials can hardly be considered impressive.

In Antidepressant Outcome Studies Drug Treated Patients Report No More Improvement in Their Depression Than Placebo Treated Subjects (Thase, M.E., et al., 1999).

Patients, in rating their *perceived* improvement (generally more modest than *prescriber* rated improvement of the same patients), report that recovery was no better for those on the drug than those on placebo. Family doctors would be better off dispensing inert placebos to their depressed patients rather than antidepressants, since those on the antidepressant drug are not likely to report more improvement on the drug than those on sugar pills. Those on placebos would be just as satisfied with their treatment as those on the drug. Moreover, because of drug side effects, patients on placebo would have greater "drug" compliance than patients on antidepressants. The placebo would be less costly than the antidepressants, the placebo patients would not have the adverse side effects of antidepressants and, without side effects, these depressed patients would not require the prescription of other drugs to treat antidepressant drug side effects.

Before recommending placebo substitution as a strategy for family doctors in treating depression, we have to remember that since the placebo as well as the antidepressant patients are not learning anything from their treatment, these patients will and do have a high *depression relapse* rate. Moreover, at the end of the *acute* treatment phase of the antidepressant clinical trials, drug *and* placebo patients are *still* mildly depressed.

In All Antidepressant Drug Outcome Studies The Response Rate is 50% for The Drug and 32% for Placebo (Steinbrueck, S.M., et al., 1983).

If my arithmetic serves me, this response rate difference means that one would have to give *six* depressed patients antidepressants to be sure that *one* patient had something more than a placebo response. I must repeat that the difference observed between drug and placebo is between the drug and an *inert* placebo and not the more appropriate *active* placebo. The latter is important since the prescriber/rater in the outcome studies would be "blinder" in the active versus the inert placebo studies and less likely to unconsciously favor the drug or the placebo as the case might be.

One must admit that the power of the drug over (*inert*) placebo is certainly not very robust, which is a word I have heard "promoters" use when confronted with this research finding. In evaluating the difference between drug and placebo, the word robust is a little too strong and the word *weak* would be more appropriate to describe the power differential between the antidepressant and inert placebo in treating depression.

When we see results such as these on how minimally effective the antidepressant is in treating depression, we must question if there is indeed a *drug* effect in addition to the *placebo* effect. If a physician had to give six people with infections antibiotic drugs in order to be sure that one had more than a placebo effect, antibiotics would simply not be utilized in health care today. However, antibiotics are used because they *are* substantially more powerful than placebo in treating infections.

What About the Newer Antidepressants—Are They More Effective?

Under its Evidence-based Practice Program, the Agency for Health Care Policy and Research (AHCPR, 2002) has been developing scientific information on health to be used by agencies and organizations to form clinical practice guidelines, quality improvement and performance measures for a variety of health problems, including major depression.

In the late 1980s, the U.S. Department of Health and Human Services sponsored guidelines for the treatment of major depression. In the 1990s, there was an explosion of newer antidepressant drugs on the market, especially the SSRI and related antidepressants, and AHCPR commissioned a research project to address the efficacy of the *newer* pharmacotherapies for the depressive disorders and for individuals with recurrent or refractory depression. AHCPR constructed this study with the newer drugs because psychiatrists *believed* the newer drugs were more *powerful* in treating depression than the first generation drugs.

The study searched the literature from January 1980 to January 1998 to capture literature relevant to *newer* released antidepressants such as Prozac, Paxil, Zoloft,

Effexor and others. The study reviewed randomized controlled trials that lasted at least six weeks, compared a "newer" antidepressant to another antidepressant (newer or older), or placebo in patients with a depressive disorder and studies which had a clinical outcome. Reviewers identified 338 studies/trials that met their criteria for inclusion in the review.

Antidepressant response rates were defined as a 50% or greater improvement in symptoms as assessed by an accepted depression symptoms rating scale or a rating of much or very much improved by a global assessment method. It is interesting and telling that the study group, all believers in the value of antidepressants, did not even compare differential *remission* rates between antidepressants and placebo, since remission is so rare in these drug clinical trials.

More than three hundred randomized trials evaluated newer drugs to treat depression. The largest number of comparisons (N=206) were between *newer* and *older* antidepressants. Over one hundred studies compared the efficiency of newer antidepressants versus placebo. More than 90% of the trials were short duration (six to eight weeks) and used double-blind, placebo-controlled methodology.

After the final selection, more than eighty studies prove *newer* antidepressant drugs, as the older antidepressant drugs, were more efficacious than (inert) placebo for treating adults with major depression. *Response rates were 50% for active treatment* compared to 32% for placebo, which is exactly the same outcome for the older antidepressants versus placebo.

Despite the hopes of many psychiatrists and other drug "proponents," the newer antidepressants were no more effective than the first generation antidepressants. For patients who had recovered from major depression (the report did not give the percentage of patients remitting on drug or placebo), continued treatment with a newer antidepressant for at least six months beyond the acute treatment phase decreased the relapse by only 20%. These are hardly impressive figures for the power of these drugs or the need to stay on these drugs even if there is improvement.

Is the Antidepressant Quicker Than Psychotherapy?

There is some scientific literature suggesting that when there *is* a positive response to the antidepressant, it occurs sooner than the response to psychotherapy; however, therapy catches up quickly, and there are some studies that suggest that pharmacotherapy and psychotherapy are apparently of equal effectiveness in treating depression. There was one major NIMH study that *seemed* to suggest that drug treatment is more effective than psychotherapy in treating cases of *severe* depression (Elkin, Shea et al., 1986). However, there are also a number of studies showing that Cognitive Behavioral Therapy (CBT) is substantially more effective than drugs in treating depression. For example, a meta-analysis of fifty-six outcome studies found that psychotherapy had a substantially greater impact (mean effect size of 1.22) on depression than drug therapy (mean effect size = .61) in unipolar depression (Steinbreuk, et al., 1983). The effect size difference means that psychotherapy had about *twice* the power of reducing depression as did the drug.

The official position of the American Psychiatric Association is that *combined* therapy (drugs and psychotherapy) is more effective than either alone. However, the American Psychiatric Association's own committee review of twelve studies concluded there was *no* demonstrable relationship between *endogenous* depression (one without an *apparent* cause) and treatment outcome (Zimmerman & Spitzer, 1989)— that is, drug therapy was no more effective than psychotherapy for *severe* depression. It is obvious to me that the average psychiatric practitioner's standard of care (and also NIMH) in treating depression is quite different even from that officially endorsed by the parent organization. However, in the above case the APA guidelines for depression treatment came from the scientific research rather than prescriber belief.

The Emperor's New Drugs

Question: *"When is an Antidepressant Drug Not an Antidepressant Drug?"*

Answer: *"When the Antidepressant Drug is an Antidepressant Drug."*

We call an antihypertensive drug an antihypertensive drug because the drug reduces blood pressure substantially better than a placebo. Typically these are inert placebos, but even with an inert placebo the drug is substantially more effective than the placebo in reducing blood pressure. Most other drugs have no effect on blood pressure (e.g., statins, antibiotics and others), and perhaps a few drugs have some effect on lowering blood pressure but not to the same extent as antihypertensive drugs. Therefore, we would not refer to these other drugs as antihypertensives.

With Active Placebo

Let's turn to antidepressant outcome studies in which improvement of depression on the antidepressant was compared with the improvement of similarly depressed patients on an active, non-antidepressant drug rather than an inert placebo. These active drugs, unlike inert placebos, have side effects similar to some of the side effects of antidepressants (dry mouth, for example) and these side effects make it more difficult for those rating improvement to know *which subjects are on the antidepressant and which are on the active (non-antidepressant) drug.* With this experimental design we are strengthening the blind and thus improving the objectivity of the patient ratings by the raters. This design better allows the determination of an *antidepressant* drug effect beyond a "placebo" effect. If the antidepressant has a substantial drug effect on depression then the antidepressant should have a greater antidepressant effect than the active non-antidepressant drug.

Let us consider some compelling evidence. Greensburg and Fisher (1989) found that the effect of antidepressant medication is smaller when it is compared to an *active* placebo than when it is compared to an *inert* placebo (Greenburg & Fisher, 1997). Remember that the critical difference between active and inert placebos is the presence of pharmacological side effects, which reduces the transparency of the "blind". Data from other studies indicate that most participants in studies of antidepressants are able to deduce whether they have been assigned to drug or placebo (Blashki, et al., 1986).

To test this hypothesis, one study (Kirsch, J. and Saperstein, G., 1998) reported on *four* controlled antidepressant drug studies in which improvement on the antidepressant was compared to similarly depressed subjects receiving an active but *non-antidepressant* drug. These active comparison medications were amylobartitone (a sedative drug), liothyronine (a drug that treats hypothyroidism) lithium (a mood stabilizer that treats bipolar disorder) and adinazolam (a benzodiazepine that treats anxiety). These drugs individually may have some effect on depression in an ancillary way (the sedative drug, for example), but individually these drugs should *not* have anywhere near the *antidepressant* effect as the antidepressant. Right? Of course, but let's look at the results. *The antidepressant was no better than the other non-antidepressant drugs in treating depression.*

Since these drugs were all equally effective in treating depression should we call all of the drugs antidepressants, or should we *not* call *any* of these drugs antidepressants? From this data I think none of these drugs, including the antidepressants, should be called antidepressants. These five drugs have unique physiological effects on many bodily systems, yet all of them are equally as effective in treating depression as are the licensed drugs to treat depression. Of all *possible* explanations it seems most reasonable to ascribe the improvement on these five drugs to placebo effects. We know for a fact that many people with depression *do* get better on antidepressants, but in examining the evidence as a whole, a case has not been made for a *drug* effect beyond a *placebo* effect.

Under the Freedom of Information Act, Kirsch secured clinical trial data for the six most widely prescribed SSRI antidepressants approved between 1987 and 1999. There were 47 FDA submitted placebo-controlled short-term efficacy trials for Prozac (5 trials), Paxil (16), Zoloft (7), Effexor (6), Serzone (8) and Celexa (5), which involved 6,944 drug-treated and the same number of inert placebo-treated patients (Kirsch, J., 2002). These were the antidepressant, placebo-controlled studies that were *submitted* to the FDA. The data does not include those studies with "negative" findings that were *not submitted* to the FDA.

All study patients met criteria for clinical depression. The prescribing psychiatrists rated depressed antidepressant and inert placebo-control patients (13,888 patients in all) on the 17 or 21 item HAM-D (Hamilton Depression) scale, which provided the single measure for clinical improvement.

In 22 of the 46 clinical trials (48%), the difference in drug and placebo groups on improvement was *not significantly different*. This statistic, 48% of all FDA submitted clinical trials found no differential improvement between drug and placebo cases, is the most serious indictment in the whole study of antidepressant ineffectiveness in treating depression. The drug companies *have* to know how ineffective these drugs are in treating depression. Several of the drugs had major difficulty getting approval, yet the drug companies have continued to market these drugs to general physicians as a powerful (and as a sole) treatment of depression.

In the Kirsch study there were no expected dose/effects response in these patients receiving antidepressants. Patients on the *lowest* dose did as well (or badly) as those on the *highest* doses, which is *exactly* what one might expect from a drug with only *placebo* value.

It is, of course, highly unusual in general medicine for a drug *not* to have the expected dose/effects response in patients. In the absence of the expected dose/effects response one looks at the possibility of an inert drug with placebo effects only. Obviously the Kirsch data suggest the drug does *not* treat depression. Knowing there is no dose/effects response, one can imagine all of the physician workshop hours conducted by drug company staff telling physicians to increase the dose when the patient is not responding or change to another antidepressant.

Overall in the Kirsch study, the drug/placebo improvement difference was less than two points on the HAM-D scale; the range was from a 3-point drug/placebo difference for Effexor to a 1-point difference for Prozac. As intimated in FDA memoranda (Langhren, 1998; Leber. 1998), the *clinical significance* of the differences is questionable.

In the Kirsch study, the best measure of improvement (i.e., studies in which all drug and placebo patients completed the trial) found that the placebo duplicated 85% of the drug response.

Bias

The data in the Kirsch study suggests that if there *is* a drug effect it is clinically negligible. The clinical trials, as we have seen are biased in favor of the drug. For example, all trials used a placebo washout period. All subjects were first put on placebo for a five to ten day period and those who improved more than 20% on the HAM-D measure were *eliminated* from the study, which stacks the selection process in favor of the drug treated subjects.

The FDA requires positive findings from at least *two* controlled clinical trials for a drug to gain FDA approval, but the total number of trials can vary. For example, Celexa's *two* controlled trials were positive (in favor of the antidepressant), but on *three* other clinical trials there was no drug-placebo difference! Despite this outcome, Celexa received FDA approval.

Kirsch reports that in 25 trials the experimental design allowed the use of chloral hydrate (a sedative) in addition to the antidepressant if needed. Moreover, it is almost impossible to maintain the blind with inert placebos since placebos do not have the physiological side effects that antidepressants have. Penetrance of the blind was important because the prescribers (also the monitors) of the placebo and antidepressant patients were conducting the ratings on the HAM-D Scale for all patients. Given that in these drug trials patients tend to report *smaller* differences than clinicians (Moncrieff, 2001), one wonders how the pattern of results in these clinical trials would have looked if the *patients* – and not just the prescribers – had rated their improvement.

Kirsch et al., noted that at least six trials allowed replacement of drug nonresponders, an obvious bias and serious compromise of scientific objectivity in these trials.

The writer does not see evidence that a drug effect (beyond a placebo effect) has been established for antidepressants in treating clinical depression. Even if the small difference observed between drug and placebo is a *real* difference, it would mean as I said earlier one would have to treat six depressed patients with drugs to be sure that *one* of the six had more than a placebo response.

Of all *intent-to-treat* patients in the above FDA clinical trials, the positive drug response rate was only 42%, that is, of 100 depressed patients on the drug only 42 would meet criteria for improvement.

Those depressed patients in the clinical trials such as in the above are very unlike patients in a typical primary care group of patients. Only about 15% of patients in a typical primary care clinic would even qualify to participate in most antidepressant trials (Zimmerman, Mattia & Posternak, 2002), suggesting that the real world outcome for drug treatment of depression would be *lower* than that found in the clinical trials.

<u>Longer Treatment</u>?

Some might believe that longer-term drug treatment might favor drug outcome. FDA staff psychiatrists continue to say this when commenting on the marginal drug effects in short-term clinical trials. However, data from the National Institute of Mental Health Collaborative Depression Study does not support this belief. An eighteen-month follow-up data from that multisite trial (Shea et al, 1992) found patients assigned to placebo (plus clinical management) had intent-to-treat outcome comparable to that in the drug condition with clinical management.

Other research suggests that *longer* treatment does not *lower* relapse following drug withdrawal (Viguera, Baldessarini & Friedberg, 1998). Despite this research evidence to the contrary, psychiatrists and other physicians are recommending that many depressed patients should stay on these drugs *for a lifetime*. Lifetime drug maintenance does not appear warranted since even with maintenance antidepressant treatment the published literature suggests that up to 33% of *remitted* patients experience a return of depressive symptoms (Byrne & Rothschild, 1998) while on antidepressant medication.

SSRIs and Anxiety Disorders

The clinical efficacy of SSRIs in treating various anxiety disorders for which these drugs have FDA approval is no better than their record in treating depression.

In one study (Bellew, 2001), 36% of patients receiving Paxil for generalized anxiety disorder (GAD) achieved remission (as defined by the study) versus 23% for those receiving inert placebo, a 13% difference in favor of the drug.

There is a host of literature in addition to the above referenced Kirsch study that suggests antidepressant drugs for the treatment of depression and some of the anxiety disorders should not have been given FDA approval. These drugs are simply not very effective in treating depression or anxiety beyond their placebo value.

Marginal Effect

Dr. Thomas Laughren, head of the FDA's psychiatric drug division, made the following concessions at a Houston conference (2000): "there is a certain amount of myth" in the claimed efficacy of psychotropic drugs that have shown only marginal effect above placebo. "We don't know how effective they are, only that in clinical trials, they demonstrated somewhat greater efficacy than placebo." He then acknowledged: "There isn't any standard for what effect size is required to get a psychiatric drug on the market . . . we have never, in my experience, not approved a drug because of a finding that the effect size is too marginal."

Excluding Subjects

To obtain even a marginal effect above placebo, 60% to 85% of clinical trial patients who are most likely to be prescribed antidepressant drugs are *excluded* by the eligibility criteria. That's the finding of a Brown University analysis of 31 antidepressant trials published from 1994 to 1998 (Brown University). Only 15% of 346 depressed patients who were evaluated in a Rhode Island hospital psychiatric clinic would have met the eligibility requirements of a standard drug trial. Such a selection process inevitably skews the results, thereby invalidating the published findings and claims about the efficacy of antidepressants. Zimmerman expressed concern: "If antidepressants are, in fact, not effective for some of these large subgroups of depressed individuals, their prescription incurs an unjustifiable exposure of risks and side effects, and alternative treatments need to be considered" (Zimmerman, 2002).

Dr. Laughren at the conference also argued "that if the patients in clinical trials don't resemble the patients who are later prescribed these drugs . . . what relevance do the trials have for clinical care?" Dr. Laughren, that is a very good question.

Dr. Laughren was quite right in his remarks at the conference. The FDA has not established an "effect size" for antidepressants or indeed all drugs. An effect size is a statistic that represents the power of an independent variable such as a drug, medical procedure or indeed any program on any dependent variable, e.g., improvement in depression, blood pressure, cholesterol, reading improvement due to remedial reading instruction and the like.

On these and other dependent variables we take a pre-treatment baseline measure (e.g., HAM-D depression scores, blood pressure, reading grade level) and take a post-treatment measure to determine how much, if any, improvement has occurred due to the treatment (i.e., the independent variable) given the subjects.

For example, in looking at improved reading due to an afterschool one hour remedial reading program, we might randomly assign poor readers to either the remedial program or to a one hour afterschool basketball program and determine which program has the more powerful effect on post-treatment improvement of reading.

Something has a pretty good effect size if the improvement is what statisticians call one standard deviation or better above the mean, or an effect size of 1.00 or better. Antidepressants in clinical trials have an effect size *far below* 1.00 standard deviations. For example, Greenberg (Greenberg and Borstein, 1994) in nine controlled

Prozac outcome studies showed only a modest mean effect size of 0.39 in comparison with controls on patient-rated measures. That finding is comparable to the improvement found in patients on a wait-list with no treatment (Dobson, K.S., 1989). As a contrast to drugs in treating depression, the Dobson study just referred to found in 19 CBT depression treatment studies, CBT had an effect size range from 0.67 to 2.87, with a mean effect size of 1.60.

Dr. Laughren is quite right, the FDA needs to establish minimum effect size for all drug approval, not just antidepressants. The present FDA standard, two positive clinical trials in which the drug proved superior to inert placebo, is simply not enough for drug approval.

Drug-depression researchers have accepted a *lower* standard for the most part because the drug is only marginally effective. In the above Prozac-Paxil study, for example, the average seven week HAM-D score in both groups would still reflect a patient who following treatment can still be characterized as mildly depressed. Is this an example of effective treatment? No, but this is the best that drug treatment has to offer so psychiatry and the drug industry go with it.

Goal of Depression Treatment: Recovery

Drugs are not effective treatment for either anxiety or depression. The problem with depression is not simply to get rid of it — an exercise program, a sugar pill or an antidepressant will often do it temporarily. The goal is to keep it from returning, which requires the learning of cognitive, coping or problem solving skills by the patient to gain and maintain normal mood. It would be wonderful if a pill could do this, but it cannot. Persons with stress/anxiety or mood/depression need information and instruction to learn a variety of *coping* skills up to and including cognitive therapy when needed.

A major theme of this book is that despite current practice to the contrary, there should be no *one* approach to treating depression with either drugs or psychotherapy. The clinician-therapist has to understand not just depression but *this* depression in *this* individual. By understanding how depression fits into *this* individual's life the therapist knows best how to treat it. Moreover, do general physicians have the appropriate knowledge of the pertinent issues to effectively treat these mental health problems?

If the patient's depression is arising primarily from an adverse life event (a job loss, e.g.), rather than depression engendering personality traits, the focus should be on helping the patient to better resolve and master the depressogenic adverse life event the patient is facing. The decision to focus on the life event or the patient's mental organization (or both and to what degree) is a *clinical* decision that is perhaps as much an art as a science, a clinical decision that draws upon the clinician's knowledge and broad experience in treating depression.

Pleasant Activity Therapy (PAT)

We know that depressed people as a group show a very limited capacity to engage in behaviors of a pleasurable nature. Pleasant Activity Therapy attempts to help the patient regain the ability to re-constitute day to day pleasurable activities in their lives. The depression dissipates as the patient is helped to increase the patient's repertoire of daily pleasurable activities. Mood improves as pleasurable activities increase in frequency.

The Research: PAT vs. Drug Treatment

In research studies on Pleasant Activity Therapy (Wilson, 1982), depressed patients were randomly assigned to a tricyclic antidepressant or placebo and to one of three psychological therapies (pleasant activity therapy, relaxation therapy, or minimal contact) for a two-month period. Significant improvements were noted on most measures for all of the treatments at termination, and the results were maintained at six-month follow-up. Pleasant activity therapy plus placebo was shown to be just as effective as pleasant activity therapy plus the antidepressant on patient-rated measures of outcome. At midtreatment, pleasant activity therapy (PAT) resulted in better outcomes than minimal contact. Minimal interpersonal contact does not seem to address the core of the depressive disorder but PAT appears to. Moreover, this study is consistent with many studies in the literature that behavioral interventions with depression when combined with drugs are no more effective than the behavioral interventions alone (Antonuccio, David, et al., 1984).

Perceived Benefits of Antidepressant Drugs

There is of course a great difference between a real vs. a *perceived* benefit of something. The growth of the antidepressant drug industry has been nothing short of phenomenal and its thirteen billion dollars a year bill to society attests to the enormous *perceived benefits* of these drugs by physicians and patients alike.

The *real* benefits of these drugs as shown through scientifically controlled research demonstrates that the clinical value of these drugs is marginal at best. On the basis of these antidepressant outcome studies, one could hardly anticipate much of an economic future for these drugs.

Physicians

Obviously the growth of the antidepressant industry has been fueled by something more than the scientific foundation upon which any drug or medical procedure *should* be based. Unlike the tonic Geritol which had widespread public acceptance through advertising despite little scientific merit, the antidepressant industry has been able to capture the imagination of most medical practitioners who perceive enormous benefit of these drugs for a growing number of their patients. Geritol appealed to the imagination of the users ("This will make me better and feel good."), but physicians had no "stake" in the product and probably discouraged the use of Geritol by some of their patients. Not so for antidepressant drugs; the physician becomes a willing and even *eager* partner of the drug company when the topic comes up during office visits.

I certainly knew without any research that these drugs are enormously popular with most physicians, but I wanted to obtain some data on the use of these drugs by physicians. I decided to survey a group of physicians in Wichita, Kansas about the use of these drugs in their medical practices.

Survey Indications of Perceived Benefits

I developed the following survey (see Figure 1) and sent it out to over 100 family practice and other non-psychiatric physicians and received returns from 31 physicians for a return rate of about 20%. Figure I also presents the data, the percentage of those responding in a certain way on each item, including the range of responses for each item. Questions #11 through #15 required a rating by the physician from 1 to 5 on a strongly disagree (1) to strong agreement (5) dimension involving various attitudes about these drugs (e.g., SSRI and related antidepressants are fairly benign in side effects).

I certainly did not discover anything new or revolutionary about the results but I did find the data of interest and reflecting much of what we suspect about antidepressant prescribing patterns. However, as the reader will learn, a few unexpected "twists" emerged in the data.

Survey of Wichita Primary Care Treatment of Depression/Anxiety

	# Yes	**# No**
Do you treat patients with stress (anxiety) and mood (depression) as their primary problems?	27	4
	Averages	**Range**
What percentage of the time have you used drugs when patients presented with such?	68%	10-100%
Of your drug treated patients with stress and mood problems, what % of the time have you referred your patients to psychologists or other behavioral health professionals for psychotherapy?	33%	5-100%
What percentage of your (psychotropic) drug treated patients do well on drugs alone?	61%	10-90%
In treating depression, how often do you use SSRI and related antidepressants?	83%	50-100%
What percent of your total patients are placed on antidepressants/anxiolytics drugs?	21%	5-75%
With patients who are on an SSRI antidepressant, how frequently have you had to:		
a. increase the dosage?	34%	10-75%
b. add a second or third antidepressant?	10%	5-30%
c. add an anxiolytic drug?	12%	5-40%
What percentage of your psychotropic drug treated patients are on two or more psychotropic drug classes (antidepressants, anxiolytics, antipsychotic, antimanic) at the same time?	22%	0-50%

	# Yes	# No
Based on your experience, how much more powerful are antidepressants than inert placebos in treating depression?	60%	25-95%
When do you prescribe drugs to treat the side effects of SSRI type antidepressants?		
a. when the patient begins to have difficulty sleeping	17%	0-90%
b. when the patient gets anxious/restless	13%	0-80%
c. when the patient has decreased sexual libido	15%	0-60%
d. when the patient gains weight	5%	0-60%

For the following items, please choose the number that best reflects your opinion.

Disagree---Agree

1 2 3 4 5

	Averages	Range
SSRI and related antidepressants are fairly benign in side effects?	3.72	2-5
Depression is primarily a chemical imbalance in the brain?	3.75	2-5
Current generation antidepressants are more effective than tricyclic antidepressants?	3.75	2-5
Withdrawing from antidepressants poses no serious problems for the patient?	2.41	1-4
I feel pressured by patients to prescribe these drugs.	4.06	1-5

Figure I, Preferred Mental Health Management, Inc., December 3, 2003

Prescribing Antidepressants

Close to 90% of these physicians used antidepressants to treat the stress and mood problems of their patients (Question #1).

When patients showed up with stress and mood problems, about 68% of the time these physicians prescribed antidepressants, with a range of from 10 to 100% (Question #2).

Referral

In item #3, I was looking for the amount of referral to behavioral health specialists when their patients had stress or mood problems. An average of one third of such patients are referred to behavioral health specialists (a range of from 5-100%). Actual referral may be somewhat less than reported and perhaps most referrals are to psychiatrists rather than non-physician behavioral health specialists when drug-treated patients do not improve.

The Minority is Significant

These physicians believed that as a group about 61% of patients on these drugs did well, with a range of from 10 to 90%. The results on several items suggest that despite wide acceptance of antidepressants by physicians as a whole, there is a minority of 8 to 10% who seem not to have joined the bandwagon and do not routinely prescribe these drugs.

Let's hope some of these non-prescribing physicians with a more "psychological" bent to their attitudes than their peers have not bought the biological disease concept of depression and perhaps see the disease model as too simplified for the facts.

SSRI Use vs. Tricyclics

In our physician survey, question #6, as expected, showed 83% of these prescribing physicians used SSRI and related antidepressants (rather than the earlier tricyclics such as Elavil). This is an expected finding because these are the drugs that are heavily advertised and the ones pushed by drug detail men and women.

The answer to question #6 is consistent with some of PMHM's other research which showed that in one benefit plan, 22% in the plan received one or more prescriptions for an antidepressant or related drug in the year. The reader will notice that at least one physician had 75% of all of his patients on such drugs! I think the drug company should give this physician an award. All of us are potential users of these drugs since all of us have down moods from time to time and periods of high stress.

Drug Efficacy

In a disguised way Question #7 gets at drug efficacy problems, although this may not be apparent to the reader. I take these drug dosage *increases* and drug *additions* as indications that the patient had not been responding to drug therapy. Why would a physician increase the dosage or add another drug if the patient were doing well?

The reader should not look at a placebo recovery too narrowly or to think of it as not a *real* recovery. It *is* a real recovery or improvement at least temporarily. With hope renewed the antidepressant drug user may now be able to deal with problems that he or she avoided earlier; just as there is a "snowballing" down in depression, snowballing can occur on the *upside* as well. Placebo-like drug cures are sufficient for some people, but we know that often the core problem of the depression has not been addressed and placebo and drug "cures" are subject to high relapse.

Question #8 addresses the efficacy problem as well. The survey physicians estimated that 22% of their (antidepressant) drug treated patients were on drugs from two drug classes. At least one physician had a high of 50% of these patients were on drugs from two drug classes.

Physicians who prescribe these drugs *have* to believe that these drugs are indeed powerful. It was not a surprise to learn that the average physician in the survey believed that these drugs were 60% *more* powerful than placebo, with a range of 29 to 95%.

Drugs for Side Effects

Question #10 assesses the prescriber's predilection to prescribe other drugs to treat the adverse side effects of SSRI antidepressants. One can see from the data in question #10 that drugs used to treat SSRI side effects are not a rare event. Sleep difficulty, anxiousness, decreased sexual libido/ performance problems, and weight gain are not unusual drug induced events, and these physicians as a group aggressively treat these side effects when these side effects emerge. The survey responses at the upper range of these drug-induced symptoms (90%, 80%, 60%, and 60%) suggest that some of these physicians treat these side effect symptoms very aggressively with other drugs.

The very aggressive treatment with other drugs for SSRI induced adverse symptoms is comparable to physician behavior in treating drug-induced side effects in other areas of medicine. Certainly this is true for cancer and many other illnesses — even though depression, unlike cancer, for example, has effective *non*-drug forms of treatment. However, these behavioral treatments of depression are not within the repertoire or experience of these physicians. Instead of discontinuing the drug when there are drug induced side effects, the physician does what he knows best, that is, give another drug.

In view of the frequency of antidepressant drug induced side effects, one might think it difficult for these physicians to maintain a belief that these drugs have tolerable side effects, and that, unlike tricyclic antidepressants, the SSRI drugs are quite benign. This is a good case of cognitive dissonance, the person verbalizing one way but behaving differently. In this case these physicians might say these drugs have benign side effects but their prescribing behavior might reflect something else.

<u>Prevailing Attitudes</u>

The remaining questions in the physician survey, questions #11 through #15, were designed to tap prevailing attitudes about these drugs by these physicians. The survey request was to answer these questions on a four point scale from strongly disagree (1) to strongly agree (4).

These physicians, on question #15 ("SSRI and related antidepressants are fairly benign in side effects"), had an average score of 3.72 (and a range of 2 to 5), which is in the direction of seeing these drugs as fairly *benign* in their side effects. It seems that these physicians have, as a group, bought the propaganda but apparently at least some may have some reservations about the propaganda.

On question #12 ("Depression is primarily a chemical imbalance in the brain."), again the group as a whole is very favorable toward endorsing this concept (Average of 3.75, range of 2 to 5), but again a few have some reservations about totally committing themselves to this conventional wisdom. The belief in the chemical imbalance theory of depression is important to these (and other) physicians because it "justifies" drug treatment as the sole treatment of depression.

Reservations and Prescribing Behavior

These physicians, on question #13 ("Current generation antidepressants are more effective than tricyclic antidepressants."), appear to think that SSRIs are more effective than tricyclics in treating depression (3.75 and a range of 2 to 5), but again these physicians are not uniformly convinced of this. However, latent reservations about the superiority of SSRI effectiveness does not spill over into their prescribing behavior. PMHM data suggest that of all antidepressants prescribed, about 65% are SSRI and related drugs.

Withdrawal

In answering question #14 ("Withdrawing from antidepressants poses no serious problems for the patient."), these physicians, as a group, seem to have much more of a problem accepting this particular conventional attitude than with the other four items in this section of the survey. The average on this item was 2.41 (and a range of responses of 1 through 4), which unlike the other answers in this section of the survey is in the direction of *mild* to *moderate* disagreement. Perhaps a number of these physicians have had some personal difficulty in getting some of their patients off these drugs, and they may well have had some exposure to the "serotonin syndrome" that comes up in the medical literature from time to time.

Pressure to Prescribe

These physicians were very close together in their response to item #15 ("I feel pressured by patients to prescribe these drugs."), which produced a fairly high level of agreement in their average score of 4.06 and a range of responses from 1 to 5. This item confirms what one might expect; patients in general have a very high regard for these drugs and their effectiveness in treating these problems, and as our survey suggests perhaps a higher regard for these drugs than do their *prescribing* physicians. I believe if these physicians *had* a better understanding of the limited effectiveness of these drugs, these physicians might be more successful about dissuading their use among their patients. However, these physicians simply have too many professional, regulatory, and other groups extolling the virtue of these drugs, groups that encourage physicians to prescribe these drugs as the sole treatment of these problems.

Again, this physician survey suggests that these physicians *do* have some reservations about these drugs as the sole way of treating depression. And, at least theoretically, these physicians might seem receptive to education about these drugs, which might change their prescribing behavior of these drugs. However, what current entity will provide these physicians with such education?

No Benefits

Over the past fifteen years, there has been accumulating scientific evidence in the community about the ineffectiveness and dangerousness of these SSRI antidepressants for treating depression and anxiety. We have seen that, although FDA-submitted depression clinical trials are flawed and biased in favor of the drug, the results of almost half these clinical trials in recent years show no superiority of the drug over inert placebo in treating depression. And, as noted, these results do not include the *unpublished* and unsubmitted clinical trials.

It is time to begin to enlighten covered members and benefit plan physicians on the inappropriate and overuse of these drugs and to offer and arrange alternative *behavioral* interventions for these problems.

Many payers are reluctant to do anything in this area, but the costs are becoming so high — and drug treatment of these problems so poor — that payers will *have* to do something about the problem. The drug model is wasting too many dollars toward providing ineffective and inappropriate treatment of these problems.

CHAPTER V

ANTIDEPRESSANTS: AS SAFE AS THEY SAY?

A major reason for the expanding use of current generation antidepressants has been the belief promoted by the pharmaceutical industry that SSRI and other current generation antidepressants have fewer and more benign side effects than the earlier tricyclic antidepressants such as Elavil.

SSRIs More Benign Than Earlier Antidepressants?

It is true that SSRI and related antidepressants have a lower *lethality* rate than the tricyclics in an overdose situation (either purposeful or accidental). Lower lethality simply means that it is much more difficult to kill oneself through overdose on Prozac-type drugs than antidepressants such as Elavil.

<u>Overdose a Liability</u>

Years ago when tricyclics were in vogue, general physicians rarely treated their depressed patients with antidepressant drugs. Instead they referred these patients to psychiatrists or psychologists for treatment. The possibility of a suicide through an overdose of prescribed tricyclics by the prescribing non-psychiatric physician put a restraining influence on non-referred treatment. In referring to the specialist the general physician also transferred the liability surrounding the patient to other professionals.

Unrestrained Physicians

From a general physician under the restraining influence of liability prescribing a tricyclic antidepressant, we have gone from perhaps 10% of antidepressant use by non-psychiatric physicians to the current 80% or more use of these drugs by an array of non-psychiatric physicians. In one recent plan, PMHM examined the prescribers of these drugs in the benefit plan. The physicians prescribing antidepressants included oncologists, podiatrists and even dentists! A major reason for this change is the marketing inspired belief that the newer antidepressants have more benign and less serious side effects than the earlier tricyclic drugs.

Armed with these drugs the general physician has surplanted psychiatrists, psychologists and clinical social workers as the *primary* mental health provider in society today. I can think of no greater marketing achievement than the marketing of SSRI antidepressants to physicians and consumers as drugs with fairly benign side effects. Now general physicians who are not specialists in mental health or mental disorders can "safely" prescribe antidepressant drugs.

<u>Wide Spectrum Use</u>

Another equally important factor in fueling the expansion of the general physician's drug treatment role in mental health is that current generation antidepressants have come to be seen as *wide spectrum drugs* to treat a growing list of anxiety and depressive disorders among others.

In earlier days the tricyclics were seen as drugs for depression; the benzodiazepines (e.g., Valium) were drugs to treat anxiety. Of course, the benzodiazepines are highly addictive and supposedly limited to short-term use. Moreover, many patients present with both depressive and anxiety symptoms, and it takes an experienced clinician to identify the primary disorder for focussed and appropriate treatment. General physicians could not (and cannot) make the appropriate differential diagnosis in cases with mixed symptoms, and physicians were reluctant to diagnose and prescribe for the disorder.

However, with SSRI and related antidepressants, there is no longer *any* reluctance to experiment in mental health treatment since these drugs have FDA approval for a broad range of both depressive and anxiety disorders. The conventional attitude is that these drugs are good for whatever ails you mentally. The need for correct differential diagnosis is moot, and the doctor can proceed with SSRI pharmacotherapy without any hesitation.

Why have SSRI antidepressants gained FDA approval for treatment of a dozen or so different diseases? The answer is that these drugs do not treat *any* of these disorders very well. SSRIs are a little better than sugar pills as we have seen in treating these disorders in Random Clinical Trials (RCTs) and are probably much less effective in the real world for patients who see their primary care physician and who do not have a diagnosis by a psychiatrist or psychologist.

When Maria visits the physician with a variety of distressing symptoms, the physician does not *have* to make a diagnosis, does not *have* to choose between one or two classes of drugs (antidepressants and benzodiazepines) as earlier. The doctor can now prescribe an SSRI antidepressant and check on Maria a month from now no matter what kind a disorder she has or doesn't have.

The above treatment paradigm is the way it is *expected* to work, but it does not seem to work that way in the real world. In the actual world (from my company's pharmacy research data) those persons prescribed an antidepressant are typically on 1.5 different antidepressants during the year. And of those prescribed an antidepressant, about 40% are also prescribed a benzodiazepine (Valium or Xanax, e.g.,).

Shotgun Approach

We have a pharmacological *shotgun* approach to treating mental health problems in the physician's office, and the dangerous benzodiazepines are as much alive in the physician's office today as they were years ago. There is frequent use by PCPs of multiple antidepressants, frequent dosage increases when the patient is not doing well, the adding of Xanax-type drugs because "placebo" recovery or improvement does not cover all cases.

Physicians Not Trained

With introduction of the SSRI antidepressant in 1987 (Prozac), family physicians crossed the line and without training became *mental health* professionals. The profession of psychiatry, the National Institute of Mental Health (NIMH) and other segments of society encouraged this new role for the family doctor as we have seen.

The senior drug company officials at the House oversite hearing (see Chapter VI) said over and over how complex and serious depression is, how it can be and often is a life-threatening disease, and that it must be treated. I did not hear anyone say, "Since it is such a serious and dangerous disease, why are you marketing these drugs to pediatricians, family physicians and other non-psychiatric physicians as the sole treatment of depression by physicians who do not have adequate training to diagnose and treat mental disorders?"

This is the *one* area that family physicians, with support of the drug companies, the FDA, and other groups, have claimed as their own. Until their patient has had at least *two* antidepressant drug failures, which is the guideline recommended by NIMH, these physicians are not expected to refer the patient.

To support their drug treatment of depression, physicians have to maintain their conviction that depression is a *biological* disease; that depression is a chemical imbalance in the brain, that the *right* antidepressant defines its effective treatment, and other personal or family factors can be essentially ignored in its effective treatment.

The research has shown that one class of antidepressants is no better or worse than the others in terms of effectiveness. This does not dissuade these physicians in the least from experimenting with several antidepressants and related drugs until they find the *right* drugs or combination to treat *this* patient's depression. Each drug treated patient is in a sense an *experiment* for the antidepressant prescribing physician.

A Quick Fix for the Untrained?

Undoubtedly general physicians treating depression with drugs alone have been confronted frequently by the failure of the "magic" to work. Perhaps they have been hearing about CBT and the use of CBT to prevent relapse following drug treatment. Incidentally, you never hear of research studies using drugs to reduce relapse *following* initial treatment by CBT.

These physicians also seem to think CBT is simple. I have noticed a trend for nurses to go to CBT workshops presented by psychologists or practicing CBT therapists and then "performing CBT" with drug-treated patients, often with the insurance companies paying for such treatment. I certainly question such a practice. Mental health should *not* be a sideline practiced by non-mental health professionals.

The World of Side Effects

It would be wonderful if powerful disease treating drugs had no side effects, but there is no drug without risks or side effects. As a patient or a physician we must look at any drug or health procedure in terms of its benefit/risk ratio. As the benefit of a drug or procedure increases we can accept increasing risk with increasing benefit, especially when there are no alternative treatments available.

Life saving surgery is a good trade off for a fairly low incidence of brain damage secondary to general anesthesia. A patient not fully informed or knowledgeable about *either* side of the equation cannot make an informed decision.

With the limited benefits of SSRIs, we should certainly not be prepared to accept anything more than *minimal* risk, especially since there are proven non-drug treatments available. The whole of society is misinformed about the benefits (i.e., effectiveness) of antidepressants and the ten million or so people taking these drugs at any one time are totally misinformed about their benefit. In assessing any drug or medical procedure the starting point is an evaluation of benefit. If benefit is minimal there is no point in evaluating risk, the drug or procedure is simply not worthwhile. However, when there are *perceived* benefits, we will have to look at side effects.

What About Antidepressant Side Effects?

"Proponents" of antidepressants have not only misinformed the general public on the very limited *effectiveness* of these drugs, but "proponents" also have succeeded in successfully minimizing the perception of the adverse side effects of these drugs. Prescribing physicians and users have come to believe that these drugs, as a class, have minimal and tolerable side effects. Although the truth is otherwise, the *perception* that these drugs have mild and tolerable side effects continues to play an important role in the drug's increasing popularity over the past fifteen years.

Reporting the Facts

The unfavorable side effects of these drugs are substantially greater than the drug company and the prescribing physician tell us. When a new antidepressant drug appears on the scene, the adverse side effects are usually limited to those that were reported on drug-treated, depressed clinical trial subjects in the FDA-submitted studies. The key word here is "as reported."

Compared to Tricyclics

In studies comparing SSRIs to first generation tricyclic antidepressants, SSRIs had higher rates of diarrhea (10% greater), nausea (10% greater), insomnia (7%) and headache (3%). Tricyclics had higher rates of dry mouth, constipation (12%), dizziness (11%), blurred vision (4%) and tremors (4%). Nine uncommon (less than

1%) but serious adverse effects were definitely associated with the SSRIs: bradycardia, bleeding, granulocytopenia, seizures, hyponatremia, hepatotoxicity, serotonin syndrome, extrapyramydal effects, and mania in unipolar depression (Kiev, Ari, 1997).

Despite the conventional understanding that *newer* antidepressants have fewer side effects than older drugs, participants discontinued treatment at similar rates for newer and older antidepressants. These discontinuations have been due to lack of effect, adverse effects, or other reasons.

These "reported" side effects are typically fewer and occur at lower frequencies than later side effects of the same drug reported by physicians and patients during periods of longer use. For example, the early SSRI antidepressants diminished sexual libido is reported as one or two percent of trial subjects (and thus reported to prescribing physicians), but later research and clinical practice finds that over half of antidepressant subjects experienced sexual interest/performance problems (Clayton, A.H., et al., 2002). A six to eight week drug clinical trial is simply not long enough for some side effects to appear or for subjects to become aware of some side effects.

Do the side effect profiles in marketing communications perhaps reflect the *patient* reported side effects from the clinical trials rather than the more accurate side effect picture determined by more long-term users? I think you can answer this question as well as I can.

<u>See Side Effects as Part of Disorder?</u>

Some subjects experience drug-induced side effects but do not report these side effects for one reason or another. For example, the subject on an antidepressant may experience a symptom or behavior change (e.g., difficulty sleeping or decreased sexual interest) but may see this as a part of the disorder and will not report it without prompting. Given a checklist of possible side effect symptoms, the drug treated patients will report more adverse drug side effects than when they report without prompts.

We certainly don't want to manufacture "side effects" through a subject's normal suggestibility, which is a danger of the checklist approach. However, we do not want to *underreport* a drug's side effects as the drug companies are now doing.

The side effect profile of SSRI and related antidepressants as well as the major problem patients have in withdrawing from these drugs are far from benign. The increasing popularity of these drugs is testimony to the fact society has a very distorted perception both of the drug's efficacy and the risks involved for the patient using these drugs. Why do we have such a distortion of the true side effect profile of these drugs?

Confusion: Symptom or Side Effect

Physician prescribers and patients as mentioned above often misattribute drug side effects to assumed consequences of the condition the drug is supposedly treating. Developing side effects are often misinterpreted as a deepening of the depression, and these undiagnosed side effects become an occasion for increasing dosages or adding another drug.

For example, insomnia is a frequent concomitant of depression, but insomnia is also a frequently observed adverse side effect of these drugs. We know this because many patients on antidepressants who do not have impaired sleep as a presenting symptom *develop* sleep impairment secondary to the antidepressant. Many depressed patients *do* present with impaired sleep and when prescribed an antidepressant, may then have their *subsequent* sleep impairment increased as a consequence of the drug and not the depression. In this case the physician prescriber may now see the impaired sleep not as a side effect but as a "deepening" of the depression and may, as a result, increase the dosage, add a tricyclic antidepressant (which is more sedating), or perhaps give Ambien to help the patient sleep.

Multiple Drugs, Multiple Side Effects

It is not unusual to see patients on SSRIs taking three to five other drugs such as Ambien, Xanax (for drug induced anxiety), Viagra (for sexual side effects) and Topomax (for weight gain) to address *some* of the side effects of SSRIs. Prescribing drugs to chase symptoms/and or side effects, which my company has seen in *every* pharmacy plan it has examined, is not a rare event. One might see this prescribing pattern as comical if it were not for the tragic aspects for the patients taking these drugs. I don't think this problem (by prescribers and patients) of confusing side effects with pathology has gotten the attention it deserves either in the professional literature or in the popular press.

Unfortunately, the vast majority of patients on these drugs have no idea about the difference between their basic mental health problems and the "mental health" problems secondary to the drugs that are, ironically, caused by the chemical imbalances initiated by the drug.

The typical prescribing physician probably has no better ability than the patient does to make this differentiation. Many times we have a situation of the blind leading the blind. When there is a drug approach to treating mental disorders, there is a decided "tropism" to change the medication if the patient is not doing well.

When one of these patients is not doing well for any reason (e.g., the basic mental health problem or drug side effects or both), it is not surprising to find the patient on four or more additional drugs. When side effects occur, especially when there may be several drug side effects operating simultaneously, it is best to gradually withdraw *all* drugs from the patient to determine who is the "real" patient beneath all of the side effects of the various drugs.

Physicians and many psychiatrists unfortunately no longer think that the environment or unfavorable life events or disordered behavior or, indeed, that the patient's personality/patterns of thinking have *any* effects on the patient's disorder. If the drug-treated patient is not doing well, the prescriber often fails to look at the patient and his or her life and instead looks to a drug answer for the patient's problems. The belief that depression is a biologically based disease leads to ignoring very real situational or behavior problems. The lack of evidence that drugs are the solution for these problems has not affected prescribing behavior. Drug treatment of depression continues despite the absence of any evidence to support such an approach to treating these problems.

Are SSRI Antidepressants Addictive?

Certainly the benzodiazepines are addictive in that there is drug habituation (to continue the same effect requires increasing dosages) and serious side effects on abrupt withdrawal from these drugs. The rebound phenomena that can occur includes an intensification of symptoms during the withdrawal phase. For example, withdrawal from Xanax for treating panic attacks increases the frequency of panic attacks over what they were prior to the treatment (Consumer Reports, 2004). Many people each year on benzodiazepines have to be detoxed in the hospital.

After chronic use of anxiolytics there should *never* be abrupt termination from these drugs because of the risk of seizures and other health hazards. People get hooked on these drugs because of habituation and withdrawal effects when they attempt to cut down on the frequency of use. I am sure many physicians finally help their addictive patients to safely discontinue their benzodiazepines, but the physicians may transfer these patients to a "safer" SSRI antidepressant.

The SSRI antidepressants are not habituating. Unlike heroin or anxiolytics, the SSRI user does not require an increasing dosage of an SSRI to obtain the same effect. However, a drug does not have to be *habituating* in order to be addictive, for example cigarettes. The antidepressant believers are quick to say that these SSRI drugs are not habit forming, but speaking out of the other side of their mouth they also say, "Don't discontinue these drugs abruptly."

If the "believers" say these drugs are not addicting, they should look at the thousands of users who have often tried to get off them. Sometime people have severe withdrawal effects after only a few days of drug use. Even with tapering of the drug, withdrawal effects, as we will see, can occur a month or more after last use. These withdrawal effects will quickly subside if the drugs are restarted, which is characteristic of addictive phenomena.

Withdrawing from Benzodiazepines and Antidepressants

Withdrawal of these drugs should be under a physician's supervision. Professor C. Heather Ashton, DM, FRCP of the University of Newcastle, Division of Psychiatry, recommends the following guidelines for long-term benzodiazepine users also taking antidepressants and wish to withdraw from both drugs.

1. Complete the benzodiazepine withdrawal before starting to taper your antidepressants.
2. Allow at least 4 weeks after stopping your benzodiazepines before starting on antidepressant withdrawal.
3. Consult your doctor before starting to withdraw the antidepressant and agree on a tapering schedule.
4. Antidepressant withdrawal must be gradual to avoid withdrawal effects.

a. Make each dose reduction as small as possible, e.g., by halving the tablets or using a liquid preparation.
b. If smaller doses are not available, reduce by taking a tablet every other day, then every third day, etc.
c. Allow one to two weeks between each dosage reduction.
d. If withdrawal symptoms are severe, increase the dosage slightly (e.g., to the dose at your last reduction). When symptoms have settled, resume withdrawal at a slower rate.

5. With slow tapering, as outlined above, withdrawal symptoms from antidepressants are usually absent, or if they occur, are mild and short-lived.

From Dr. Ashton's recommendations it is apparent that those on both a benzodiazepine *and* an antidepressant have double trouble, especially in discontinuing both. From PMHM's research at least half of those on antidepressants take a benzodiazepine as well. The SSRI antidepressants were touted as treating anxiety as well as depression, which relieved general physicians from using the "dangerous" benzodiazepines for anxiety. However, the benzodiazepines are brought in the back door when the SSRI antidepressants fail to do their job.

<u>Withdrawal Symptoms</u>

The marketing folks at the drug companies have been fighting a rear guard action for many years in denying the existence of SSRI withdrawal side effects. The companies have attributed the "side effects" to a *re-emergence* of the depression. The drug companies do not want these drugs to be seen as addictive or dangerous in any way, because that would be incompatible with their marketing to family physicians. Actually, when the drug companies see these withdrawal effects as "re-emergence of the depression" it does not speak very well for the drug's efficacy. When pressed the believers bring out the "fact" that depression is a chronic, relapsing disease, which in many cases requires *lifetime* drug maintenance.

Symptoms of depression are totally different from drug withdrawal effects. Many physicians, including many psychiatrists, fail to pick up the difference and frequently prescribe other drugs to treat these misinterpreted withdrawal or side effects as the primary depression. Common withdrawal symptoms include nausea, abdominal pain, diarrhea, sleep disturbance, insomnia, vivid dreams, nightmares, general somatic distress (sweating, lethargy, headaches) and affective symptoms (low mood, anxiety, irritability). A few of the foregoing side effects can be "depressive" symptoms as well. However, other withdrawal symptoms include such bodily sensations as dizziness/lightheadedness, various sensory abnormalities including numbness, paraesthesia, electric-shock-like sensations, and what is called akathesia/agitation, which has been implicated in causing violent behavior.

Depression certainly affects the whole person but not to the extent as in the above, especially in the variety and magnitude of the organ systems involved. The withdrawal symptoms imply that the whole nervous system — not just the brain, but the peripheral nervous system (the sensory and motor systems), the autonomic nervous system and hormonal system are involved.

What's in a Name?

The drug companies prefer the term Discontinuation Syndrome rather than Withdrawal Syndrome and some researchers (perhaps those more allied with the drug companies) tend to prefer the first designation. By using the term Discontinuation Syndrome, "proponents" do not blame the drug. They blame the precipitous withdrawal *from* the drug. SSRI antidepressants are not equally subject to withdrawal side effects, perhaps because each antidepressant may vary in their half-life, that is, how long the drugs stay around in the system. Paxil, which has a very short half-life, is known to have marked withdrawal effects. Lesser effects are found for Zoloft (sertraline) and Prozac because of their longer half-life. Here are some cases of withdrawal effects culled from websites.

> Mrs. A., a 29 year old married lady with a moderate depressive disorder, was switched to paroxetine by her general practitioner after an initial prescription of dothiepin. She found the tricyclic dothiepin too sedating and after a week or so of this medication requested a change. After two weeks on paroxetine (Paxil) 20 mg daily a consultant psychiatrist who increased the dose to 40 mg daily reviewed her. The patient suffered a dystonic reaction to procyclidine. The paroxetine was discontinued. Unfortunately the dystonic reaction persisted when off all

> medication and required further medical admission and the re-prescription of procyclidine. The depression continued unabated and a tricyclic was started with some improvement in mood. Seven months after the paroxetine had been stopped, tardive dystonia was noted to be present and to vary with anxiety levels, body posture, alertness, and emotional state. (Green, Ben)

Mrs. A may have had some problems prior to her drug therapy, but to me it sounds as if her original problems don't compare with the problems her "treatment" gave her. Don't forget that in addition to the quality care issues, there are also significant costs involved in these iatrogenic (physician caused) issues.

> A 35-year-old man (Mr. B) was prescribed paroxetine (Paxil) 30 mg daily for depression. The depression resolved and the paroxetine was continued at the same dose for two years. The medication was discontinued in a staged way, with reductions to 20, then 10 mgs, managed over six weeks or so. Symptoms of withdrawal occurred throughout this period and were comprised of vivid nightmares, lability of mood, irritability, hypersexuality, episodic lightheadedness, and episodic electric shock like sensations, glove paraesthesiae, and ataxia. These symptoms ended two weeks after the withdrawal regime was finished. Nevertheless the patient continued to describe problems of an episodic nature well after the paroxetine had been discontinued. These episodes, lasting hours to days at a time, consisted of paraesthesias, dizziness, mild ataxia, and slurred speech. These episodes have occurred intermittently throughout twelve months of follow-up during which time the patient has been drug-free. There were no focal neurological signs or any features suggestive of progressive neurological disease, nor was there a family history of neurological disease.

So much for the "correcting of the chemical imbalance theory." Despite drug tapering this patient continued to have side effects *twelve months* after he had been drug free. Considering the patient's withdrawal symptoms, I doubt that the patient's original depression was as disabling to him as the horror he experienced during his withdrawal.

> Mrs. C., a 29-year-old mother of one, became ill with depression when her son was aged eight months. She was suicidal and required hospital admission when she was started on fluoxetine (Prozac) 20 mg daily. The antidepressant worked well and her mood was restored within four weeks of admission. She was discharged home, but commented that her sleep was occasionally disturbed by bad dreams and she was aware of twitching when in the bed. She was kept on the fluoxetine (Prozac) for a further twelve months and at outpatient reviews mentioned that nocturnal twitching still occasionally disturbed her sleep. She said that her husband had started to sleep separately, because he was 'tired of being kicked' in the middle of the night. The fluoxetine was discontinued eighteen months after the admission. Mrs. C described no worsening of her mood and was euthymic (normal) at outpatient review. However, she was distressed to report that her nocturnal twitching, which took the form of sudden myoclonic jerks of her limbs, had actually worsened off fluoxetine. During the day these abnormal involuntary movements were less marked and more easily disguised, but nonetheless were a problem for the patient. At follow-up eight months after discontinuation the untoward myoclonic jerks were continuing. There are no focal neurological signs or any features suggestive of progressive neurological disease, nor was there a family history of neurological disease.

Apparently Mrs. C's physicians did not pick up the fact that her nightmares and muscle twitching were Prozac side effects and not depressive phenomena. Finally someone got the idea that they were seeing drug side effects, and Prozac was discontinued after eighteen months. Her myoclonic jerks of her limbs had actually worsened when she was off Prozac, which is not a rare event. Her myoclonic jerks were not the result of her depression worsening; I have never seen a depressed patient who had myoclonic jerks as a part of the depression.

> Mrs. D., a 49-year-old health professional was prescribed 20 mg paroxetine (Paxil) daily in April 2000 for a depressive disorder. This relieved the depression, but after three months the patient started to develop paresthesiae in the right hand, and some weeks later experienced her fingers being 'fumbly'. She visited her GP and complained that although her mood was satisfactory there were

unpleasant side effects. He asked her to reduce the dose to 10 mg daily. Mrs. D began to experience painful, restless legs at night and vivid dreams. The tingling in her hand spread into her body and head. After a week of the 10 mg dose the patient discontinued the paroxetine altogether in the belief that the paroxetine would be out of her system in a few days and her symptoms would subside. The symptoms, however, persisted. She took a week off work, but the following symptoms persisted for the next three months:

- paraesthesia in hands and feet spreading up arms and legs intermittently
- stiffness in calf muscles
- unsteadiness on her feet with wide gait
- clumsy fingers
- loose bowels
- disinhibited mood

These symptoms appeared worse at the end of the day, following heavy physical work, and with even small amounts of alcohol. By December, four months after discontinuing the paroxetine most of the symptoms had reduced in severity to near normal.

The above is such a contrast to the magazine and television ads that show the before and after images of the sad person being transformed by the drug into a picture of happiness.

Mrs. E., a 48-year-old woman was prescribed citalopram (Celexa) by her GP for eleven months. The indication for the prescription was chronic anxiety. For fifteen months following the discontinuation of this therapy she suffered headaches and dizziness. She also complained of a fluttering sensation across her scalp. To date there has been little improvement.

If Mrs. E. was not anxious before, she certainly is now. Sometimes the magic pill just doesn't work. Will she learn from that? Will she try another miracle cure?

GlaxoSmithKline (Paxil) Modifies Label—Under Duress?

A California lawsuit against GSK charged the company with a failure to warn about the possible dangers of Paxil withdrawal. The suit was said to be resolved in January of 2002 but, as usual, the terms of the agreement/settlement were not announced. However, later GSK did modify its Paxil label, which may have been one of the terms of the agreement. Peter Briggin, M.D., who provided expert testimony for the plaintiff, was told on good authority that it was likely that the lawsuit caused both the drug company and the FDA to strengthen the label with regard to Paxil withdrawal effects.

GSK Precautions

On December 14, 2001, GSK added information to its label regarding withdrawal from Paxil (also sold as Seroxat in England).

GSK still maintains that the reactions reported in patients after the clinical trials may have no causal relationship to the drug and the side effects are generally self-limiting, a familiar refrain.

Dr. Briggin stressed the importance of "anxiety" and "agitation" mentioned on the label in association with Paxil withdrawal. Briggin and others have stressed that "anxiety" and "agitation" can contribute to aggressive, violent or suicidal behavior, but the label makes no mention of any danger of aggression, violent or suicidal behavior during Paxil withdrawal. In the modified Paxil label warning, however, GSK still refers to discontinuation effects rather than withdrawal effects.

The Violent World of Psychiatric Drugs

For a number of years many people and groups have expressed concerns about psychiatric drugs in general as a primary cause of violence in society today. The following case examples of violent behavior of persons on psychiatric drugs come from the Citizens Commission on Human Rights (CCHR) International, which is said to have a data base of hundreds of cases of violence by psychotropic drug using patients during the past fifteen years.

1. On March 6, 1985, Atlanta postal worker, Steven W. Brownlee, pulled a pistol from his pocket and shot and killed a supervisor and a clerk.

Another clerk was wounded. Brownlee had received treatment and psychotropic drugs at the Grady Memorial Psychiatric Unit.

2. On November 20, 1986, 14-year-old Rod Mathews beat a classmate to death with a bat in the woods near his home in Canton, Massachusetts. He had been prescribed Ritalin since the third grade.

3. William Cruse was charged with killing six people in a shooting rampage on April 23, 1987, in Palm Bay, Florida. Cruse had been seeing a Kentucky psychiatrist and stated he had been taking psychiatric drugs for several years.

4. Bartley Dobben killed his two young children on November 26, 1987, by casting them in a 1,300-degree foundry ladle. He had been placed on a regimen of psychiatric drugs in 1985.

5. On May 20, 1988, Laurie Dann walked into a Winnetka, Illinois second grade classroom carrying three pistols and began shooting innocent little children, killing one and wounding five others before killing herself. Subsequent blood tests revealed that both Lithium and the antidepressant Anafranil were in her bloodstream at the time the murder was committed.

6. On September 26, 1988, 19-year-old James Wilson took a .22 caliber revolver into an elementary school in Greenwood, South Carolina, and started shooting school children, killing two 8-year-old girls and wounding seven other children and two teachers. Wilson had been in and out of the hands of psychiatrists for years, and, within eight months of the killings, he had been on several psychiatric drugs which can generate violent behavior. Since the age of 14 he had been given psychiatric drugs, including Xanax, Valium, Thorazine and Haldol.

7. On January 17, 1989, Patrick Purdy opened fire on a schoolyard full of young children in Stockton, California. During his vicious and unprovoked assault, Purdy killed five school children and wounded 30 others before killing himself. During the two years prior to the murders of the Stockton children, Purdy had been on two strong psychiatric drugs.

8. On April 28, 1992, Kenneth Sequin drugged his two children, aged 7 and 5, took them to a pond, slashed their wrists and dumped their bodies in the water. He then drove home and killed his wife with an ax while she slept. He was on Prozac at the time.

9. In November 1992, Lynwood Drake III, in San Luis Obispo and Morro Bay, California, shot and killed six people with a handgun before he killed himself. Metabolized Prozac and Valium were both found in his system.

10. In December 1993, Steven Leith of Chelsea, Michigan, walked back into a school meeting and fatally shot the school superintendent and wounded two others including a fellow teacher. He was on Prozac at the time of the shootings.

11. 16-year-old Brian Pruitt, who fatally stabbed his grandparents in 1995, had a history of psychiatric treatment and had been prescribed psychiatric drugs.

12. On November 3, 1995, Sergeant Steven B. Christian, a 25 year commended veteran of the Dallas police force drove to a police sub-station and seriously wounded an officer outside in his attempt to get inside and shoot others. Christian was shot and killed by two fellow Dallas police officers. The autopsy revealed high levels of an antidepressant in his blood.

13. In Connecticut on March 6, 1998, Mathew Beck, a lottery accountant, reported promptly to his job, hung up his coat and methodically gunned down four of his bosses, one of whom he chased through a parking lot before he turned the gun on himself. Beck had been seeing a psychiatrist and taking three types of "medication".

14. On May 28, 1998, Brynn Hartman murdered her husband, comic Phil Hartman and then committed suicide. She had been prescribed and had been taking the antidepressant drug Zoloft, which the coroner found in her system along with alcohol and cocaine.

15. On February 19, 1996, ten-year-old Timmy Becton grabbed his three-year-old niece as a shield and aimed a shotgun at a Sheriff's deputy who had accompanied a truant officer to his Florida home. Becton had been taken to a psychiatrist in January and had been put on a psychiatric drug.

16. While on vacation, on May 25, 1997, in Las Vegas, 18-year-old Jeremy Strohmeyer raped and murdered a seven-year-old girl in the ladies rest room in a casino. He had been diagnosed with ADD and prescribed Dexedrine. He had begun taking the drug a week before the killing.

17. On September 27, 1997, 16-year-old Sam Manzie raped and strangled another boy to death. At the time of the killing the younger boy had been selling candy door to door for the local PTA. Manzie was under psychiatric "care" and was being "medicated".

18. On May 21, 1998, 14-year-old Kip Kinkel shot and killed his parents and then went on a wild shooting spree at his Springfield, Oregon, high school that left two dead and twenty-two injured. He was reportedly taking Prozac and Ritalin and had been attending "anger management" classes.

19. On April 20, 1999, Eric Harris, one of two Colorado high school seniors who went on a deadly rampage, entered his school shooting students and faculty and setting off explosives. 12 students and one teacher were killed, along with the two gunmen who ended the rampage by killing themselves, while 23 others were wounded. A toxicology report revealed Luvox, an antidepressant, in Harris' system.

20. On May 4, 1999, Steven Allen Abrams rammed his car into a preschool playground in Costa Mesa, California, killing two and injuring five. He had been placed on probation in 1994, which required him to see a psychiatrist and take Lithium.

In a few of the above cases antidepressants were specifically mentioned. However, the above killers were on a wide variety of psychiatric drugs such as the atypical antipsychotics, mood stabilizers (for bipolar disorder), stimulants (e.g., Ritalin), anxiolytic drugs (e.g., Xanax) and, of course, a variety of antidepressants, including the SSRI and related antidepressants. Many people and groups will accept the above case examples as proof of the connection between the drugs and violence. Although I am sure we could come up with case examples of violent acts by persons who have never been on psychiatric drugs, these examples, even if they are not proof, indicate we need to vigorously pursue the answers to such an important question.

The Link

As a clinician I find the link between these drugs and violence to partly come from the bizarre quality of these violent episodes. An example of this bizarreness is case number four, in which the father killed his young children by casting them in a 1,300-degree foundry ladle. Many serial killers, most of whom are not on psychiatric drugs, can and do perform horrendous acts that give them pleasure. Yet at least these despicable acts could be seen as "rational" as opposed to a psychotic person who kills in irrational ways on the basis of a delusion. For example, the delusional person might have killed his neighbor whom he believed to be on the payroll of the F.B.I.

The Sociopathic Difference

Serial killers are generally correctly diagnosed as Sociopathic, an Axis II Disorder. The serial killer has no conscience, no sense of right or wrong, and he is therefore not internally deterred in any way from doing whatever it is that gives him/her pleasure. The general public has a tendency to confuse mental disorder with the predatory behavior of sociopathic people and believes the killer must have been mentally deranged to commit such a horrendous act. However, these sociopathic killers are not psychotic; they are of sound mind even though their behavior is not modified by a working conscience.

Sociopaths rarely go to a psychiatrist on their own. Sociopaths only come to the attention of mental health professionals when they are forced to by the courts because of various antisocial behaviors. There is no psychiatric drug that will give such individuals a normally operating conscience or the ability to modify their own self-interest or pleasure because of the anticipated pain of others. However, this fact does not keep modern psychiatry and the drug companies from pursuing or trying a drug that will curb sociopathic behavior.

Depression Not Primary Problem in Personality Disorders

If the depression or anxiety is *primary* and not a malformation of the person's personality, the patient can do well in their life and in their relationships when successfully treated for depression or an anxiety disorder. Unlike the patient with a *primary* depression, the personality disorder's whole personality is defective. "Cure" would require a complete *overhaul* of the personality. Unfortunately, the personality cannot be overhauled despite what some mental health professionals want to believe.

Personality disorders are not free of periods of stress or low mood because of their maladaptive ways of relating to others. But what gets them into trouble with others is the *personality* problem, not the stress or mood problems secondary to their maladaptive personality. These personality disorders cannot be cured but often their problems can be *managed* by a competent therapist who is very knowledgeable of the personality disorder. To manage the personality disordered person's behavior, a therapeutic alliance with the patient must be obtained and sustained. However, we have to accept the fact that no *drug* will cure these personality disorders or even their "depression" or "anxiety".

Axis II

There is no scientific evidence that drugs provide effective treatment of patients with a personality disorder. Personality disorders, including but not limited to the sociopaths, are called Axis II disorders in the DSM-V classification of the mental disorders and are not rare. However, as a behavioral health reviewer and manager I rarely see psychiatrists using an Axis II diagnosis. Generally the psychiatrists prefer a diagnosis such as MDD (Major Depressive Disorder) for patients who have one of the Axis II disorders.

As a reviewer, I have wondered if the psychiatrist is so diagnostically naive that he or she fails to recognize the primacy of the personality disorder diagnosis or if he/she knows the correct diagnosis but is creating another diagnosis for insurance purposes? Whichever way it is, many psychiatrists are treating these personality disorders *as if* the patient had a mental disorder that is treatable with drugs (such as schizophrenia or bipolar disorder). As a reviewer, I note that these patients are typically put on antidepressants, mood stabilizers, anixolytics and at times atypical antipsychotics, alone or more typically in combination. However, there are *no scientifically controlled drug outcome studies that show that these or any psychiatric drugs are effective with these kinds of patients.*

Defense

Many psychiatrists defend their drug prescribing with these patients by saying in their clinical experience (anecdotal evidence) they have found drugs to be effective with these patients. However, such "evidence" is no evidence at all. If psychiatrists *believe* these drugs are effective with personality disorders, why not conduct scientifically controlled studies to test this belief. In the absence of such studies drug treatment of personality disorders *cannot* be defended. Even if the psychiatrist *says* that depression is depression irrespective of the presence or absence of a personality disorder, we can safely say a primary depression is *not* the same as the "depression" in a personality disorder.

The "depression" of the latter is more akin to unhappiness than to a primary depression. Treating unhappiness with drugs is not appropriate treatment and does not address the core problems giving rise to the pseudodepression.

The Danger of Polypharmacy

Modern psychiatry uses a polypharmacy approach in treating a variety of mental disorders. This polypharmacy is driven not by science but by clinical hunches and anecdotal evidence (e.g., "I added a mood stabilizer to my schizophrenic patient and, boy, did she sure do well."). Science and not wish fulfillment must guide drug treatment.

I am quite sure that polypharmacy was quite prevalent in the group of the above twenty cases of violent behavior. Again, when the patient is not doing well — and these patients could not have been doing well prior to their violence —typically the first and last response of most prescribers is to increase the dosage or add a second or third (or fourth) medication.

The modern psychiatrists have only one tool (i.e., drugs). If the patient is not doing well, the response is to bring out the tool and add another drug. The question of the dangerousness of psychiatric drugs is compounded when the patient is on two or more drugs. It is possible that neither drug is dangerous alone, but in *combination* these drugs may well be dangerous. The dangerousness may have occurred not from the drugs the patient was on, but from the improper withdrawal of a *previous* drug.

Most of the above twenty cases of violence were *voluntary* patients who were being treated by psychiatrists or general physicians. The lack of more comprehensive treatment may have played a role in the subsequent violent behavior. Insight into these violent people could have been gained if, during their incarceration following their crimes, they could have been studied with psychological testing/assessment during and after being withdrawn from their psychiatric drugs. Psychological testing needs to be done to determine what the personality structure was *prior* to drug treatment.

It is important to understand these twenty individuals and other violent crime perpetrators who are on psychotropic medication to determine from their history and behavior the level of conscience development of these persons. The nature of the violent acts suggests that at the time of the crime, normal conscience or superego functions were not operating in these individuals. Was this result a product of the person, the drugs alone or the two in combination? Did psychiatric drugs or other factors compromise their superego functions, or did the individuals lack adequate superego development prior to their violent acts? If psychiatric drugs *did* indeed compromise superego operations of these persons, allowing the violent behavior to emerge, studies should be done to determine the critical factors in this emergence.

The Andrea Yates Case—A Look at Polypharmacy

This case of the Houston, Texas mother who killed her five children is pertinent to our discussion. The case is a good example of the failure of modern mental health treatment. The modern model is drug treatment and when the patient does not do well, polypharmacy. This treatment model neglects the patient and the patient's environment. The newspaper accounts of the trial, Andrea's history, family life and her extensive psychiatric and mental health drug history gave insight into her life and to her as a person. Her psychiatric drug history was characterized by *multiple* medications from a variety of drug classes, often two SSRI antidepressants concurrently, an anxiolytic drug from time to time, mood stabilizers, atypical antipsychotics and perhaps drugs to treat the side effects of these same drugs. She may also have had agitation/akathisia from the SSRIs and other adverse side effects that may have been seen as side effects and/or symptoms of her basic pathology.

She was first treated as a post-partum depression with antidepressants, probably SSRIs, but her mental disorder worsened with each subsequent pregnancy and birth. Her pharmacotherapy soon broadened to include *all* of the drug classes. These types of cases have become more typical in recent years as psychiatry moved to an almost exclusive reliance on the drug treatment of mental disorders. If Andrea also had some "therapy" from time to time, it seemed to be adjunctive and subordinate to the role drugs played in her treatment.

From media reports no definitive diagnosis can be made, but from the array of medications she was on, it is likely her psychiatrists suspected a psychotic disorder. The possible psychotic disorders are MDD (Major Depressive Disorder with psychosis), schizophrenia, schizoaffective type, bipolar disorder, anxiety disorder, dependent personality or some combination of the above. What the correct diagnosis was is unknown.

Earlier in my career I was often called upon to assess such problem cases. Now with the expansion of psychiatric medications — and the sheer number of drugs that patients are now taking — the diagnostic task is made more difficult because of the problem in separating the *pathology* from the drug *side effects*. When I come across such a situation I have often recommended starting over, that is, *withdraw* the patient from *all* psychiatric drugs and find out *who* the patient really is before proceeding with further treatment.

With Andrea, however, the correct label was not so important as an understanding of the *psychosocial* factors that were operating in her life and that were seemingly ignored in her treatment. Her treatment seemed to be the search for the perfect chemical cocktail that would stabilize her and would make her accept her role in life.

The key to understanding Andrea's problems, which is necessary to plan effective treatment, was to understand not chemical imbalances but to understand the relevant *psychosocial* factors operating. Andrea was a baby-making machine, probably with a dependent personality. She was married to a husband in a fundamentalist Christian church tradition that was likely to be "coercing" her to have more babies.

This "diagnosis" was based on publicly disseminated information. I did not have access to any psychological testing of the patient, nor was there any evidence that there was any psychological assessment of the patient. If it had existed, psychological testing *could* have been very productive. What is important to see here is my attempt to understand what the patient was going through in order to develop a treatment plan that could be revised with increasing understanding of the patient and the conflicts in her life?

I apologize to her psychiatrists for doing this post-mortem since it is always much easier to be an astute diagnostician in hindsight than at the time events are unfolding. Nor do I envy the psychiatrists who treated Andrea because she and her situation were very difficult. Still someone should have told her husband and the minister, "Look, if she has more babies she will either kill herself or kill them." I suspect Andrea was between a rock and a hard place in which she saw no way out.

The case indicates to me that psychiatry has to turn away from a reliance on the biological/disease approach that results in polypharmacy and return to looking at the whole individual and treating the whole person.

Discounting the Danger

Moreover, the cases of violence of patients on SSRIs involve not only suicide but also homicide, especially very brutal homicides. It is difficult to believe that someone with a serious depression alone can work around their conscience and commit murderous acts without the imposition of some type of brain dysfunction secondary to drugs. Depressed people are much more likely to be violent toward *themselves* than toward others. With murder one must look for an explanation *other* than depression.

The antidepressant believers often say that the patient was really a bipolar disorder and the SSRI unmasked a bipolar disorder. It is difficult to accept this theory. Many people including Phase I normal subjects on SSRIs have reported feelings of rage and aggressive urges to do harm to themselves (e.g., cut off their arm) and to harm others; fortunately, these antidepressant users were somehow able to suppress the urge.

Psychiatrists, with a few exceptions, discount the issue of dangerousness with regard to these drugs, on the other side some detractors want to ban *all* psychiatric drugs but there is a rational middle ground. Certainly these drugs *cause* chemical imbalances (we must forget the claim that they restore brain chemical balance). All such drugs without exception and in varying degrees produce *dysfunction* in the brain. These drugs all impair *cognitive* functions such as alertness, attentional capacity, concentration, and problem solving, but these *cognitive* impairments do not in themselves preclude the use and effectiveness of drugs in treating various mental disorders. I suspect that in schizophrenia and correctly diagnosed bipolar cases the brain dysfunction arising from the mental disorder is greater than the brain dysfunction produced by the drug. I suspect these psychotic patients experience *improved* brain function rather than a net loss of brain functioning ability when taking appropriate medication.

Schizophrenia is a very broad disorder. It can range from individuals who spend most of their life in mental hospitals on psychiatric drugs, to the other extreme, the very bright schizophrenics who are able to carry out fairly normal professional and social lives without drugs or mental health treatment of any kind. I have seen such "well functioning" schizophrenics in my day-to-day life and relationships. The eminent psychiatrist, Harry Stack Sullivan, who was noted for the interpersonal theory of schizophrenia, was said to have been schizophrenic and was not, to my knowledge, on psychiatric drugs.

Disclaimer

Peter Briggin and many groups are opposed to *all* psychiatric drugs and, in this, I definitely part company with them. I do not believe that many schizophrenic patients, accurately diagnosed cases of bipolar disorder and ADD or ADHD can be treated competently and successfully without *appropriate* psychiatric medications. Cognitive therapy and environmental manipulation are very powerful treatments for a variety of mental disorders, including the psychoses, but these non-drug treatments cannot replace drugs in treating the disorders I mentioned above. Appropriate *behavioral* interventions are necessary but not *sufficient* treatments for the *psychotic* disorders and for the disorders that require stimulant medication. According to the DSM Major Depressive Disorder (MDD) is one of the *psychotic* disorders, but I do not see a unipolar depression (MDD) as a psychotic disorder. However, if Dr. John gives Mary an antidepressant he is "telling" Mary, or any of you who have taken these drugs, that you are and she is psychotic.

Many schizophrenics, however, require and function much better on the earlier and present day atypical antipsychotics. If I ever returned to treating schizophrenics, I would not try to do so without the use of antipsychotic drugs in most cases. We should be prepared to accept some serious risks *when* the drug benefits justify such risks. The antipsychotic drugs have the risk of tardive dyskinesia, a very serious neuromotor disorder, but I believe the benefits of the drug in most cases outweigh such risks.

An Alert in Psychiatric Diagnosis

We certainly cannot prove anything scientifically from case studies alone, just as we cannot use testimonials to prove that a drug such as an SSRI is effective. However, we do know that people in general are *very* predictable in their behavior, whether the person is a Mike Tyson or a church going fundamentalist. We simply do not tend to depart very far from our "chosen" or beaten path.

When I observe in a patient a drastic change in behavior, an act that is inconsistent with the way the individual has behaved throughout his or her life, I tend to look for some type of *brain or toxic condition* to "explain" the behavior change.

The behavior is simply incompatible with the personality structure-organization of the individual. When this happens I look for some type of brain abnormality (sub-clinical seizures, organic dementia, drugs or other) to account for the behavior change. Brain dysfunction can occur not only secondary to neurological diseases but brain dysfunction also can and does happen with most, if not all, psychiatric drugs. You will read later that the akathesia/agitation found in the SSRI antidepressants with some patients is believed to be a cause of violent behavior.

For example, I was asked by a neurologist to see one of his hospitalized male patients, a man in his middle sixties who had some sort of emotional or brain difficulties. I interviewed Ed, took a history and found that in the recent past Ed had been putting pressure on his wife for both of them to take up nudism. This is not unusual in itself, and is not in itself indicative of any type of pathology, but it was very unusual for *this* individual and extremely uncharacteristic of the kind of path Ed had taken during his whole life. It was so uncharacteristic that I could not attribute the change to emotional factors and I came to the conclusion that some type of brain abnormality was operating to account for Ed's behavior change and other recent problems.

I expressed this clinical opinion to the referring neurologist in a written consult, then conducted neuropsychological testing in the hospital and diagnosed an early progressive dementia of the Alzheimer's type. An apparent personality change may be caused by brain changes that are compromising behavior. The brain changes can arise from neurological disease or *drugs* that cause brain dysfunction.

When you read about these cases of violence (murder, suicide or both) by persons taking SSRI or related drugs there seem to be common themes including the lack of any type of prior violent history. There is no question that these types of crimes occur in individuals not taking SSRI antidepressants or other drugs. The question is not the crime itself, but the consistency or lack of consistency between the crime and the *personality* of the individual committing the crime. To understand violent crimes and those who commit them we need a deeper understanding of these individuals and their patterns of behavior prior to the violence.

Comprehensive Treatment

I subscribe to comprehensive treatment of mental health problems by highly trained behavioral health specialists—not nurses, general physicians, psychiatrists with drugs alone, physician's assistants, counselors or marriage/family therapists and the like. Psychiatric drugs should only be prescribed when these drugs have been proven to be effective in treating the disorder at hand. Drug treatment based on clinical hunch should not be allowed, but clinical hunches can and should be subjected to controlled scientific tests, which is the *only* way these and similar questions can be answered.

Since psychiatrists as a group have turned away from behavioral interventions (except through referral), there is no potential for them to provide comprehensive treatment or to make enlightened decisions on whether drugs are or are not required. I am sure that using psychiatric drugs can be very seductive. The prescriber can become so enamoured of these drugs that the prescribers become blind to all non-drug considerations. When psychologists become trained and licensed to prescribe behavioral drugs they will be subjected to the same pressures. However, I hope that psychologists will be able to bring science and rationality to the endeavor and curtail the rampant prescribing abuses that are unfortunately quite prevalent today.

Psychiatric drug prescribing has gotten well beyond the science supporting it. Much of the psychiatric drug prescribing is non-productive and, what is worse, results in adverse side effects that add further cognitive burdens to the patient.

There is no doubt that in a number of the above twenty cases psychiatric drugs played a major, causal role in the person's violent outbursts. We simply do not expect homicidal and sadistic behavior from persons with a normal brain and a primary depression. Moreover, one does not expect violent behavior toward others from over-conscientious and perfectionistic individuals. Others, criminally sociopathic and predatory individuals *are* capable of such violent and sadistic outbursts, but as adults they are not very likely to look for professional help on their own or to take psychiatric drugs.

We know that certain of these drugs undermine inhibition, which could well be a factor in such violent behavior, but drug effects that undermine *normal superego control*, would seem a more plausible explanation for these violent episodes. With these drugs there can be a dulling of feeling, which a patient of mine described as a "rag doll" effect, which could allow violent acts to emerge in basically non-violent people.

Antidepressants and Suicide

Over the past ten years or so there have been increasing reports of a possible link between SSRI antidepressants and suicide. An earlier review of the literature of Prozac and violence found no substance to these reports, but continuing reports persisted. Dr. Jonathan O. Cole, a Harvard psychiatrist, who has suggested a link between the two, believes the drug companies haven't adequately investigated the problem. No one has done the large-scale studies to resolve the issue. If such a link were proven, however, it should indeed be the end of the antidepressant industry.

Cole and his Harvard colleagues, nearly ten years ago, reported on early cases of extreme agitation among patients taking Prozac and other selective serotonin reuptake inhibitor antidepressants.

"SSRI" Suicide

According to a court document in support of a lawsuit brought by the family of Matthew Miller, a Missouri teenager — Miller, 13, had been taking Zoloft, a chemical cousin of Prozac, for only a week when he hanged himself in his bedroom closet July 28, 1997. Again, suicide does not and should not occur when hope had to be alive (after starting on a drug) for this teenager. I am clinically certain this drug caused the boy's suicide.

Dr. David Healy, a British researcher who was the family's chief expert witness (we will hear more from Dr. Healy later) said there is adequate evidence that Zoloft caused the youth to commit suicide. However, a lawyer on the side of Pfizer, Inc., the maker of Zoloft, said there is no credible scientific evidence of a connection between the drug and suicide. Pfizer was able to marshal scientific "experts" on the other side to support its case.

Depressed and suicidal patients usually do not commit suicide in the *depths* of their depression probably because of depleted energy and difficulty planning. Most professionals are aware that in a depressed patient's *sudden* improvement of mood the risk of suicide may *increase* rather than decrease. Ironically, when a depressed person comes up with a plan to kill him or herself, the plan itself can be an instant "cure" of the depression. Such a depressed person with a suicide plan *now* has a way out. There is now no reason to be depressed.

Knowing this, a number of mental health professionals have expressed the idea that since SSRIs are serotonin enhancers, the increased energy level better enables the depressed person to carry out the act. The increased energy may be why we see many suicides early in antidepressant therapy. I have heard this many times, but I have never thought much of this idea. For one, it implies that there *is* efficacy in SSRI treatment of depression, which is very questionable. For another, psychiatrists used to give the depressed patient an amphetamine drug for a short period of time as a mood "booster," but there was no evidence that these amphetamine drugs increased the potential for suicide in these depressed patients. Moreover, tricyclic antidepressants never had the reputation of *inducing* suicide as the current antidepressant drugs do.

Six or so years ago I did not think there was a relationship between SSRIs and violence. However, since reviewing the scientific literature I have changed my mind. The drug companies take the position that it was the person's *depression* and mental makeup rather than the drug that caused the violence, but such a theory is not proof.

As noted above, when tricyclic antidepressants were in common use there was *never* any suspicion that these drugs may be a cause for violence.

I am especially concerned about the violence that comes about only shortly after the drug has been initiated or when there are dosage increases. If the suicide occurred only in children I might tend to discount the connection, but these events are not restricted to children. If we are given a pill we are given a dose of hope — whether a drug or a sugar pill — and when we have some hope, even false hope, we are less likely to kill ourselves until all hope is abandoned.

As a clinician and diagnostician it just does not make any sense to me for suicide to occur so early in drug treatment when hope *has* to be alive. In all my years of treating depressed patients, I had only one suicide and this did not occur at the *initiation* of my treatment. In this case at our first session I could easily see the patient's great risk of suicide. The patient's father had committed suicide with a handgun, and I had the foreboding thought that the patient would do the same one day because she had all of the earmarks of a potential suicide, including several "failures" at therapy in the past. Two months into therapy my patient killed herself with a gun. Lest the believers and promoters of antidepressants say I killed my patient because I did not put her on antidepressants, she *was* on antidepressants and other drugs from her psychiatrist. I did not believe at the time that in this case the drugs had anything to do with her suicide, but in retrospect I am now not so sure.

SSRI Antidepressants and Suicide-Clinical Trial Database

If antidepressants are indeed antidepressants, that is, that they do indeed treat depression, then those treated with antidepressants *should* have a *lower* rate of suicidality than those treated with placebo. However, the exact opposite is true. How can we legitimately call a drug an antidepressant if the drug does *not* reduce suicide in depressed patients? In fact, there is overwhelming evidence that SSRI and related antidepressants induce suicide in many patients who take them.

A psychiatrist, Dr. Arif Kahn and colleagues (Kahn, A. et al, 2000), using the FDA clinical trial database from 1985-2000, tracked the successful suicides/suicide attempts of placebo and investigational drug cases in these trials. First, these clinical trials *exclude* actively suicidal subjects from being included in any clinical trial and, because of this exclusion, one would expect *fewer* suicides and suicide attempts in these highly selected depressed populations. The investigators looked at the suicidality numbers of these clinical trial cases against the population base rate of 11 suicides per 100,000 population annually. The clinical trial sample consisted of over 71,604 people receiving placebo or investigational drugs such as atypical antipsychotics, SSRI and related antidepressants, Valproate (Depakeote) and the benzodiazepine alprazolam (Xanax).

Clinical trial subjects were not characteristic of the population as a whole and we can expect that *trial* subjects would have a *higher* rate of suicidality than the population as a whole. The reader would be somewhat alarmed by the number of expected completed suicides in the following (investigational) drug groups.

The investigators found on the basis of the clinical trial data a projected 752/100,000 successful suicides for those treated with atypical antipsychotics (Risperdal, Zyprexa, and Seroquel).

There were 718/100,000 projected successful suicides for those on SSRI antidepressants (Prozac, Zoloft, Paxil, Luvox and Celexa) for the treatment of depression.

For the treatment of Social Anxiety Disorder (SAD) there were 425/100,000 projected completed suicides on those treated with Serzone, Remeron and Wellbutrin/Zyban (all SSRI type antidepressants). Social Anxiety Disorder tends to be a relatively self-limiting problem, and very few suicides would be expected in this group.

Anticipated or projected suicides for those on Depakote, for the treatment of Obsessive Compulsive Disorder (OCD), were136/100,000.

Kahn found that suicide rates were higher in the trials *taken as a whole* for those assigned to placebo versus the investigational drug (1,750/100,000), but because of differential time on the drug versus placebo Kahn could not assume an *anti-suicidal effect* of the medication. In the case of drug clinical trials for depression and anxiety, suicide rates were in fact *higher* among those on the drug versus those on placebo. However, Kahn did not find a statistically significant difference. The Kahn data supports my theory that the SSRI and related antidepressants *are* more dangerous than the atypical antipsychotic drugs. In Kahn's projected suicides for the two drug classes (atypicals and antidepressants), the projected number of suicides per 100,000 of those on SSRIs was only 4% *less* than for those on atypicals, which are prescribed for a population with a higher base rate for suicidal behavior.

Those who have treated both groups "know" that the suicide rate is substantially higher for patients whose problems are treated with atypicals than patients treated with SSRIs alone. The differences in terms of impulsiveness and volatility between these two groups are quite large; therefore, the SSRI suicide drug effect is substantially greater than the suicide drug effect of the atypicals.

In Stride

Of course from such data one cannot hope to convince SSRI "proponents" that their SSRIs are not 100% safe. Anything that comes along that questions the safety and efficacy of SSRIs is taken in stride by the "proponents" who have a ready answer to address any bit of reality or bad news.

In addressing this seemingly "bad news," the proponents say, "Yes, but many patients on atypicals have major depression and depressive episodes. This is why the two groups have comparable suicide rates."

I might retort by saying, "If that is true why wouldn't the depressed group on antidepressants have a substantially *lower* number of suicides than the group on atypical antipsychotics?"

NIMH Response

As could be anticipated, the Kahn findings did not sit very well with either the FDA or the National Institute of Mental Health. One of the NIMH psychiatrists, in defending antidepressant drug use in the face of the drug's suicide rates and their marginal clinical values, said that these drugs treat depression very well *but apparently they do not treat suicide.* Is it difficult to believe that a rational mind could say this, especially a mental health professional? This is an excellent example of the "logic" of the "believer."

One must keep in mind that even some emotionally normal people become suicidal on these antidepressants in Phase One studies. The benefits of antidepressants do not justify their use in treating depression and, when combined with some dangerous side effects, mandate that the FDA should withdraw licensure of these drugs.

The Story of David Healy

As noted above, in recent years there has been increasing concern from some SSRI users, some psychiatrists and researchers questioning the basic safety of SSRI antidepressants and related drugs. Writers such as psychiatrist Peter Briggen (and numerous court cases) implicating SSRI antidepressants as causing violence have raised serious concerns about the safety of these drugs. Peter Briggen sees the SSRIs as much more dangerous than the drugs they were supposed to replace. Despite the growing warnings to the contrary, antidepressants continue to carve out a growing market share of users at all age levels.

Dr. David Healy has impeccable credentials as a researcher in psychopharmacology. In January of 2000 he was director of the University of Wales College of Medicine, in the Department of Psychological Medicine. Several years ago, as a part of some investigational research, Dr. Healy gave a popular SSRI antidepressant and a non-seratonin antidepressant to normal, non-depressed nurses and other hospital staff in what the industry calls a Phase I study. This is the first step in evaluating each new drug, giving the drug to *normal* people not patients, to observe its effects and safety.

Dr. Healy found that the SSRI made some absolutely normal people better than well, but it also made two of these volunteer subjects acutely suicidal. I do not believe the Phase I studies of the SSRIs have become public since none of this data had become public prior to Dr. Healy's report. Dr. Healy was an expert witness on several legal actions against the drug companies in which people had committed homicide or suicide while they had been taking SSRI antidepressants. Under the rules of discovery, he was able to see the Phase I data on GSK's drug, Seroxat, better known as Paxil in this country.

Dr. Healy's lengthy correspondence to the Medicines Control Agency was an attempt to alert the MCA about the dangers of SSRI antidepressants found in his own research and the research of others. Here we see in this correspondence the whistleblower at work, and how the world (in this case the MCA) tends to respond to the whistleblower's "unwelcome" news.

MCA responded by defending itself and the status quo. Since Dr. Healy is a respected researcher, the MCA correspondence to him was very professional and matter of fact, responding with alternative explanations but between the lines you know the MCA is saying, "For God's sake, get off my back."

Dr. Healy is a bearer of bad news: mistakes have been made. But the thought of going back or providing a remedy would be just too much to ask. The thought "We would look bad," and "We were snookered by the drug companies" would be just too much to admit and too painful for the MCA or the FDA to accept gracefully.

The MCA, a defender of itself and a defender of the drug industry, does not want to hear that these drugs should never have been approved because they are unsafe. The fact that these drugs are not efficacious is not BAD news to the MCA/FDA — they can always fall back on the *better than a placebo* argument. The BAD news is that these drugs are *dangerous*.

Dr. Healy's research seems to have been critical in the MCA's ultimate warning against the use of Paxil in treating children (also in FDA's warning). This warning was the first chink in the armor of the antidepressant drug industry, and I believe there is much more to come, but there will be much "kicking and screaming along the way."

Healy's Letter to MCA's Dr. Raine

Let's look at Dr. Healy trying to make his case to MCA in a letter to Dr. Raine on the dangers of SSRI antidepressant drugs in June 2000.

> *You may or may not have heard that yesterday in Cheyenne, Wyoming a* ***Court*** *found* ***GlaxoSmithKline*** *guilty on several accounts including the count that* ***Paroxetine can cause suicidality****, that it specifically did so and* ***contributed to the wrongful*** *death of Don and Rita Schell as well as Deborah and Alyssa Tobin* ***and that the*** *company had* ***been responsible for a failure to test and a failure to warn.*** *You may also be aware of a verdict in the Hawkins case in New South Wales some weeks ago where a Supreme Court Judge made it clear that in his opinion* ***Mr. David Hawkins would not have murdered his wife but for the influence of Sertraline****.*
>
> *In the course of my work as an expert witness in Tobin versus SmithKline I got the chance to look at SmithKline's healthy volunteer database in Harlow. Their characterization of this for you was that: 'There were no reports of suicidal thoughts in any of the volunteer studies. There were few reports of 'emotional lability', however these reactions were not found to be related to suicidal thoughts or behaviour. Some volunteers reported anxiety, nervousness and agitation while taking paroxetine, however the most commonly reported adverse events were nausea, diarrhoea, drowsiness and agitation while taking paroxetine.'*
>
> *What I found was that approximately 25% of the volunteers in the studies that I reviewed which were all of the healthy volunteer studies done prior to the filing of this drug for registration in the US and in the UK – 34 studies approximately in all. These yielded a* ***25% agitation, nervousness/akathisia rate****. Some of the multiple dose studies in healthy volunteers lasting 2-3 weeks yielded an up to 85% withdrawal rate in the volunteers.*
>
> *All of their healthy volunteer studies were supposed to have been made available to me but not all were. Of the* ***ones that were missing*** *there was trace correspondence left in one indicating that* ***the investigator had never witnessed such a level of problems in a study with healthy***

> ***volunteers**. Another study was a single dose study which in a dose dependent fashion yielded a 75% rate of severe adverse events most of which involved the central nervous system. There were other disturbing indications from one of the other missing studies.*
>
> ***Volunteers who had participated in the programme went on to suicidal acts.** The relationship between their intake of paroxetine and later suicidal acts is a matter about which neither you nor SmithKline Beecham should be sanguine.*
>
> *These studies were for the most part done on company employees. **None of the studies bar the missing ones were done by investigators with a background in psychiatry**. The investigators were general physicians with a primary interest in gastrointestinal problems who could not have been expected to detect mental problems of this sort that have concerned me and I would have thought should concern you.*
>
> *My testimony in this case also bore witness to **sealed studies and other unreported data**. It commented on the Montgomery Baldwin Study, which yielded a projected rate of **45 suicide attempts** in a group of recurrent brief depressive disordered patients on paro-setine per annum **versus 12 on placebo**. The figures were not statistically significant in great part one has to suggest because **the company had terminated the study early**. This termination and subsequent non-publication I would imagine the jury will have found and others will find significant.*

In the coming years we will probably see the Phase I SSRI data emerge to public view. Further litigation may be needed, but this data *will* emerge. The drug companies have already begun to put their spin on the data — agitation/suicidal thoughts are less likely to occur in depressed patients (with "depressed" brains) than in the normal people in Phase I volunteers. Yet, the vast majority of SSRI users resemble *normal* Phase I volunteers rather than patients.

Agitation

The agitation or akathisia, as it is called by some, is considered by Dr. Healy and others to be the side effect of most concern. The agitation can occur during use or during discontinuation or tapered withdrawal. Dr. Healy believes that agitation occurs in up to 25% of the volunteers exposed to Paxil or other SSRIs in multiple-dose studies. These are hardly rare events. He also discovered that there was one actual suicide in GSK's volunteer panel, which happened some weeks after drug discontinuation.

One of Healy's volunteers took several weeks to recover her equilibrium following the adverse experience on the drug. In the volunteer study the suicidality that emerged with the drug disappeared once the drug was stopped, but the volunteers were said to have been left with impaired self-confidence, dysphasia and nervousness for weeks after. How long these adverse events can last after drug discontinuation is anyone's guess. Dr. Healy reports that he has observed these adverse experiences lasting upwards of three months following drug discontinuation.

His review of the GSK health volunteer Phase I data found results much as in his own study. These drug withdrawal side effects are simply that, drug side effects and not manifestations of the "disorder" that the drug is *supposed* to treat. Patients and most prescribing physicians do not know this and in general patients are often misinterpreting their drug side effects as their emotional problems. Moreover, the withdrawal side effects are locking in some patients to continue the drug permanently, which the drug company might refer to as the "perfect" drug.

Glenmullen Testimony

It is a rare psychiatrist who has a realistic appreciation of the serious risks involved in the use of SSRI and related antidepressants, but one gave testimony at the FDA hearing. What he had to say is worth reporting here.

> Joseph Glenmullen, M.D.
>
> DR. GLENMULLEN: I am Joe Glenmullen. I am a psychiatrist and clinical instructor in Psychiatry at Harvard Medical School and the author of Prozac Blacklash, which describes my experience seeing patients become suicidal on SSRIs.

> I am here at my own expense because there is a specific side effect of SSRIs called akathisis that can make some patients so agitated that they feel death would be a welcome relief.
>
> This side effect is so well established that it is clearly described with SSRIs in the Diagnostic and Statistical Manual, the DSM, the American Psychiatric Association's official diagnostic manual.
>
> If you look at the transcript of the FDA hearing on this very side effect 10 years ago, you will see the FDA saying repeatedly we don't know what to do, we need more research. It is a tragedy to be here 10 years later and hear the FDA saying the same thing.
>
> The industry's response to this side effect has been to blame the underlying psychiatric conditions of patients, to dismiss legitimate medical case reports as anecdotes, and to scare the media away from the subject, claiming that it would frighten patients away from treatment.
>
> Indeed, there is a prevailing authoritarian attitude doesn't [sic] warn patients, you might scare them.
>
> Well, I prescribe SSRIs and I warn patients, and they are not frightened away from treatment. Let's stop blaming patient's underlying psychiatric conditions. Let's stop blaming the victims and deal with this very real side effect. Thank you."

Dr. Glenmullen is quite right; ten years have passed and the FDA is still doing the same thing, saying we need more studies. The FDA, as Dr. Glenmullen says, is still placing the blame not on the drug, but on the underlying depression. He tends to believe that truth in advertising is the answer — *warn* the patient in advance about the akathisia, — but, despite the fact that he probably uses these drugs safely in his practice, he still has to my mind an exaggerated picture of their efficacy.

In my experience, when people ask their doctor to take them off a drug they *are* better and feel confident about going it alone. These antidepressant drug-treated patients who are better may not make it in the long run because they have not learned to master problems in their life. In general, suicide during drug withdrawal (discontinuation) is *not* depression and suicide soon after SSRI initiation is *not* from depression.

As noted elsewhere, my company's data found some patients on four to five different antidepressants during the year. I suspect withdrawal effects play an important role in this. A patient may cut down the dosage of an SSRI, experience withdrawal effects, think they are getting worse, increase the dose or ask their physician to change to another antidepressant or add a second antidepressant. In such a situation a patient can have withdrawal effects from two or more SSRIs at the same time.

In Dr. Healy's attempt to alert the MCA about the dangers of SSRIs, he suggested they review the Montgomery study conduced in 1992/1993. This was a placebo controlled Paxil study that yielded a projected annual rate of 45 suicide attempts in the Paxil treated group versus 12 suicide attempts in the placebo group.

One study examining FDA antidepressant clinical trial data demonstrated no difference in either successful or attempted suicides in the drug and placebo groups (Khan, A. et al., 2000). I take this as an indictment of the drug since any drug *claiming* antidepressant effects *must* reduce suicide, which antidepressants do not. In the Khan study, as in the Montgomery study, the clinical trial data shows a *higher* rate of suicide for those on the drug than those on placebo. However, the difference did not reach statistical significance.

Placebo Run-In Period Skews Data

As one can imagine in all of the submitted antidepressant clinical trials there were a number of suicides during the placebo run-in period, a period *before* the subjects were either placed on the drug or assigned to placebo. However, there is some evidence that the industry assigned these suicides with those occurring during the *treatment* phase of the study to the placebo group, which inappropriately increased the number of suicides in the placebo group occurring during the drug-placebo treatment phase.

The suicide comparison *should* have been limited to the drug and placebo *treatment* groups, not *before* randomization into the two treatment groups. Dr. Healy has presented information revealing that when certain industry data are readjusted to a proper comparison, suicides during the *treatment* phase occurred substantially more often in those on the drugs than in those on placebo.

<u>GSK Figures Indicate</u>

Figures used by GlaxoSmithKline in its legal trials indicated that 1.52 percent of patients taking Paxil either committed or attempted suicide versus 1.44 percent of patients on placebo (probably not a statistically significant difference). David Healy believes, however, that the company's suicide figures for patients on placebo were inflated. These people were not really on placebo, but were in the "run-in" phase of the clinical trial. In looking at the data this way, Healy believes that suicides and attempted suicides increased *ninefold* in the Paxil versus the placebo group. There is growing evidence as in the above that a number of suicides *are* drug induced.

I would recommend that the FDA have an outside, unbiased research group go back and re-examine *all* of the clinical trial data, including all of the SSRI Phase I data.

In these recent reports of SSRI induced suicides I believe we are just seeing the tip of the iceberg — more will appear in the near future. As I edit this section in January 2005, the media has just announced that previously suppressed Eli Lilly memos from the late 1980s on Prozac induced suicides have recently come to light.

Serotonin Syndrome

<u>Excess Serotonin</u>

There have been about thirteen cases published in the literature on a condition that arises because of possible excessive Serotonin levels, which is a condition restricted to the SSRI antidepressants such as Prozac and Paxil. The incidences are apparently more widespread than those reported in the literature. An SSRI dose increase, the addition of another SSRI or a number of non-antidepressant drugs that increase Serotonin levels often precipitate the syndrome. Over half of these cases require detoxification and stabilization in a hospital while the patient is being withdrawn from the drug(s). Other drugs that are Serotonin antagonists (e.g., propandol) may be used with benefit to the problem. About 10% of the cases can be stabilized within 24 hours and almost all cases within 96 hours.

The first was described in 1987. In these earlier years I suspect the syndrome was often misdiagnosed — unfortunately, there is no reason to think this has changed. The syndrome is characterized by changes in mental status, confusion or disorientation, agitation or irritability, coma or unresponsiveness. Autonomic nervous symptom changes include fever or hyperthermia, diaphoresis (heavy sweating), sinus tachycardia, hypertension, prolonged dilation or restriction of the pupils, nausea, etc. There may be a multitude of neuromuscular changes including myoclonic jerks, muscle rigidity, restlessness or hyperactivity, tremor, ataxia or incoordination and others.

Companies Play Down Side Effects

Websites

Go to Eli Lilly's website for Prozac and GlaxoSmithKline's website for Paxil. These companies play down the drug's respective side effects. Eli Lilly describes the side effect profile of Prozac as mild, while GlaxoSmithKline's describe Paxil's side effects as mild to moderate. Prozac's side effects as described by Eli Lilly include nausea, difficulty sleeping, drowsiness, anxiety, nervousness, weakness, loss of appetite, tremors, dry mouth, sweating, decreased sex drive, and impotence. These side effects are said to go away within a few weeks of starting treatment and, according to Eli Lilly, are not serious enough to cause people to stop taking Prozac.

The maker of Paxil describes its side effects as mild to moderate and they "may" fade or disappear completely over time. In looking at the advertising of these and other antidepressant drugs, I have noticed that the word "may" is very popular. For example, you *may* have a chemical imbalance, the drug *may* correct a chemical imbalance and, as in the above, the side effects *may* disappear completely over time. For Paxil, side effects are said to include nausea, injury, infection, diarrhea, constipation, decreased appetite, sleepiness, dizziness, yawning, sweating, abnormal vision, and sexual side effects.

The above side effects of Prozac and Paxil, although described as mild or moderate but tolerable, have certainly very widespread effects on the central nervous system and autonomic nervous systems. These look like the side effects as reported by subjects in the original clinical trials. However, let's contrast the side effects of Prozac and Paxil as reported on their respective websites with the side effects of both drugs from a research study by Kiev and Feiger, 1997, which was a comparison of Paxil and Prozac during a seven week trial.

Table 1 presents the most frequently reported adverse events for subjects on Prozac and Paxil.

Table 1. Most Frequently Reported Adverse Events Associated With Fluovoxamine and Paroxetine Treatment (> 10% for Either Treatment Group) (Intent-to-Treat Safety Sample

	Number (Percentage) of Patients Reporting Event			
	Paroxetine N = 30		Fluvoxamine N = 30	
Adverse Event	N	%	N	%
Headache	17	57	12	40
Nausea	14	47	11	37
Sweating	10	33	3	10
Somnolence	9	30	12	40
Diarrhea	9	30	4	13
Dry mouth	8	27	11	37
Dizziness	8	27	6	20
Impotence[a]	3	21	2	14
Ejaculatory abnormality[a]	3	21	1	7
Insomnia	6	20	9	30
Nervousness	5	17	4	13
Libido decrease	5	17	4	13
Dream abnormality	5	17	0	0
Asthenia	4	13	7	23
Constipation	4	13	2	7
Dyspepsia	4	13	7	23
Anxiety	4	13	2	7
Tremor	4	13	3	10
Depersonalization	2	7	4	13
Palpitations	1	3	4	13
Flatulence	1	3	4	13
Dysmenorrhea[b]	0	0	3	19

[a] Percentage based on male patients only; N = 14 in both groups
[b] Percentage based on female patients only; N = 16 in both groups

Kiev, A. & Feiger, A. "A Double-Blind Comparision of Prozac (Fluvoxamine) and Paxil (Paroxetine) in the Treatment of Depressed Outpatients." The Journal of Clinical Psychiatry*, 58:4, 146-152, April, 1997. Physicians Postgraduate Press.* Adapted/Reprinted by permission.

The authors considered the above side effects as tolerable, but even in this acute trial the frequency of these adverse events are substantially greater than what the company websites would suggest. For Paxil (paroxetine), ten side effects had frequencies 20% or greater (including headache, nausea, somnolence, impotence, insomnia and others). For Prozac (Fluoxetine) eight side effects (including headache, nausea, insomnia, somnolence) had frequencies of 20% or greater.

Side Effects Add to the Burden of Depression

The depressed patient is *already* quite distressed, discouraged and feeling helpless and hopeless. The addition of *any* of the above side effects is an unnecessary strain on already stressed individuals.

The acceptance of side effects of this nature for antidepressant drugs may be a carry over from drug side effects in treating "medical" conditions (e.g., hypertension) to drug side effects in treating mental disorders such as anxiety or depression. The effect is not the same nor should the two be considered equivalent. In the former the drug side effects do not *worsen* what is being treated, but antidepressant drug side effects such as insomnia, headache, anxiety, nausea and others *do* add to the burden of the depressed person.

Benefit/Risk Study

The antidepressant "believer" will tell me that the benefits of the antidepressant far exceed the adverse events but, as I have noted, the benefit of the antidepressant is minimal at best.

The Kiev and Feiger study on "benefits" actually reveals the risks of antidepressant drugs. The major findings of the study determined that neither Prozac nor Paxil had the advantage over the other in side effects. Again, all depression is self-limiting over time, that is, any group of clinically depressed patients will get better on their own without any treatment. However, of 81 clinically depressed outpatients who volunteered to participate in the Kiev and Feiger study, 21 patients or 26% were *discontinued* prior to receiving the drug because they did not meet participation criteria; 6 or 7% had a placebo response, 3 withdrew consent, 3 were non-compliant, 2 had abnormal laboratory test results, or had medication sensitivity (N=1). We have here a biased selection of depressed subjects in an already biased sample (not all depressed patients were allowed into the study). Moreover, a total of 18 patients or 30% in the intent to treat population *failed* to complete the study. Two patients in the Prozac group and 4 patients in the Paxil group or 10% withdrew due to adverse events. The high attrition rate does *not* sound like tolerable and mild side effects.

These studies use a technique of carrying forward the last measurement for study non-completers in measuring improvement. If a subject quit the study *after* the three-week assessment, for example, any improvement noted at week three was carried over automatically to the fourth, fifth, sixth, and seventh week for measurement purposes. This non-completer could have gotten much worse or much better in the remaining weeks; the actual outcome for any subject is unknown.

SSRI Sexual Side Effects

Decreased sexual desire and impaired orgasmic capacity are common side effects of these drugs. Earlier about 1 or 2% of SSRI users were thought to have these sexual side effects but, currently, the generally accepted revised frequency is 40% or more. It is difficult to get an exact figure. There can be some degree of sexual dysfunction not reported because it is below the threshold of the patient's awareness and not all cases of sexual dysfunction are reported to the reviewers.

A caller to my behavioral health company said she stopped taking antidepressants recently because she had simply gotten tired of "feeling like a rag doll," i.e., having no feelings. It seems unwise to give a patient whose sexual interest is probably already compromised by emotional problems a pill that compromises sexual interest/performance further. The "proponent," has a ready answer; give another pill to take care of the sexual side effects. Unfortunately this strategy characterizes much of health care thinking today.

Viagra – An Antidepressant?

Physicians, as I mentioned earlier, are using Viagra to treat the sexual side effects of SSRI antidepressants and also as an adjunct to antidepressants in treating depression. Many psychiatrists and other physicians are prescribing Viagra, at around $10 a pill, for treating some of the adverse sexual side effects of antidepressants for approximately 40% of those males taking antidepressants.

One psychiatrist took the managed care industry to task for not authorizing payment for Viagra to treat the sexual side effects of SSRI antidepressants (Pomerantz, Jay M, 2003). My published response to the article Pomerantz wrote said that not only did I *support* the policy but also recommended that managed care *not* reimburse for drugs to treat the *other* side effects of SSRIs. I do not find it prudent to pay for drugs to treat the side effects of drugs that have little if any clinical value.

Dr. Pomerantz, in the same article, also recommended that Viagra should be reimbursed for treating the decreased libido and erectile dysfunction arising secondarily from the depression itself.

Viagra is also being promoted as a "primary" treatment of depression in men and women who are also being treated with antidepressant drugs. This use of Viagra will likely proliferate because Viagra is *much more effective* than antidepressants in treating depression. In one study (Seidman, S.N., 1998) using mild to moderately depressed males in a placebo-controlled research design, 73% of Viagra treated males' depression improved while only 14% of the placebo-controls improved. From this data, Viagra in depressed males is much more powerful than *antidepressants* in treating depression, and Pfizer (the maker of Viagra) may well be gearing up to market it to depressed males as an "antidepressant." Fewer males take antidepressants than females but these depressed males might be more likely to take Viagra than an antidepressant.

Before the reader goes to buy Pfizer stock, Viagra should not be used as an "antidepressant" because the drug addresses only a *symptom* (albeit an important symptom) of depression. With such an approach you would need ten or more drugs to treat the many symptoms of depression. Remember that there are proven non-drug alternative treatments for depression. If in depression the mood problem is often secondary to dysfunctional thinking and if we used Viagra to treat depression, we might well have the same relapse as that found in antidepressants.

Viagra is *supposed* to be used for *organically* caused impotency but from my experience and knowledge of the field of sexual impotency, I would estimate a majority of males taking Viagra do *not* have an organic disease underlying the impotency. Most of these men have *performance anxiety* as the cause of their ED, and their *performance anxiety* can be more appropriately treated by non-drug therapy.

On the other hand, another use of SSRI antidepressants is to cure premature ejaculation! SSRIs have a frequent side effect involving delay or prevention of orgasms in women and men. Physicians, being aware of this, have been prescribing SSRIs in a nonstandard use to male patients complaining of premature ejaculation, however one may define it. In this practice we have a drug to treat a non-disease that is a problem that can generally be resolved by a few sessions with a psychologist who treats anxiety. I once had a male patient who wanted to be able to sustain sexual intercourse for thirty minutes (would he be a case for an SSRI?). I told him I *could* teach him how to do it, but I said "Why do you *want* to do it and do you really *want* to do it?"

Sexual Dysfunction

The drug companies are concerned about antidepressant treatment-emergent sexual dysfunction (SD) because of its effect on drug noncompliance. Many women taking antidepressants seem to accept the drug induced sexual dysfunction as the price they pay for their improved mood but others discontinue drugs because of this problem.

Should We Call This a Benefit?

There are reports by a number of women treated with SSRI antidepressants having unexpected orgasms while taking the drugs. One woman while shopping alone in a store experienced an orgasm, which seemingly came from nowhere. Needless to say it must have been startling and the woman reportedly stopped using the drug immediately even though she said she did enjoy the experience.

A psychiatrist and other colleagues of the Department of Psychiatric Medicine at the University of Virginia conducted an observational study of the frequency of antidepressant-induced sexual dysfunction at 1,101 primary care clinics in the United States (Clayton, A.H., 2002). The researchers studied the incidence of sexual dysfunction on eight of the most widely used current generation antidepressant drugs. Of a target population of 6,297 patients, the researchers selected 802 patients who were *least* likely to have sexual dysfunction from *non-drug causes* and who had never been on psychiatric drugs other than antidepressants. Patients had to have been on one of the eight antidepressants for at least three months for inclusion in the study. Clayton found the prevalence of sexual dysfunction in the study group to be 37%, ranging from 22% in bupropion induced sexual dysfunction to 43% for Paxil.

Real World Variables

Prior to the study, the participating physicians in the above study had estimated the incidence of antidepressant sexual dysfunction to be about 20%, which is a little more than half the rate the study found. Some researchers estimate the rate to be from 50 to 70% in the real world. This estimate is made because patients are often on more than one psychotropic drug unlike the Clayton study. Moreover, some of the study subjects may have been switched from another antidepressant because of drug induced sexual dysfunction. The researchers also noted that PCPs tend to use *lower* doses of antidepressants than psychiatrists, resulting in a lower incidence of sexual dysfunction.

The most common sexual dysfunction side effects in the Clayton study were erectile dysfunction, diminished libido and delayed/alternated or absent orgasm.

In another study (Salerian, A.J., et al., 2000), the researchers retrospectively looked at 31 women and 61 men with psychotropic-induced sexual dysfunction. Of these patients, 64 were on SSRIs, 8 on TCAs, 36 on other antidepressants, 20 on benzodiazepines, 20 on mood stabilizers, 4 on stimulants, 4 on narcotics and 9 on atypical antipsychotics. Interestingly 62 (68%) of these 92 subjects with drug induced sexual dysfunction were receiving more than one of these drugs.

There were no significant differences between men and women on various measures of sexual improvement, except for sexual arousal, which favored the men. Patients on SSRIs demonstrated less improvement in their sexual performance than those on the other drugs. Again, another example of the SSRI's low side effect profile!

None of the commentators on the problem of drug-induced sexual dysfunction ever recommend the rational solution to the problem, i.e., of tapering the patient off the antidepressant and discontinue the drug. Even if the physician does not refer the patient for psychotherapy, the return of the patient's sexual capacity and sexual pleasure should help the depression everything else being equal.

Most of those who comment on the drug-induced sexual problem raise a number of possibilities but generally settle on the drug sildenafil (Viagra) as a treatment for treatment-emergent sexual dysfunction. Fava and Rankin, (2002) found

9 of 10 men were cured of the SSRI induced sexual dysfunction problem by Viagra, although one of the ten had adverse side effects from Viagra.

The Cost of Treating the Sexual Side Effects

In several articles on Viagra to treat treatment-emergent sexual dysfunction, no authority brought up the *cost* of Viagra to treat these cases (or even question the *desirability* of using Viagra in this way). Just think of the financial cost. Let's say the drug companies keep 15 million of us on an SSRI during the year, which from the above translates to about 5.25 million of us with drug-induced sexual dysfunction. Put in an average of two sexual encounters per week, at $10.00 per pill, which translates to 273 sexual encounters per person per year or $2,730 per person or $14.3 billion dollars per year to treat the sexual side effects of antidepressants! The researchers making the Viagra recommendations can do the arithmetic, but apparently cost is *never* a consideration. Moreover, the 14.3 billion dollar costs to treat sexual side effects of SSRI antidepressants would be more than the SSRI drug costs themselves.

I suspect most of the 40% treated with SSRI antidepressants who experienced impaired sexuality due to the drug never see this as drug induced and accept it as another indication of their "emotional problems." This is sad, but all too true.

If you think Viagra *should* be used as an antidepressant since it is more effective as an antidepressant than Prozac, one should keep in mind that a drug *should* have some relationship to the disease or condition it is treating. For Viagra to be considered an antidepressant we would have to re-define depression as "an insufficient blood supply to the genitals."

Certainly the accepted conviction that antidepressant drugs have very tolerable side effects *cannot* be supported by the facts, yet this conventional wisdom prevails.

Patients are not told that there can be a major problem getting off these drugs and that often the primary drug requires one or more drugs to address adverse side effects. The incidence of side effects are underestimated by the industry and prescribers. Therefore, many patients prescribed these drugs are not given adequate information on the benefits/risks of the drug or alternative treatments available for the patient to make an informed decision.

Drug Treatment Side Effects Diagnosed as the Disorder

Most of my readers will have been aware that the new Jane Pauley Show began on television in September of 2004. In television interviews and on her show, Ms. Pauley announced that she has bipolar disorder. On her show and in her book, Skywriting, she talks about her illness and some of the circumstances around her diagnosis and treatment. I admit I was skeptical about her diagnosis. After reading her book to learn more about her situation and ruminating about whether or not I wanted to intervene in her mental health affairs, I wrote a letter to her on September 2, 2004. I made these points in that letter:

- You did not meet criteria for a diagnosable bipolar disorder or clinical depression. A stress management approach such as Cognitive Behavior Therapy would be the most effective way to help you manage your stress.
- Your "illness" was *drug* induced, it was not a part of you as a person.

  You had adverse side effects from the *steroids* you were taking for hives. Steroid treatment can produce psychotic-like symptoms such as in your case.

  You also had an adverse reaction to antidepressant drugs, which can cause suicidal ideation or attempts. Moreover, antidepressant drugs do *not* treat depression, which from your history I do not think you have had.
- Although certain drugs are needed to treat correctly diagnosed bipolar disorder, bipolar disorder is overdiagnosed and your diagnosis is a case in point.
- What are the indicators of your misdiagnosis?

  —The DSM-IV™ states bipolar issues must *never* be diagnosed when it arises from a medical condition or medical procedure (e.g., your steroid treatment).

  —When you had a psychotic reaction to steroids and were seemingly in a "manic" state, you described it as if you were aware that your experiences were "abnormal," which does *not* sound like a *true* manic state.

  —Your personality traits, being creative and shy, are *normal* ones, not indicative of *any* mental illness.

—Neither stress nor depression is a disease. All of us experience these stress/mood problems to some degree or other, but your history of hives suggests a core problem with *stress-anxiety* that may need *appropriate* intervention.

- You are not alone in having been misdiagnosed as having bipolar disorder. There are tens of thousands of individuals like yourself and bipolar illness has become the fad diagnosis of our generation.
- Your psychiatrist probably told you that the steroid treatment uncovered a pre-existing bipolar illness, but such reasoning is simply hokum, not science.
- Find out if you *are* bipolar and if not consider discontinuing the lithium and any other psychotropic drugs you are undoubtedly taking.

I would rather see Jane Pauley become a poster child against *misdiagnosis* in psychiatry than to become a poster child *for* bipolar disorder.

Patients prescribed these antidepressant drugs put trust in their prescribing physicians. Patients do not realize that many times they are putting confidence in a family physician whose knowledge of these matters is generally limited to marketing materials from the drug companies and drug company sponsored workshops on drug treatment of depression and other mental disorders.

I am sure patients are not told to watch out for any periods of agitation with aggressive or destructive urges, which should be perceived as a side effect of the drug and not a worsening of their problem. We have, then, a physician with very limited understanding of mental disorder and human behavior, one who believes that depression is simply a *biological* disease that can be corrected with an SSRI antidepressant whose side effects are very mild and tolerable.

The same physician would not *dare* to treat other serious medical conditions without specialist referral, but when it comes to the vast majority of mental health problems, the physician has accepted the propaganda that most of these problems are responsive to a pill alone.

Miscellaneous Adverse Effects

Do Antidepressants Cause Breast Cancer?

It has been known for some time that antidepressant drugs in clinically relevant human dosages cause tumor growth in mice and rats. For example, one rodent study (Brandes, L.J., 1992) found that eight of twenty Elavil or Prozac-treated mice developed fibrosarcoma tumors by day five as compared to saline controls (P less than 0.002). Studies of results in humans are a little more mixed. In one large study (Kelly, J. P., 1999) involving over ten thousand women, the researchers found *no* relationship between breast cancer and antidepressant use overall; however, when the researchers looked at the SSRI antidepressants they *did* find a slightly increased risk in women who had taken an SSRI in the previous year — a result they called "non reassuring." In another study (Cotterchio, M., et al., 2000) comparing 700 women diagnosed with breast cancer from 1995-1996 to a random sample of non-breast cancer women, the researchers found that women who had used tricyclic antidepressants for more than two years had twice the risk of developing breast cancer. The researchers also found that women who had used the newer antidepressants had a *seven-fold* breast cancer risk. Despite the negative studies the issue is very much alive and bears further investigation. I doubt, however, that of the many female antidepressant users there are not many who are aware that there is a question of *any* such risk of these drugs.

As Safe as They Say?

Antidepressant drugs have grown in popularity partly because users have been told that these drugs are safe and have few and tolerable side effects. Non-psychiatric physicians are the most frequent prescribers of these drugs because they, too, have been told by drug detail men – and the FDA – that these drugs are safe and much safer than the Elavil-type drugs. Physicians have accepted the propaganda rather than the reality, which has been presented in this chapter. I believe these drugs *are* unsafe, especially the SSRI and related antidepressants, and will *one day* be pulled from the market. I believe the *truth* will eventually win out over the marketing, suppression of evidence and spindoctoring that has characterized the industry and the "proponents" of these drugs.

Chapter VI

EVALUATING THE RISK: ANTIDEPRESSANTS FOR CHILDREN

How Prevalent are These SSRI and Other Atypical Antidepressants Prescribed in Pediatric Mental Health Problems?

This is Crazy – Prozac for Babies?

In 1994, 3,000 prescriptions for fluoxetine hydrochloride (Prozac) were written for children *under one year of age* (JAMA, 2000). The 3,000 Prozac treated infants occurred in 1994, and there has probably been an increase in its use in the intervening years.

Three-Year-Old Child

Recently a mother of a three-year-old child called PMHM because her child's pediatrician recommended an antidepressant drug for her child for behavior problems. Although not opposed, she wanted a second opinion. How many times do such mothers routinely go along with such recommendations without question? I am concerned there are more cases than we would like to think. It is true some physicians might question the sanity of prescribing antidepressants for a three-year-old. However, in view of accepted thought about these drugs and depression, our physician could make a "good" case for his or her actions. Nor is three the youngest age prescribed an antidepressant, remember the youngest is one month and perhaps earlier.

The Cost of Giving Children Drugs

In the pediatric population, approximately 10.8 million total prescriptions were dispensed for all of the drugs under consideration, representing a substantial 7% of the total antidepressant market in 2002. The younger group (one to eleven-year-olds) accounted for approximately 2.7 million prescriptions while the adolescent population accounted for 8.1 million prescriptions. In terms of dollar amount, at an estimated average price of $72.00 per prescription, total pediatric sales would be 777 million dollars in 2002.

If one takes pharmaceutical company profits at about 18% of revenues, the net profit to the drug industry in pediatric sales alone would be $158 million annually and rising. Net profit on total sales of 13 billion would be 2.3 billion dollars for the industry, which is not a small piece of change. Do you think the industry, with such profits, will try to influence the scientific and political process involved over such matters that were before the FDA committee in 2004?

Dr. Gianna Rigoni presented testimony at the FDA hearing on Pediatric and Adolescent Antidepressant Drug Use in the United States. Dr. Rigoni found that there were 900,000 physician office visits that involved antidepressants in the younger pediatric population in 2002. Office visits for adolescents involving these products were 2.6 million in 2002. I made an estimate of total office charges to dispense these drugs to all youth. I took an average non-psychiatric physician office visit of $72.00 per visit and an average psychiatrist office visit of $99.00 (a "discounted" visit).

I "guestimated" psychiatrist office visits at 35% of the total, which would come to 1,225,000 psychiatrist office visits or $121,275,000 in psychiatrist revenues. Non-psychiatric physician office visits for antidepressant pediatric use would total 2,275,000 visits. These visits, at an average office charge of $72.00 per visit, would result in general physician antidepressant office revenues of $163,800,000 annually in 2002.

The conventional wisdom says that drug treatment of mental health problems is cheaper than specialist (psychotherapy or family therapy) treatment of these problems in the case of children, adolescents and adults. To determine value and setting aside for the moment the question of risk and dangerousness, we have to determine the efficacy of these drugs in treating childhood depression.

Did anyone ask "Should non-psychiatric physicians have sole responsibility for the diagnosis and treatment of children with a variety of mental health disorders?" I used *mental health disorders* rather than childhood depression since I doubt all of the children on antidepressants would have a diagnosable depressive disorder.

A Higher Cost

The pediatric use of these drugs is appalling. First, prescribing these drugs to a child implies that something is being done to help the child, which is untrue. Second, the problems in the family and the environment that are helping to give rise to the "depression" or maladjustment are completely ignored. Finally, the parental attention is directed to non-existent chemical imbalances and implies that the drug will correct the problem.

Studies show that SSRI antidepressants impair a child's growth. Further, because of their widespread effects on brain mechanisms one can anticipate negative effects on the developing brain. We do not know if these drugs cause permanent harm in children with regard to learning capacity, emotional development, socialization, and empathic capacity, but the probability is strong. Antidepressant drugs cause major brain dysfunction/alteration (shown in the withdrawal effects) if not permanent brain damage. The fact that Prozac alone is now approved for pediatric use does not make it any safer than its cousins.

About half of the school shooters were on SSRI antidepressant drugs and other drugs. Press reports suggested that these boys were quite dysfunctional in a number of ways and, without exception, parents seemed to have been concerned about their child's behavior and had sought professional help. SSRIs are contributory if not causative in these cases of violence. We also know that an SSRI antidepressant is not effective therapy with depressed children.

The prescribing doctor or psychiatrist *thought* that something was being done — the parents and perhaps schoolteachers also *thought* something definitive was being done for the disturbed child — but actually the drug was a non-treatment. Child mental health problems require more. Unfortunately, the SSRI may have been more than just a non-treatment and may have played a causative role in the subsequent violent acts of some of these school shooters.

The problem with child mental health treatment is the almost exclusive use of drugs to treat the whole range of child mental health problems today. It is now rarer for a child with mental health problems *not* to be treated with drugs than it is to be treated with drugs.

The thinking among "believers" is that if the drug is effective in treating *adult* depression, it *should* treat child depression as well. But it does not. The body of research (antidepressant outcome studies of depressed children) weakens any argument that antidepressants have *any* efficaciousness. Children on antidepressants have been exposed to the possibility of cognitive impairing and/or other adverse side effects of the drugs when there has been no scientific evidence of their efficacy.

Prozac for Depression and Obsessive Compulsive Disorder

For years psychiatrists and general physicians have used SSRIs in off-label use to treat childhood "depression" and a wide range of child anxiety disorders. In addition, these drugs have also been used with a broad spectrum of child behavior problems that went beyond diagnosable anxiety or depression. Antidepressants are routinely used with conduct disordered children. Again, there have been no outcome studies of the use of SSRIs with these or other groups to determine efficacy. Such a lack of proof does not deter their use nonetheless. There were almost a *dozen* double-blind, placebo-controlled antidepressant outcome studies with depressed youth and the results found no differential effectiveness of the drug over placebo (Sommers-Flanagan, et al. 1996). These scientific findings had no influence on the prescribing patterns of antidepressants with children, however.

In January of 2003, the Food and Drug Administration approved Prozac to treat children and adolescents seven to seventeen years of age for depression and Obsessive-Compulsive Disorder (OCD). According to the National Institute of Mental Health (NIMH) depression affects 2.5% of children and roughly 8% of adolescents in the United States. OCD affects about 2% of the population, and typically emerges during early childhood or early adolescence.

Eli Lily finally came up with two clinical trials in which the drug-treated depressed children improved in a statistically significant way over the placebo-treated children and two positive clinical trials with OCD children. The announcement did not specify how *superior* the drug treated groups were over the placebo groups. However, I suspected the difference was comparable to the adult depression outcome studies and my initial impression proved incorrect. I was wrong, they are worse.

Prior to Prozac's recently gained FDA approval none of the depression outcome studies found *any* of these drugs to be more effective than placebo in treating childhood depression. The American Psychiatric Association (the Division of Adolescent Psychiatry) has *never* recommended drug therapy as the sole treatment of childhood depression. Family therapy has always been seen as the *primary* method of treating child problems.

With no more information than the above there would be absolutely no justification for the use of Prozac with depressed or OCD children despite the FDA approval. We do not know how powerful the drug is in treating these disorders. We don't know how many clinical trials *failed* before a difference was demonstrated. More importantly, although there is no doubt that these drugs are *cognitively* impairing in the short-term, we do not know if there are long-term negative effects on the developing brain of Prozac using children. Data on any long-term detrimental effects on the brain will come one day.

The FDA announcement seems to imply that Prozac is an answer to these major child mental health problems. There is simply no drug that will address depression in children because of the important role that *psychosocial* factors play in mental health problems in children.

In the pediatric Prozac announcement the FDA reported that the common side effects associated with Prozac use in children and adolescents were similar to those experienced by adults. Side effects include nausea, tiredness, nervousness, dizziness, and difficulty concentrating, many of which sound *cognitively* impairing. In addition, one clinical trial showed that after nineteen weeks of treatment the average drug treated children gained about 1.1 cm *less* in height (about a half an inch) and about one kg. *less* in weight (about two pounds) than the children treated with placebo. Lilly agreed to conduct a post marketing study to further evaluate any potential impact of the drug on long-term growth in children. From these preliminary Prozac growth effects data, how could one get an ethical researcher to conduct such a study? It is deplorable to ask parents to volunteer their children for such a study when preliminary data suggest the drug's growth suppression.

Prozac – More Effective than CBT?

In early August of 2004, the media made a great deal out of a pre-published announcement of a research study allegedly showing that Prozac was more effective than cognitive therapy for childhood depression, although *combination* therapy was said to be more effective than either alone. My company, at the time of this announcement, had been working with a Pharmacy Benefit Consulting firm. One of their principals, hearing of this Prozac study, sent me a copy of the research conclusions for my comment, since I had said that most of the research favored Cognitive Behavioral Treatment (CBT) over combination therapy (drugs and therapy) for depression. The following are the main points from my e-mail response to his inquiry.

- MOST of the counseling work needs to be done with the *parents* as typically the child's depressed mood arises not from maladaptive patterns of thinking, as in many adults, but in *adverse* environmental and family issues. In most cases it is not the *parents* who are causing the child's depression, but the *parents* are in the *best* position to impact the child's mental health.
- There was no difference in *remission* rates between drug and placebo (which is consistent with the adult trials). There was also no difference in a 50% or more reduction in symptoms (which is the standard used for adult trials). There *was* a statistically significant difference between the two on a *30%* reduction of symptoms, but such a small reduction is hardly impressive.
- Only these two out of about 12 ***published*** clinical trials with depressed youngsters showed *any* superiority of the drug over placebo. When active rather than inert placebos are used, there is no differential improvement in children on the drug versus those on active placebo.
- The Prozac trials used much more of a mixed bag of depressed children than found in adult trials: 15% of the subjects had ADD and 22% were said to have had conduct problems. ADD and conduct disorder are in themselves unrelated to depression.
- Correctly diagnosed ADD or ADHD children require Ritalin according to my clinical experience. Conduct-disordered children get unhappy, not depressed, when their wants are thwarted; these conduct disordered children are deficient in the conscientiousness and other traits that make many of us prone to developing a depression.
- If CBT was no more effective than placebo, how could it when combined with the drug be more effective than the drug alone? How can something that is ineffective in treating something when combined with X be more effective than X alone? It doesn't make any sense and the only sense I can make of the data is that CBT *without* major parental guidance in child treatment is not very effective, which is something that is not new to most mental health professionals who treat children.

- At PMHM we seem to be able to treat both depression and anxiety without drugs. When our depressed callers mention drugs for children we typically get them to accept therapy first and say that drugs can be added later if needed. We rarely if ever have to add drugs for anxiety and depression.

FDA Hearing

The four hundred-page transcript from the FDA's February, 2004 hearing questions SSRI antidepressant use with children. The United Kingdom's equivalent of the FDA had ruled that these drugs, with the exception of Prozac, were *contraindicated* in the treatment of childhood depression both because of lack of demonstrated efficacy and the risk of drug-induced suicide.

Prozac was excluded from the British warning — and the United States warning as well — because it alone of all of the SSRIs had been approved for the treatment of childhood depression. As we have already seen, Prozac just squeaked by in gaining FDA approval for use with children. The other antidepressant drugs had been used to treat childhood depression through off-label use since all of these drugs had approval for treating adults.

The following excerpts from the testimony will give the reader a flavor of what took place. The excerpts from the several sides of the argument give the reader a view of the several forces and counterforces that were operating at the hearing. I am only presenting bits of the testimony but interested readers might read all of it at *www.fda.gov-ohrms-dockets-ac*-04.

<u>Expert Testimony</u>

With this preface in mind, let's look at the FDA testimony of Irving Kirsch and David Antonuccio, two research psychologists who have published a great deal of research in this area.

> "DR. KIRSCH: My name is Irving Kirsch. Baum, Hedlund has paid for my air tickets. I decided to come before knowing that.
>
> Dr. David Antonuccio, Amanda Drews, and I are reviewing the published literature evaluating the efficacy of antidepressants in

depressed children. A total of 12 randomized, controlled clinical trials have been published.

Two-thirds of these trials failed to find any significant benefit of medication over inert placebo. Only 4 trials reported significant differences, and these did so only on clinician-rated measures, not on patient-rated measures.

When the data from these trials are combined, the placebo response is found to be 87 percent of the drug response. This means that the drug effect is only 13 percent of the drug response. This is not a clinically significant effect.

Many children get better when given antidepressants, but the data indicate that this is largely a placebo effect. These conclusions are consistent with those found in 7 previous published reviews.

To summarize, the published clinical trial data show that the therapeutic benefits of antidepressants for children are negligible at best.

DR. ANTONUCCIO: These results were drawn from studies with design flaws that typically favor the study drug. For example, they frequently exclude placebo responders before random assignment, rely on ratings by clinicians who have a vested interest in the outcome, and are likely to publication bias and file drawer problems meaning that many studies with negative results do not get published. Adding unpublished studies, most of which have negative results, will surely shrink the difference between antidepressants and placebo even further.

In order to evaluate the cost effectiveness of antidepressant use in children, the committee must consider the benefits, as well as the risks. Clinically meaningful benefits have not been adequately demonstrated in depressed children, therefore, no extra risk is warranted.

An increased risk of suicidal behavior is certainly not justified by these minimal benefits. Neither are the established increased risks of

> other commonly reported side effects, which include agitation, insomnia, and gastrointestinal problems.
>
> The highest possible standard should be applied to scientific data involving drug treatment of children, because children are essentially involuntary patients. Those of you on the committee who are parents know this to be true because when your children have prescription medication for something that ails them, you make them take it as prescribed whether they want to or not.
>
> Children given antidepressant medication often do get better, but so do children given placebo. Thus, the clinical data suggest the improvement is due primarily, if not entirely, with placebo effect.
>
> Please be careful to ensure that our children are not exposed to risk without commensurate benefit."

In reading the above one might think how "proponents" deal with such data about the ineffectiveness of antidepressants in treating depression. The answer is drug "proponents" completely ignore it.

<u>Findings Clear</u>

Kirsch and Antonuccio put their findings very clearly. At best there is a negligible benefit of drug over placebo even though these trials are biased in favor of the drug. With negligible or no benefit, even minimal risk cannot be justified. Kirsch and Antonuccio remark that their recent review of the antidepressant clinical trials gave conclusions that were consistent with those found in *seven* previous published reviews. The British recommendation that these drugs (except for Prozac) are contraindicated in treating pediatric depression came from an examination of the evidence of both the risk and the benefits of these drugs with depressed children.

The Medicines and Healthcare Products Regulatory Agency (MHRA) found six SSRI and atypical antidepressants *contraindicated* for pediatric use including Seroxat (Paxil in the United States), Effexor (Venlafaxine), Lustral (Sertraline), Apramil (Citalopram), Cipralex (Escitalopram) and Faverine (Fluvoxamine). Prozac escaped the ban because of its FDA approval for treating childhood depression. The

British said that only 1 in 10 depressed children would benefit from being on Prozac. As we would expect, the Prozac clinical trials demonstrated growth suppression of the drug treated relative to the placebo treated children.

In the 1990s it was standard practice for the FDA, once approving an antidepressant drug for adults, to write the drug company and request trials dealing with safety issues for children. The FDA asked for the trials because it was understood that the drug would be used with children as well even though not so licensed. The first major Seroxat (Paxil) trial in children was completed in 1996, but the results were not published until 2001. Data was also gathered in 1996 after a trial of Pfizer's Lustral showed that 9% of depressed children on the drug became suicidal (Boseley, Sarah, 2003). Other drug trials that did not give favorable results were neither published nor sent to the FDA or the MHRA. Did any of these unpublished child drug trials hide any suicides?

Dr. Solomon Iyasu, from the FAA's Division of Pediatric Drug Development, reviewed the adverse events for paroxetine (Paxil) and citalopram (Celexa). Dr. Iyasu presented the adverse event reports received by FDA as mandated by the Best Pharmaceuticals for Children Act. This is a voluntary reporting system to the FDA, which includes adverse events reported by providers, pharmacies, consumers, and pharmaceutical manufactures. These reports are for a one-year period.

Paxil is the second most frequently prescribed drug for depressed children. Pediatric patients accounted for approximately 3.5 percent of the total United States prescriptions of Paxil between July 2002 and June 2003. Dr. Iyasu related that there were 17,000 adult and pediatric reports of adverse events for Paxil both domestic and foreign, received by the FDA. For the above period there were 127 unduplicated pediatric adverse event reports. Ten percent of the reports included outcomes of death (13). One third ended up in hospitals or at emergency rooms. In looking at 68 adverse (psychiatric) events there were nine completed suicide attempts, 17 suicide attempts, and suicidal ideation in 11 patients. Other psychiatric symptoms included mania, impulsively, disinhibition, obsessive behavior, etc.

In one of the 9 completed suicides there was a discontinuation or decrease of dose involved. Five of the 17 suicide attempts occurred during discontinuation or decreased dose. Two out of the 4 homicides occurred during drug changes as did 3 out of the 8 for the aggression/hostility/homicidal ideation. Suicidal/homicidal events can occur at *all* phases of drug therapy.

Drug treatment ranged from fourteen days to one year. Moreover, the aggression is across the board both self and other directed.

FDA: Paxil May Be Linked to Suicide in Kids

The FDA finally acted based on data obtained in Great Britain which was evaluated by the Medicine Control Agency (MCA). In June of 2003, the Food and Drug Administration warned physicians to stop giving the antidepressant Paxil to children. Paxil, of course, had *never* been approved to treat childhood depression, but the FDA was aware that it and other SSRI antidepressants were routinely prescribed for children. The FDA warned not to stop Paxil suddenly but to taper its use under medical supervision to avoid rebound side effects such as abnormal dreams and shock-like sensations.

Prior to the above hearing and following the British, the FDA gave a public warning about these drugs while continuing the study of the issue, hence the above hearing. In the FDA Paxil warning, the FDA *was not* showing its independence, because the prior British Paxil warning could not have gone unnoticed by the FDA; it *had* to act.

There were about ten family members who testified about what they believe to have been SSRI antidepressant induced violence (suicide or homicide) of a family member. As an example, I will only report the following case.

Terri Williams and Jacob

> MS. WILLIAMS: My son, Jacob Williams, was born on October the 15th, 1986. Jacob was an exceptional athlete who participated in football on both the varsity and junior varsity football teams in his school.
>
> In September of 2000, Jacob experienced a loss of interest in his school activities. He maintained his interest in football; however, there was a conflict with his grades and his attendance.

As a result of this issue, his father and I attended a conference at his school on October the 11th, 2000 with various representatives from the school. The school administrator suggested that Jacob may be depressed and that we should seek medical help.

I contacted Jacob's pediatrician and made an appointment for 3:45 that afternoon. On October 11, 2000, his pediatrician prescribed 10 milligrams of Prozac, which was increased to 20 milligrams three weeks later.

Shortly after starting the initial dose, Jacob began to complain of having strange dreams, which he had said were bad. Shortly after the dosage was increased, I began to notice an aggressive behavior, which had not been there before. Jacob also became destructive and destroyed some of his favorite things.

His friends would later tell me they had noticed the same behavioral change. He also showed a verbal aggression and short temper, which had not been present before.

When questioned about this behavior, he stated I don't know what is making me do this. At this time, I thought this could be a part of normal adolescent behavior and did not pursue the matter any further.

On December the 5th, 2000, I discovered Jacob's body hanging from the rafter in our attic. He had hung [sic] himself with his own belt. A letter was placed on the ladder leading up to our attic thanking us for giving him 14 years of a happy life.

Something had to have gone wrong in the thinking process to bring this about. Had I known that this was a potential side effect, suicide, I would have never allowed my son to take the drug Prozac. Thank you.

What We Can Learn From the Williams

One cannot definitively determine the harmfulness of a drug from a case example — nor for that matter the efficacy of a drug from such anecdotal evidence — because there are too many unknown factors and uncontrolled variables. However, there is much to be learned from the above tragic case about the many problems that exist today in the antidepressant industry.

The school administrator "suggested that Jacob may be depressed and that we should seek medical help," which may be read, "He needs antidepressant medication." We don't know much about what problems Jacob was encountering in his life or in his adjustment when his problems came to the attention of the school. The school was correct in being concerned but, even with the subsequent suicide, we cannot say that the diagnosis of depression was correct. The loss of interest in his school activities and a conflict about his grades and activities *could* have been related to depression. However, the problems may have had other sources, e.g., he could have fallen in love but was unable to approach his love object. Jacob is said to have continued his interest in football. If he were depressed, this continued interest in football certainly lessened the severity of the depression and reduced suicide potential. A behavioral health professional with diagnostic expertise to evaluate Jacob and discover what it was about Jacob, his life, family and peer relationships that might be the cause of his symptoms was needed to define the problem before any treatment was initiated. Instead it was decided that he was depressed and needed an antidepressant to address the biology of his depression, i.e., a possible chemical imbalance.

Psychosocial and other personal-environmental factors are completely ignored when we take a very simple, medical (drug) solution to the problem. Whether or not you think that Prozac killed the child, this is an example of the search for the simple solution for a child's mental health problems, a path that is unfortunately the dominant one in society today.

Twenty-five years ago Jacob's pediatrician would have referred Jacob and his family to a *behavioral health* professional for diagnosis and treatment. Those days are gone now. In Jacob's case the school had bought into the antidepressant conventional wisdom as did Jacob's pediatrician and Jacob's parents. If even *one* of the entities had not bought into the simple solution Jacob might still be alive today.

The Eli Lilly defense would have attributed Jacob's adverse drug side effects to his depression, the bad dreams, recent aggressive and destructive behavior, and the agitation but, we really don't know if Jacob *had* a diagnosable depression. I know it is difficult for lay persons and some psychiatrists to believe that suicide can arise from sources *other* than depression but it can and does. For example, a teen suicide often generates one or more suicides in the peer group. The reader may remember the 800 or so suicides in the Jim Jones cult; did all those people have a chemical imbalance and a Major Depressive Disorder? We do know that whatever Jacob had or did not have, depression is not treated effectively by antidepressant medication.

Parent Has a Critical Role

It is as wrong to blame the parents for a child's depression as it is to blame depression on a chemical imbalance? Whatever the source of the child's depression, the parents have a critical role to play in the child's recovery. The best child therapy is conducted not with the *child* but with the *parents*. We need an expert who knows the child and the nature of his/her problems to be able to provide competent understanding and guidance to the child's parents and school. In modern psychiatry today about the only role the parents have is to see that the child takes his or her medications as ordered. A few parents have not bought the conventional simplistic solution and insist on treatment other than drug treatment. Unfortunately these parents are far from being in the majority for we presently have more than one million children a year on antidepressants.

Jacob probably had very treatable problems. He had problems that definitely needed attention and his prognosis could have been very good. The behavioral expressions of the akathisia, the recent aggressiveness, short-temper and destructiveness were due to the *drug* and not to his personality make-up. He maintained a good feeling for his parents to the end. He thanked his parents for giving him "fourteen years of a happy life."

Although the drugs are dangerous to both adults and children (whether or not they have diagnosable depression or other problems), the immaturity of children makes them *more* vulnerable to these violence releasing drugs than adults. Kids have less experience dealing with adversity and temporary emotional set backs than adults. Problem solving skills are less well developed in youth than in those with more experience. With some maturity adults are more likely to have a "this too will pass" attitude, which reduces the impulsivity of youth.

In addition to a direct harm to the users, a strong negative of the drug approach is that it keeps or delays troubled people from getting proven help for their problems from *trained* professionals.

Mack Refused

A retired police officer (Richard Mack, page 135 of the transcript) also testified to the committee. He said that he and his wife refused a school recommendation to put his second grader on drugs to control the son's behavior. In retrospect, Mr. Mack felt he had made the right decision, saying his son turned out just fine.

Mr. Mack was a sheriff in a small town in Arizona and was aware that the community had an abnormally high rate of teen suicide and violence. He said one thing the community could not ignore was the circumstantial evidence that the common denominator in all of these cases was that the victims or perpetrators were all on SSRIs. Certainly such evidence is not proof of a relationship between drug and violence but any scientist would say that the possibility needs very serious investigation.

In addition to the police officer's awareness of the high incident of co-existing SSRI use and violence, there was another commonality Mr. Mack did not observe or mention. That is that few if any of the teens in question had *any* formal psychological treatment. Since these teens were all on SSRIs, it is probable that their problems were given "mental health" treatment, that is, medication by the family physician.

The Goffs Ordeal

Marion Goff and her daughter, Alex, appeared to tell the committee about Alex's sister, Devon's experiences when she was nine years old. Senator Lincoln Chafee's wife, Stephanie, who is a friend of Mrs. Goff, also joined Mrs. Goff. I report this case because Mrs. Goff took her daughter, who had developed an obsessive-compulsive disorder very severely and suddenly, to a specialist. On the second visit the specialist prescribed Zoloft. He increased her Zoloft to 50 milligrams but it didn't help. Then her child was switched to Paxil. I will let Mrs. Goff continue her story in her own words.

> She was hospitalized and Devon's medical condition was compromised in that she had developed a cardiac arrhythmia and had to be placed on a heart monitor. She was in the hospital for one month, and she was on the heart monitor and bed rest for the entire time.

> During this time, her Paxil was increased to 20 milligrams. A few days later she was started on Zyprexa also. Devon was not getting any better; in fact her behaviors grew worse. She began hitting her head against the metal hospital bed. She threatened to jump out of the window on two occasions.
>
> On two other occasions, we found a pair of sharp scissors in her bed. Our child was never suicidal before these medications. At one point, my 9-year-old child, who weighed little more than 60 pounds, was on 30 milligrams of Paxil and 10 milligrams of Zyprexa.
>
> Our gentle daughter would now fly into a rage several times each day. It became part of our life to have my husband and myself restrain Devon at times for fear that she would truly hurt herself.
>
> During these times, she would try to inflict injury upon herself by banging her head on walls, beds, and floors. She would punch herself in the legs and arms. She grew extremely violent toward us. She would run to the silverware drawer and get a knife and attempt to stab herself.
>
> The worst moment happened when I looked in on her, in her room one night, to find her by her open second floor bedroom window with one leg out the window in a position as if she appeared she would jump.
>
> Devon is presently being treated for Lyme Disease. In summary, our experience has been one of absolute terror to watch your 9-year-old daughter suffer so much, so suddenly, and to be so lost in helping her.

SSRI treatment was the only treatment that Devon received and the litany of the serious adverse side effects of the drugs were much worse than the symptoms of the original condition. OCD seems likely, but her ten pound weight loss prior to treatment should have alerted the psychiatrist that there might be a medical problem in addition to the OCD.

Even though some SSRIs have FDA approval for treating OCD, these drugs treat OCD about as effectively as they treat depression, that is, not at all. Other therapies should have been tried if physical health problems had been ruled out as the source of the OCD. OCD is one of the child mental health disorders that does require direct therapeutic work with the child in addition to parent guidance/counseling.

Response Prevention Not Used

Response prevention, a behavioral therapy, *is* an effective treatment for OCD but it was not used in this case.

As an alternative to a complete ban, the FDA could rule that these drugs are contraindicated for treating depression or anxiety *unless these drugs are prescribed as a part of comprehensive mental health treatment by behavioral health specialists*, treatment that deals directly with the psychosocial factors giving rise to the mental disorder. The latter is what *should* be done but I am not naïve enough to think that the FDA will do it.

The Rider Family

In a letter I wrote to the FDA committee chairman looking into these issues, I mentioned my belief that the several entities involved, including the FDA, were perpetrating a cruel hoax on the American people. The hoax is that depression is a chemical imbalance in the brain and that it can be treated effectively by a drug alone, which can be prescribed by a family physician or a psychiatrist. The words of one of the family witnesses reflected my thoughts much more powerfully than I could do.

> MS. RIDER: My name is Dawn Rider and I am here to tell you my story, and I represent, as president of ASPIRE, more than 11,000 persons who are all named on the Eli Lilly and Prozac petition, which a copy has been given to the panel.
>
> We have been educated to believe that mental, emotional, and behavioral disorders are caused by chemical imbalances in the brain. The fact is that this is only theory, and this theory is pushed on us as if it were the absolute truth.
>
> The reality is that the best of scientists do not completely understand the complex inner actions of the myriad chemicals in our brains. Those of us who elect to believe this theory and subject ourselves to treatment become guinea pigs in an ongoing [and uncontrolled] experiment.

I know this from personal experience. I trusted our family doctor when he explained that depression is caused by a chemical imbalance. We trusted him when he determined that Paxil was right for my husband, and Prozac for my son.

We weren't educated enough at that time to ask him to provide us with the test results that proved which chemicals were being balanced.

I am not going to go into details of what happened to our family. I have given you all documentation; it's very painful. Suffice it to say that my beautiful 14-year-old son is now dead, and when we discovered the problems with these drugs, we decided it would be better for my husband to suffer through depression than end up dead like our son, and we found out that he could not get off the Paxil.

He went through over a year of hell before he was able to finally withdraw from the drug, and in the process it destroyed our marriage of over 20 years.

I say with no apology whatsoever that these SSRI drugs destroyed what was once a loving and vibrant family. Why do we believe that street drugs like heroin and LDS can have outcomes such as this, yet, we won't accept that legally prescribed drugs, working on the same neurochemicals, can result in horrific crimes against persons and property?

Why do we accept that a drug like penicillin, beneficial as it is for some, can prove fatal for others? We fail to accept that these drugs can have paradoxical effects. These drugs are not safe for everyone.

They should be labeled with the strongest of precautions and dispensed only by trained physicians who have time to adequately monitor the patient. Most doctors do not have time for this level of care.

Not Just Risk, Also Ineffective

Dawn Rider said in effect she was sold a bill of goods. Her physician told her that depression is caused by a chemical imbalance and she, like most people, trusted her physician. In retrospect she knows that what she was told was a theory but not fact. Despite learning a lot about these drugs in the interim, she still does not seem to realize that there are proven non-drug alternatives to treating these problems.

The Averys

The following example is given because even many "mental health professionals," unfortunately even many *licensed psychologists* are sending many of their depressed patients to physicians for the magical cure. But, as will be seen in the following testimony, the magic simply does not work.

> MR. AVERY: Hello. My name is Jeff Avery. My 16-year-old stepson, Brandon Ferris, committed suicide on July 22nd, 2001, about three weeks after he began taking Zoloft. Brandon was a bright and socially outgoing teen who got along well with others. He was a black-belt instructor in Tai Kwon Do, active in the church's youth group, and held a part-time job.
>
> His mother home-schooled Brandon and worked at the Tai Kwon Do School, so she was very active in Brandon's activities.
>
> In June of 2001, Brandon expressed that he was feeling down, and not his usual energetic self. It was decided that he should take some time off and see a counselor.
>
> The counselor suggested that he see a doctor. The doctor, who found no physical problems, prescribed Zoloft.
>
> Sunday, July 22nd, Brandon and I went to church. On the way home Brandon volunteered to make a cake for his mother's birthday. He asked permission to go on a boating trip. He spent the rest of the day with his friends and an older brother Randy.
>
> When he came home from his youth group meeting at 9:15, he seemed fine. At 9:45 he asked his mother about the boating trip. At 10:30 he went to check his e-mail, but his brother was using the computer. At 11 o'clock, he was found in his room hung by the neck from a belt in his

> closet. We called 911; we performed CPR to no avail. He was pronounced dead at the hospital.
>
> Reflecting on the day's events, I could not detect any indication of forethought to suicide. However, [after] later conversations with others close to Brandon, I inferred that he might have been having problems with the medication.
>
> The obvious question is what happened in Brandon's mind between 10:30 and 10:45.
>
> This was not the end of unspeakable tragedy. Five months later, Barbara, unable to cope with the loss of her youngest son, took her life.
>
> Since then I have collaborated with Brandon's biological father, Dan Ferris, to obtain information that would point to the cause of Brandon's death. We believe, after having done much research, that the drug Zoloft had a causal effect in Brandon's final actions.

<u>Zoloft the Cause</u>

I agree with Mr. Ferris that Zoloft was the cause of his son's suicide. From the history as related by the father, I doubt that a diagnosis of depression could have been sustained. He was feeling down and not his energetic self, which is typical of any teen from time to time. One cannot argue with referral to a counselor, but from the testimony we know nothing of the counselor's qualifications. Was the counselor relatively untrained and did he buy into depression as a "medical" problem and send the patient to his physician for antidepressant therapy? We do not know.

Did the counselor suspect medical problems or did he make the referral to have his patient put on antidepressant medication? In my experience lesser trained mental health providers are as enamoured of drugs for treating depression or anxiety as are psychiatrists.

<u>No Evidence of Emotional Disturbance</u>

The history as given by Mr. Ferris gives no evidence of what might be considered emotional disturbance. All indications were that of an emotionally normal teenager who was full of life and optimistic. Appearances can be deceiving and these problems of differential diagnosis are not easy. Therefore, only *well trained professionals* should be in a position to advise parents who present with "problems" as Brandon did. Since it is unusual for a male adolescent to come forward to express mental health problems, we may doubt the diagnosis of depression. Were these expressions of some sort of psychological malaise, perhaps a developing depression or did he have some type of illness that was draining his energy? He was said to be feeling down, which suggests a mood problem, but were these Brandon's words or his stepfather's words? We don't know and we don't know what Brandon told his counselor. Had he made up his mind to kill himself as a way out (of something) or was his apparent happy mood his last day quite genuine?

Energy or Drug-Induced Urges

The boy had been on Zoloft for three weeks. Antidepressant defenders would say that the drug was beginning to work and he now had sufficient energy to kill himself. Although this type of reasoning seems to be quite correct in some cases it is overused. There are reports that the boy had said that he might have been having problems with the medication, which would not be in the least unusual. Even though the evidence is of an anecdotal nature, we should not dismiss self-reports of the intense suicidal and homicidal urges experienced by a significant number of persons on SSRI and related antidepressants. These urges were reported by both persons being treated for emotional problems and some emotionally normal people in phase one studies of the drugs.

With children or adults whether to treat (a psychological problem) or not is a very important clinical decision. As professionals we can err on one side or the other. First, not all mental health problems *should* be treated. Children and adults as a group are resilient. At any stage of development, emotionally sound people encounter temporary adjustment and other problems that they are capable of resolving without the need for professional help. We know, for example, that about one-third of persons with what might appear as "serious" emotional problems often resolve the problem on their own while on a wait list for professional help. This is close to the antidepressant drug efficacy.

Interesting Omission

It is interesting that a number of people at the end of their testimony at the FDA hearing make a plea for the addition of warnings about akathisia, suicide and other serious adverse side effects of these drugs despite their bad experiences. But most do not recommend an outright *ban* of these drugs. As a group these people seem to regard these drugs as efficacious but dangerous.

What these victims are asking is that users should be closely monitored to prevent the tragic effects that came out in the testimony. The FDA will put warnings on the labels, but proper monitoring of these drugs by non-psychiatric physician prescribers will not occur unfortunately. The average physician spends about five to ten minutes with the typical patient, whether the patient has a medical or psychological problem. The typical patient is then given medication and told to return in three weeks whether the drug prescribed was an antihypertensive or an antidepressant. This pattern will not change because of an FDA warning.

FDA Finally Warns

The FDA, finally giving into science and the anguished cries of parents whose children committed suicide on these drugs, warned against use of these drugs with children (except for Prozac). The FDA also asked the drug companies to attach a warning of possible suicide effects of these drugs on adult populations. In the above testimony parents told the FDA of teenagers who hanged themselves or slashed their wrists after starting on antidepressants. Many parents told of children who had become extremely agitated or anxious shortly after starting these antidepressants and of seemingly sudden impulses that turned deadly. These are direct effects of the drugs (the akathesia/agitation) and not the effect of the depression/anxiety.

The FDA warning focuses on the appropriate *monitoring* of these drugs by the prescriber, especially at the initiation of treatment or when a dosage is increased. However, I must tell you that better monitoring of these drugs will not take care of the problem. *These drugs must be withdrawn from the market.*

The Excuse

It is a very popular notion to think that antidepressant drugs in some patients can release a pre-existing but subclinical mania but again this is just a theory. Perhaps the former theory makes these adverse effects more palatable by saying they are just releasing something that was already there. An equally plausible and a simpler explanation is that these "aberrations" are what they appear to be, that is, drug effects.

Another Excuse

The pharmaceutical companies, the FDA and other drug proponent entities typically attribute these adverse events to emergence of the underlying illness. I believe "proponents" have a more difficult time of explaining away the homicide/aggression in terms of emerging of the underlying illness. If we accept this last theory we are going to have to change our definition of depression, or the "proponents" will come up with a *subclinical* homicide gene that only *some* depressed patients have!

I am not making fun of the field of neuroscience, I have been a part of it for many years, but I am exasperated with antidepressant drug "proponents" who maintain their convictions and belief in the magic despite all evidence to the contrary. Dr. Iyasu, after reporting much of the above, reminded us that many of these reports occurred in patients with underlying psychiatric disorders, therefore, "severity of illness/disease may play a role." However, this is the FDA's *only* answer to anything that arises that might imply that these drugs have serious harmful effects. The FDA points out how unscientific it is to make a case against these drugs by isolated anecdotal evidence. Unfortunately for the "proponents," the *controlled* clinical trials show the suicidal events occurred at *twice* the rate in drug treated as those on inert placebo. How can "proponents" wiggle out of this finding?

FDA Bias

The antidepressant drug-suicide relationship was the finding of Andrew D. Mosholder, M.D., MPH, a staff member of FDA. Dr. Mosholder was asked by the FDA to examine the FDA clinical trials on children on the question of antidepressant drug-suicide relationship. The FDA did not like Dr. Mosholder's findings. The drug suicide events were *double* the placebo suicide events in the clinical trials. The FDA asked for more research while not allowing Dr. Mosholder's report to see the light of day. As of April 2004, the FDA has been in hot water over suppressing this report, and the House of Representatives had asked for hearings on the matter.

Both Ways?

"Proponents" of antidepressant drugs want to have it both ways. When anecdotal evidence suggests some *negatives* about these drugs they appeal to science about the limitations of anecdotal evidence, but when an appeal is made to the scientific evidence of harm, "proponents" ask for more research and give anecdotes to support their view. When the controlled scientific research shows the drug's limited efficacy in treating depression, drug proponents are complete skeptics and want to turn to the *anecdotal* evidence that in their mind establishes the efficacy of these drugs! I don't think we should let the FDA and the other "proponents" have it both ways. They should not be allowed to continue to use science when it serves their purposes and to use anti-science when science does not meet their propaganda needs.

Laughren

In the House hearing, Thomas Laughren, M.D., of the FDA staff spoke on the regulatory history of antidepressants and suicidality and told of current plans for the analysis of Pediatric Suicidality Data. He failed to mention that Dr. Andrew Mosholder had already reviewed and reported on the data regarding suicide from his review of the pediatric antidepressant clinical trials. He thanked the families for testifying at the hearing and reiterated that "it is very difficult to assess causality based on individual cases," when the outcome is either tragic or good. He said he would turn his attention to the controlled clinical trials.

However, Dr. Laughren prefaces his remarks by bringing up the usual antidepressant drug spin doctoring; suicide is not an infrequent occurrence in the depressed; with the beginning of convalescence, suicide risk becomes greater as the patient is energized, which allows "them to act on their suicidal ideas before the drug has had a chance to affect mood." He tells us how important it is to come to the correct conclusions. "Clearly, we don't want to miss a signal of increased risk of suicidality, because that would give us greater comfort in the use of these drugs than would be warranted. On the other hand, we don't want to reach a premature decision on the strength of the signal because that could result either in the overly conservative use of these medications."

Convenient Coding Hides Suicide Events in Trials

GlaxoSmithKline, in coding suicide events in child drug trials, had classified suicide events under the heading "emotional lability." The FDA reviewer thought this was odd and requested that the sponsoring drug company put these events under a term specific to suicidality. GSK made a second report on Paxil and suicide, which went first to the MHRA in Britain (FDA's counterpart in the United Kingdom) and shortly thereafter to FDA in May of 2003. That report indeed suggested an increased risk of suicidality associated with Paxil use with children in one of the three studies done in pediatric depression.

The MHRA essentially contraindicated the use of Paxil in pediatric depression. The FDA recommended against its use in pediatric depression, but stopped short of a contraindication and "in essence, we said that we were continuing to look at the data." The FDA issued a request to sponsors of the eight other antidepressant products to look at suicidality in their databases. The FDA asked of the sponsors a broad term "possibly suicide related" and suicide attempt. The risk ratio is the number of patients having one or more suicidal events divided by the total number of patients exposed.

Definite Risk

Paxil had three trials. For the first trial the risk ratio for the drug was 6.5 for drug and 1.1 for placebo, which Dr. Laughren saw as "definitely a signal for something." Dr. Laughren, I believe this is more than a "signal for something"— it is a signal for self-harm. The risk for the drug was 6 times the risk for placebo. We can see why the MHRA came out against the use of the drug with children. If an antihypertensive drug had a risk of self-harm at 6 times greater than placebo, do you think it would remain on the market for further study? Or would it be removed immediately? I think you know the answer. It does not matter that the other two studies were negative; the risk of harm is quite clear. Dr. Laughren is concerned that the risk was not consistent across studies; I am not.

2 Out of 100

Here is another example of the FDA's peculiar logic. With regard to efficacy questions, negative findings of efficacy (placebo subjects do as well as drug subjects) are considered meaningless to the FDA. Two positive trials obtain FDA approval for the drug even though one hundred trials may be negative. However, when it comes to *risk* the negative trials *are* very meaningful and the FDA wants to do further studies.

Suicide Issues

Of the 109 patients who had either suicide ideation or a suicide attempt (there were no successful suicides), 43% were hospitalized, 39% of those with suicidal ideation alone, and 61% of the self-harm patients were hospitalized. Among those attempting self-harm, 21% engaged in cutting behavior, there were 37 overdoses, and there were 2 cases characterized as hanging behavior or interrupted suicide attempts and one case of self burning.

Suicide events are serious. Fortunately, there were no successful suicides — partly because of the very *close monitoring* of these subjects during drug clinical trials. This level of monitoring is not present in the real world when pediatricians and family practice physicians prescribe these drugs. We have to look at the suicide/homicide potential of these drugs when they are inadequately monitored, when they are used as the sole treatment, and when these emotionally impaired children are not receiving appropriate treatment for their individual/family problems.

In evaluating the lethality of these drugs with depressed children, the FDA and the MHRA work from the same data and database. On a clinical trial of Lustral (sertraline) that was completed in 1996, a drug which was manufactured by Pfizer, 9% of depressed children on the drug became suicidal! What additional information do we need? This was not simply anecdotal evidence. This drug is dangerous.

Too Hard on Themselves?

In contrast, other studies show the placebo suicidality rate is only about 1%. Moreover, the MHRA came to their conclusion from data that was *voluntarily* submitted to them by the pharmaceutical sponsors of the various drugs, often in the form of summary data. If mistakes were made or data withheld was it likely to be in favor of the interests of the drug company or not?

One would hope that the regulator would keep a skeptical eye on the drug maker, but from reading the FDA staff testimony at the hearing I saw only naivete on the part of the regulators. This was crystallized when FDA staff tried to deal with the apparent stronger suicide signal of the drug over placebo. The staff thought that in defining suicide events of the trial subjects, the sponsors *may have been too hard on themselves!* Can you believe it? How can people of above average intelligence expect the thirteen billion-dollar a year antidepressant industry to be *too* hard on themselves?

Limited Benefit, High Risk

In reviewing the clinical trials on suicidal effects and efficacy of antidepressants with children, Dr. Robert Nelson on the FDA staff found that only 3 out of 15 studies (20%) proved the drug was superior to placebo in treating childhood depression. These included the two positive Prozac trials, for which the drug gained FDA approval, but again the difference in favor of the drug over placebo was so weak as to be virtually non-existent.

Dr. Nelson found a suicide signal in 5 out of 13 FDA clinical trials (38%) with one study showing as reported earlier a 6.5% rate for the drug versus a 1.1% for placebo, that is, a factor of 6 times greater for the drug over the placebo. The English took the same data as the above, limited or no benefit of these drugs and high risk of harm, and declared (and rightly so) that these drugs, except for Prozac, are contraindicated in the treatment of childhood depression. In assessing the dangerousness of these drugs, we have to keep in mind that in the *real world* pediatricians and other physicians, unlike the very close monitoring in the clinical trials, cannot properly monitor these drugs.

Even to an untrained researcher/statistician, the above data is quite clear and the conclusion is a no-brainer. These drugs should *not* be used with children. The English came up with the right answer, but how does the FDA handle it? "Let’s do some more studying." Since the drug companies might be too hard on themselves (according to the FDA) in overdefining a suicide event, the FDA staff wanted a Columbia University research group to study the issue and to advise the FDA on this matter. The data (which was submitted by the drug industry, which paid for the clinical trials) was quite adequate to support the British conclusion, but in the hearing the FDA was looking for wiggle room, which is blatantly protective.

Faulty Premise

Since these "proponents" want to *believe* that these drugs are effective with depression across the whole life span, the "proponents" are looking for a way to demonstrate and prove their effectiveness and safety with children.

Appeal for Legislation

In August of 2004, the media had just announced the suicide of a teenage son of a prominent and influential family. This tragic event came at a time when the FDA was "investigating" the drug suicide relationship in teen suicide. Since the family may become advocates of teen suicide prevention, and their child was likely to have been on an antidepressant drug at the time of the suicide (he was being "treated"), I decided to write the family a letter.

An educated family, such as the above, is likely to share in the conventional wisdom about depression, antidepressants, and adolescent suicide. I thought I would present an alternative view of these matters that has scientific if not popular merit. I made these points in my letter.

- From my review of the scientific research and my clinical experience, I would have strongly advised against an SSRI or related antidepressant in view of the drugs' demonstrated high suicide risk.
- The current prevailing attitude is that depression is a brain disease, a chemical imbalance in the brain. Since it is assumed to be a biological disease, "proponents" believe it requires drugs to correct the chemical imbalance. This conventional attitude reduces a very complex *biopsychosocial* public health problem to a fairly simple solution, an antidepressant drug prescription by a family doctor who has virtually no training in mental health issues.
- The problem is there is absolutely no scientific support for the chemical imbalance theory of depression and its treatment with drugs. Nonetheless, currently there are about seventeen million prescriptions of antidepressants annually for children.
- Normal people (including adolescents) have "down" moods from time to time when they encounter adverse events in their lives (such as a death in

the family). Clinical depression differs in kind, not degree, from these more minor mood problems of everyday life.

- There is a great deal of normal volatility/impulsiveness that is characteristic of the adolescent period, and because of this teenagers cannot handle adversity as well as adults, which means that emotionally *normal* as well as mentally ill teenagers can and do commit suicide. Most psychologists and some psychiatrists who have not bought into the disease model would feel very comfortable with this non-disease model of many adolescent suicides.
- The focus has been giving pills rather than teaching skills and to address youth suicide we have to replace the former by the latter. Although psychiatric drugs are indispensable for treating correctly diagnosed cases of schizophrenia, bipolar disorder and Attention Deficit Disorder, stress and mood problems (including diagnosable depression or anxiety) across the life span are most effectively treated by behavioral *interventions* by trained professionals.
- Your efforts are needed to address the problem of more kids on ineffective and dangerous SSRI and related antidepressant drugs. Help decrease the number of youth suicides caused by Prozac-type drugs as a treatment of youth mental health problems.

I would recommend that you as a public figure consider the following legislative changes:

1. Injured parties should be able to sue the FDA for damages over an approved drug. The administration had directed that alleged injured parties of medical devices or pharmaceuticals approved by the FDA *not* be allowed to sue for damages. If the FDA made no mistakes this directive would be appropriate, but the FDA *does* make mistakes and access through the courts is the *only* way that bad drugs can be removed from the market.

2. Pharmaceutical companies (by law) should be forced to publish (or make available to the public) *all* clinical drug trials that are either positive or negative. Also, *all* adverse drug reactions *must* be reported as they arise and not just those discovered during the clinical trials.

3. The FDA should be forced to eliminate the biases that favor drug over placebo in drug clinical trials. In antidepressant drug trials, for example, the current practice of the use of placebo run-ins, the use of inert rather than active placebos, the use of supplemental drugs (sedating and others) and other design faults that favor the drug over placebo must be eliminated. Moreover, the standard of a statistical significance of the drug over placebo should be raised to a *substantial* statistical difference. In antidepressant drug clinical trials versus inert placebo, drug responders (a 50% reduction of symptoms) are 50% versus 32% on inert placebo, which is *not* clinically meaningful to warrant approval.

4. Independent non-drug "proponent" researchers should determine a minimum Effect Size for the FDA to use in drug approval.

5. We need better truth in labeling and advertising throughout the pharmaceutical industry. For one thing, the drug advertising to patients and physicians must state whether the drug (1) addresses the *cause* of the health problem (e.g., an antibiotic) or (2) if it just decreases a symptom (e.g., antihypertensive drugs). With antidepressants and other drugs, the number of *remissions* and not just "responders" should be reported in all communications. The remission rate of antidepressants is so poor that it is never reported.

I have not as yet heard from the public figure mentioned in the above but I trust my comments on these matters will have given the family a broader understanding of depression, antidepressant drugs and child suicide.

Failing to Mention

Much of the research on antidepressants is financed by drug companies. I have noticed that reports of these recently completed studies seem to not distort the data so much as to consistently fail to report some important pieces of data that would have modified the research conclusions quite substantially. For example, an announcement of a recent research study might have shown that for treating OCD, the drug was found to be superior to placebo in 55% vs. 39% of the patients in the two groups, but it might fail to mention that thirty-two percent of the drug treated children had to be terminated from the study for adverse drug side effects, failure to respond or other reasons. To the average lay person or physician reading this study one might think the drug is a pretty good drug because 55% of the children got better; however, when we apply the drug drop out rate, for every 100 children in the real world given this drug only 37 of the 100 children would get better, which is less impressive than the 55% figure reported and less than the 39 of a hundred that improved on placebo.

Did the announcement fail to mention that on remission (i.e., recovery from OCD) there was *no* difference between the number of drug vs. placebo remissions, which certainly weakens the power of the drug in treating the disorder? Have the researchers also failed to report that the improvement criteria was a 50% reduction in symptoms or the difference between the drug and placebo groups on the rating measure was only two points on the 21 item OCD scale? Shouldn't the general public expect a *higher standard* from these researchers who are *supposed* to be committed to science rather than to the marketplace? I think the public and the media need to look at these drug research announcements as *marketing* announcements rather than reports of scientific findings.

When a physician gives a depressed person a pill to treat the depression, the pill gives the patient hope for the future and suicide risk from the depression is reduced substantially. We know that 32% of depressed people get better on a sugar pill alone (vs. 50% on a drug) and this message of hope has an almost immediate effect on the depressed patient's behavior and well being.

After several years of good research to the contrary, the FDA is still blaming antidepressant drug induced suicide on the *condition* and not the drug itself. Moreover, the FDA is still ignoring the fact that we have no scientific evidence that these drugs have *any* clinical value in treating childhood depression, which in itself makes moot the risk issue since if there is *no* benefit we should not tolerate *any* risk.

The House of Representatives' Hearing

In September of 2004, the House of Representatives held a hearing on antidepressant drugs and children and the FDA had a second hearing on the same topic.

Representatives from five or six drug companies spoke at the hearing. There had been some discussions recently about making the results of all drug clinical trials public since often only trials with *positive* findings get published. Most of the drug company representatives said their companies had already begun to do this. There was some discussion between the House committee members and those testifying about whether these reports should be *summaries* or the whole protocol/data.

The protocol report should be neither a summary nor the other extreme. There needs to be enough of the research design protocol and the findings for independent researchers to review the data to determine whether or not the *conclusions* were consistent with an examination of the data as a whole. Too many times drug companies in their public announcements about new drugs fail to report data that is necessary for an understanding of a drug's effectiveness.

Letters

One of the House committee members brought up "Letters to Physicians." These "letters" are supposed to give physicians further information about the drug and additional research findings to help guide drug decision making. The committee member read aloud one such letter and one can easily see how bias in favor of the drug can creep in. The letter noted that efficacy of the drug for depressed children had not been established but noted "Open Label" studies which were positive, suggesting that this research may have established efficacy. These "open label" studies are worthless in establishing efficacy. In these studies the prescriber and patient are aware that the patient is receiving the drug and there is no control (placebo) group for comparison purposes.

Drug company staff write these letters and it would be impossible for these "letters" not to be biased and self-serving of the company's interests. If the drug companies outsourced such letters to independent research psychiatrists, I am not sure the situation would be improved. Physicians are too uncritical of such correspondence from the drug companies. The situation is ripe for a watch dog group to oversee the accuracy of such transmissions from the drug company because the FDA is certainly not doing it.

FDA Approved Antidepressant for ADHD?

The drug STRATTERA™ designed to treat Attention Deficit Hyperactivity Disorder (ADHD) in both children and adults, developed by the Eli Lilly Company, maker of Prozac, is expected to be a "blockbuster" drug in the mental health field. First some background.

The Drug That Already Works - Ritalin

For thirty or more years the amphetamine, methylphenidate, better known by the brand name Ritalin, has been used as the primary drug treatment of ADD and ADHD in both children, six years and older, and adults. There have been several hundred Ritalin/placebo outcome studies that have shown substantial superiority of Ritalin over placebo in treating these children and adults. This was consistent with my clinical experience over a ten-year period of diagnosing and treating these children and some adults with therapeutic doses of Ritalin.

About half of the children now on Ritalin are *not* ADD or ADHD and Ritalin is not an appropriate therapy for these people's non-ADHD problems. If the problem *is* ADD or ADHD, then Ritalin is not only appropriate it is, in my clinical experience, clearly *indispensable* in correctly treating this disorder. I have seen not just a *mild* improvement of a correctly diagnosed child on a therapeutic dose of Ritalin. With a correct diagnosis there is a *dramatic* improvement in the child's ability to master both academic and social learning. The short-acting Ritalin takes about thirty to forty minutes before it activates, its therapeutic effects last for about four hours, and the typical child requires three dosages a day, once before school, the second after lunch and the third early evening (at least four hours *before* bedtime).

A negative to Ritalin is that being an amphetamine, it is a controlled substance. It is potentially addicting and can be abused. Some parents are fearful of Ritalin for this reason. But despite this risk, most parents are open to a trial of the medication.

Within a week if the child is correctly diagnosed and on a therapeutic dose, these parents soon see that the benefits substantially outweigh the minor risks.

Another possible negative of Ritalin was that very early it had a reputation of stunting physical growth and this idea has continued to some extent even though subsequent experience did not confirm this fear.

STRATTERA™ Approved

It was against this background that the FDA approved STRATTERA™ for the treatment of child and adult ADHD in early 2003. STRATTERA™ was expected to gain a major market share even though it is much more expensive than Ritalin. However, it does not have the stigma of being a controlled substance like Ritalin and it requires only early morning, once a day dosing (the school need not know the child is on STRATTERA™).

STRATTERA™ is one of a class of drugs called selective norepinephrine reuptake inhibitors (SNRIs), a class of drugs under investigation for treating depression and anxiety. These drugs are "cousins" to antidepressants such as Prozac, Paxil, Zoloft and other drugs, which in off-label use have been unfortunately used to treat ADHD and other behavior problems.

No Data on Adverse Brain Effects

I and other psychologists and some psychiatrists were opposed to using *any* antidepressant drug with children because of potential harm to the *developing* brain. We have no data on any long-term, adverse brain effects on the *adult* brain with chronic use. However, it seemed inappropriate to use such a drug on a *developing* brain without knowing what harm might be done. Moreover, there was a proven drug alternative, Ritalin. Undoubtedly Eli Lilly knew of the off-label use of Prozac, for example, for ADHD children and it was a no-brainer to try STRATTERA™ on these ADHD children and adults when it proved completely ineffective in treating child depression.

STRATTERA™ Risks

In the clinical trials, the STRATTERA™ treated children lost 0.4 kilograms of weight over seven weeks while the children on a sugar pill gained 1.5 kilograms.

There was also a statistically significant height gain in favor of the placebo group. It is unknown at this time whether STRATTERA™ will affect final adult height or weight.

In addition to the usual growth suppression side effects of antidepressants, I am most concerned about the drug's effects on heart rate and blood pressure. The STRATTERA™ treated children had substantially *higher* heart rate and blood pressure than those on placebo. I must say I was not reassured when Eli Lilly agreed with the FDA to monitor for any long-term growth and cardiovascular effects on these STRATTERA™ treated children. I could not imagine an ethical researcher with such preliminary research data asking parents permission to expose their children to such possible long-term dangers, especially when there is a *proven* drug to treat the problem.

Letter Ignored

From these adverse growth and cardiovascular side effects alone, I do not think the medication should have gained FDA approval. After reading advertising on STRATTERA™ and an article on it in Behavioral Health Today, May 2003, I submitted a letter to the editor with my comments on the drug and recommending that it be withdrawn from the market. The publication agreed to publish my letter and said it would appear in the next issue. A week later I received an e-mail saying the publication was not able to get my article in this issue but it would try to squeeze it in the next. Originally they asked if I would mind a rebuttal statement by someone else, and I said I would not mind. As I write this, my letter has not appeared in Behavioral Health Today. Who is surprised?

STRATTERA™ Benefits

Any drug, of course, should be reviewed in terms of a benefit/risk ratio and some drugs with high benefit outweigh the serious harm they might do to the patient. For example, some drugs for cancer are known to destroy brain cells, but these drugs are used anyway because the spreading cancer is life threatening. What about the benefits of STRATTERA™ in treating ADHD?

We know from the STRATTERA™ trials that the drug in well-diagnosed ADHD children was more effective than a placebo on measures of improvement. We know that in two clinical trials STRATTERA™ treated children did better than ADHD children on placebo, but is this enough for us or the consumer to know? We need to know how the drug compares to *Ritalin* in its effectiveness. One might tolerate some greater risk if the benefits of the new drug were *substantially* superior to a proven drug.

However, in double-blind placebo clinical trials, STRATTERA™ was also compared to methylphenidate (Ritalin). However, Eli Lilly *did not report how STRATTERA™ did against Ritalin in the clinical trials* in their official announcement of STRATTERA™.

Compared to What?

Eli Lilly was mute on the most important comparison in the clinical trials, how the new drug did against Ritalin. Someone will be able to obtain the FDA data through the Freedom of Information Act. It is likely that *STRATTERA™ did not compare at all favorably with improvement* of the subjects on Ritalin. Why? If STRATTERA™ had only proved *equally* effective to Ritalin, this fact would have been touted in the official announcement. Therefore, it is all too probable Eli Lilly did not like the findings since these facts were not announced. I am wondering what spin Eli Lilly will give on why these results were withheld when the truth comes out. My bet is that Eli Lilly will withdraw STRATTERA™ from the market one day (either voluntarily or non-voluntarily) when the truth is unraveled. The withdrawal will be either the lack of benefit of the drug in relation to Ritalin or more likely *the long-term health risks mentioned above* or both. As I write this section in January, 2005 the media has announced that STRATTERA™ has just been implicated in causing liver damage.

Twisted Logic on Antidepressant Drugs and Children's Suicide

The FDA held their recent committee meeting in Bethesda, Maryland, and the FDA is recommending pretty much what I had anticipated from their previous hearing several months ago, that is, stronger *labeling* for antidepressant drugs with children and not contraindication of the drug.

The FDA finally admitted the reality of drug suicides when they made a pre-publication announcement that some recent research found the rate of child suicide was *twice* that of those on the drug versus those not on the drug, which is consistent with the drug clinical trial data.

Warning, not Ban, to Decrease Use

The FDA has escalated a posted warning to what is called "a black box label," which some believe will discourage the use of these drugs with children. The evidence of the dangerousness of these drugs with children was so overwhelming that the FDA finally had to admit it. The FDA still played down the lack of efficacy, and made the political "black box" decision rather than an outright ban.

At the prior FDA hearing only a few months before this, the FDA was still denying the dangerousness of antidepressant drugs for children and was continuing to blast the *condition* and not the *drugs* for child suicide.

I expected the FDA to *continue* the denial because I mistakenly thought that if the FDA *ever* admitted drug induced suicides, the FDA would *have* to make these drugs contraindicated in child treatment. I was totally wrong about the extent of their willful blindness.

Restricted Damage Control

It sounds as if the FDA restricted damage control to pediatric use of Paxil. How can a drug be dangerous and require a warning for persons seventeen years of age and younger and be safe for persons eighteen years and over? Of course it cannot be. The drug is either safe or unsafe regardless of age and any warnings should be unrestricted as to age. The FDA might argue that the drug has been *approved* for the treatment of depression in adults, but it has not been so approved for the treatment of childhood depression. The difference, the FDA may say, is *proven* efficacy. However, we have already seen how Paxil and all of these related drugs have only *limited* efficacy at most. I did not believe the public would accept such sleight of hand on this issue.

Longer Trials Not the Answer

Most of what I know of the recent hearings (the full text will not be ready for awhile) is from the media. What the FDA is saying is that most child drug clinical trials are only *four* months and these drugs may *still turn out to be effective with longer trials*. I do not see how anyone can have the *nerve* to say such a thing and keep a straight face. If an antihypertensive cannot reduce blood pressure over placebo in the first four months, why should we think it should be effective over a longer period? There is no reason to think that if the drug and placebo groups do not pull apart in the first four months that the groups would pull apart later. Please, the acute drug biased clinical trials have found no efficacy of the drug over placebo. Why should we expect *longer* trials to show a difference?

Read the Label on the Snake Oil

The FDA goes along in this drug suicide matter as if these drugs have proven their effectiveness in treating depression in both adults and children. The FDA also acts as if there is no other treatment available to effectively treat these problems and drug treatment is our *only* path of hope. It is true that prescribers, a small army of psychiatric drug researchers, and the drug companies are telling the FDA that these drugs are indeed effective in treating depression and the whole industry is built on such testimonials (just like snake oil). However, the FDA cannot point to any *scientific evidence* to support its position to post drug warning labels rather than admitting that these drugs as a class have not demonstrated efficacy. It should withdraw them from the market or at the very least make them contraindicated (as the British have done) in treating childhood depression.

Chapter VII

WHAT'S HAPPENING ON THE ANTIDEPRESSANT DRUG CHAT LINES?

The following excerpts, taken from antidepressant chat lines of users talking about their depression and antidepressant drug experiences, give insight on what is going on in this industry with patients. I could certainly not portray it nearly as well as reports from some users. These were in no way *selected* interactions. Each story was inherently interesting, and I took a whole series from beginning to end without any omissions. I edited only for brevity's sake. I consciously kept in any of the user's *positive* expressions about their antidepressant therapy experience. So few positive comments from this group might surprise some readers.

A pill that promises a cure represents a powerful message to the patient, and such a message to a person in great distress can be very effective medicine. One must realize that in well-diagnosed depressed patients, a sugar pill has a 32% response or improvement rate—which reflects what hope can do. You may see in the following messages that most of the expectations of improvement for these patients is in the future, that these users will *one day* find the perfect pill or combination of pills that will solve *all* of their problems.

You will see that the anticipation has been dashed several times in the past use of a long litany of drugs, but despite the poor return from the drugs, the hope continues. This attests to the power and pervasiveness of the common conviction that depression is a disease caused by a chemical imbalance in the brain and an antidepressant drug is its primary treatment. Many of these patients and their doctors are unaware that there are proven alternative treatments for their problems and these patients are cut off from effective help with their problems.

This experimenting with antidepressant and anxiolytic drugs has earmarks of the 60s and 70s, in which many illegal drug users tried to come up with the perfect drug combination that would lead drug users to the Promised Land. Currently the search with *legal drugs* for the perfect chemical cocktail has approval of the establishment.

With this introduction behind us, let's get to these user testimonials:

I'm new to this depression forum, but I've posted on panic/anxiety. I was just wondering if anyone is taking the right combo of meds that has alleviated their depression/anxiety. I'm taking fluoxetine and klonopin. One of my anxiety symptoms is a spacey feeling. I've read that a combo of an SSRI plus Benzo. will eliminate this symptom. I sure would appreciate some constructive feedback.
God Bless
Fay

Fay is new to the depression forum, but I expect she will be part of it for a long time to come. She is looking for the magical pill solution to her problems.

Hi,

I also have recently come off effexor, two weeks ago. I have suffered severe nausea and have had what they call "brain shivers" this is where it feels like a wasp or bee has flown into one ear and out the other in sound terms and you get an electric sensation, sort of buzzing as well. I was and am worried by this, as I have been dizzy as well and thought that this was some other illness like a brain tumor.

I gained 4 stone over 1 year that is over 56 lbs. in American weight terms. I also get terrible "itching" all over my body and have been using pruriton antihistamines to alleviate this, this is the worst thing along with the nausea.

I really thought that I had finally lost it until I have read literally hundreds of personal testimonies about the adverse reactions to this drug. I just hope I can get some of this weight off as I have also read that this can stay after discontinuing this drug?? Oh, definite sexual dysfunction as well.
James

The Brits have accepted the drug treatment theory of depression as much as we in America have and, at times, it is a very rocky road. James has experienced much misery in going through his antidepressant drug history. One might think he might get off the boat, but he has so many interesting stories to tell and to share with other users.

I have no appetite, and all I want to do is sleep. I don't want to go out of my house; I just want to stay in bed all day under the blanket.

I don't want any phone calls, and I don't feel like talking to anyone. I don't answer the phone or the door.

I don't want to go to work anymore, and am giving up on my job and starting to lose enthusiasm and interest. I am not doing too good at work anymore – don't want to be there!!

I am married and I like to be with my husband. But all I do is sleep. I can't cook any more, no energy, so I eat cereal when I am hungry.

I also started talking in my sleep (my hubbie tells me). I talk A LOT and have been having very intense dreams mostly nightmares that last a long time, and sometimes wake up confused, and don't remember if I am married, or a kid living at home.

I am 39 and have been married for 10 years. And this morning upon waking, I thought I was in my old house with my parents in New York.

I am on Klonopin 1 mg 3 x per day, Paxil 12.5 mg 1 x per day, Vistaril .50 mg 2 x daily and Wellbutrin 300 mg per day.

Do you think the meds are causing the above symptoms or is this depression? I still feel very depressed.

Downlady

To Downlady, wherever you are.

Much of what you report is due to adverse reactions from the prescription chemical cocktails you were taking and is *not* arising from the problems you were having when you began your drug "therapy."

Some of what you report in the first several paragraphs of your message are for the most "mild" drug side effects rather than depression, but later you report some reactions that you seem to think are worsening of your depression ("...and don't remember if I am married, or a kid living at home."); the latter may reflect a *toxic psychosis* from the drugs and not your original "depression."

In describing the latter symptoms you may be undergoing an acute brain syndrome brought on by your drugs, and most likely you are open to taking other drugs to fight these adverse symptoms; however, right now the drugs *are* your problem. I would ordinarily tell you to go to your physician but he or she helped put you where you are today. Go to a physician to help you detoxify from the drugs and also see a psychologist to help you to get through this period until

you are able to "find" yourself. I would be reluctant to send you to a psychiatrist to take you off these drugs, but I am afraid that even if he or she got you off these drugs you may jump back on this same merry-go-round.

Most people reading your "tale of woe" and most physicians who prescribe these drugs to others probably thought your description described someone undergoing a very severe depression. However, I don't think so, although midway in your litany I could begin to see a "real" depression emerging. Despite reporting a host of what *could* be depressive symptoms (no appetite, all I want to do is sleep, etc.) you mention "starting to lose enthusiasm and interest." In the latter you seem to express that you are closing in on a diagnosable depression, but I suspect your *drugs* and not so much your *problems* have been pushing you toward "depression."

Hi Jim

I am finally on new meds and they seem to be working. I had a real hard time with Lithium, I had every side effect there was and even had side effects that weren't listed. I am now taking Geodon, Trileptal, Trazodone and Xanax as needed and am doing better than I have been in awhile…

Carol

Well, Carol, you seem to have all bases covered in your drug cocktail, but your basic problems are complicated by your prescriptions. Perhaps you weren't told this, but the body habituates to Xanax-type drugs. In time you will need more of the drug to get the same effect.

I have been on and off Paxil for the last 2 years and frankly it did not really help that much. Not really any side effects suffered, but I was not too happy with the results overall. It also takes up to 3 weeks to kick in and even then it only helped me minimally. Since then, I have been on a multitude of other drugs (none of which seemed to do the trick). I am going to see a second doctor tomorrow to see if I can get a different prescription. Good Luck.

Sam

Sam seems to have very good insight into the fact that these drugs have not been of help to him at all. However, he looks like he is going to keep trying

and hopes that his new doctor will offer a different prescription. What are the chances that his new doctor, after taking his medical and prescription history, will tell him; "Look, Sam, it looks as if these drugs have not helped you at all; what about trying something new and seeing a professional for non-drug treatment of your problems." This would be reasonable and sound advice based on Sam's history. I suspect, however, his new doctor will prescribe Prozac or if he or she is very daring, an MOI antidepressant.

Paxil – "It gave me my life back despite insomnia.

Didn't your doctor prescribe you a sleeping pill? Pills for side effects are the norm. Tell him to get with it.

Paxil – happy with her Paxil because no sex drive (which ironically I prefer) and sleep a lot... I love sleeping; it's like a hobby. I am currently not on Paxil because I have no job. I still sleep but my life now has a depressed angle so it's hard to enjoy sleeping. Sex? Well I am single and have tried to give up dating many times in my life so having no sex drive really helps me personally. I don't believe in God but if I did, its clear to me I am supposed to be celibate. Its ironic because I am very attractive, I just can't handle relationships like that on any level.

This is a sad case. She is happy because the drug has taken away her sex drive. Does her doctor count this one as a success? This woman has a serious, yet probably very treatable problem, but the solution won't be found in a pill.

On line chat room

. . . I lie compulsively. It started out by making up life stories to impress, but it has gone so bad that sometimes I can't differ a true story from a lie because I've said it so many times and started to believe it is true. It worries me a lot because I don't want to be like this. In fact, this problem has brought me even bigger problems. For instance, I first lied about I have a self-mutilation problem until I actually did start doing it. Same thing happened with bulimia and anorexia. I want to be happy of who I am now and want to stop lying but it comes out naturally and quite frankly I'm scared of the consequences. WHAT DO I DO?

P.S. my therapist has no idea of this… I think sharing it with her seems like a good idea, right?? Please give me some feedback if you have this problem or if you know of a way I can help myself…Thnx

p.p.s. could my meds help out with this? Are there any that could? It's a dumb question but I am curious.

The above is a good example of the "diseasing" of America, i.e., turning everything into a disease. The above individual believes that his lying arises from OCD, and he is looking for a quick fix to the problem. The lay person would think that this individual has low self-esteem. A therapist, with the same diagnosis, would keep this person in therapy for forty years without a change in behavior. A superior attitude is as likely or more likely than an inferior attitude. Whatever the cause, the focus of therapy should be on helping the patient to change his behavior—which is what he says he wants, too.

Chat room

…that I have as much luck on this as I did on Celexa, minus the dead sex thing… I tried to add Wellbutrin and that made me nothing but sick and I wasn't dealing with that. Plus it increased my appetite immediately and I don't like that at all…. I don't want to gain back what I lost on Celexa, which is almost 20 lbs.!!!

I hope I don't feel sick this week. My doctor said go right on 10 mgs and that he considers it like Celexa and I do not have to wean to it. Hope this works, where it is a newer med, I am sure he still has to learn himself. Well I am hoping and praying!!! To stay happy, for no sickness, weight gain, and a sex drive again.. Tall order!!!

Grace

Grace seems pretty committed to the pill approach even though we would hope she had learned something from her pill-seeking behavior. She is hoping that the pharmaceutical industry and God are both on her side and will work together for her salvation. I think she could achieve a lot of her goals (no sickness, no weight gain and a sex drive again) by simply *withdrawing* from her drugs. Which is worse; her original misery or the misery caused by the drugs?

Grace,

I'm positive you will find Lexapro much better than Celexa and without many of the annoying side effects.

I've been on 20 mg for about a week. I'm taking it for anxiety and feel like I'm not where I would like to be. I know the good of what Paxil did for me and I'd like to get to the same level of effectiveness with Lexapro. I think this is my one shot...if 20 mg won't do it I'll have to find another medication. I'll probably know in another two weeks.

I am not too hopeful that the above individual will find the one drug he is looking for. I don't think it really exists for whatever ails him. Down the line when he continues to fail on drug after drug perhaps his doctor will recommend ECT or perhaps a brain implant. Many patients, of course, may be looking for the easy way, but now we have many physicians and psychiatrists who also believe in the easy way, that a pill will take care of it and if not this pill another pill, etc.

Grace, I was on 10 mg of Paxil for about 4-6 weeks. I lost the ability to have an orgasm. My sex drive was still there though.

Anyway – I am now taking 10 mg of Lexapro. I've been on it almost 6 weeks. I feel that it's working extremely well. My sex drive and orgasm is back and sometimes I get a kink in my neck but its not bad. Nothing a little hot pack and massage can't help.

I found the transition from Paxil to Lexapro not that bad. I think I had 3-4 days of feeling like I almost had a flu or cold coming on. Then again – it is the season! I have much more energy now and I can actually accomplish things I couldn't do before, like eating in a restaurant. By the way – I am on it for anxiety. I was diagnosed with panic disorder.

Good Luck!

Betty

Betty, you have a very treatable problem. However, medication is not the answer, although you seem to feel your current chemical cocktail is working for you. I suspect you do have a panic disorder and, of all the anxiety disorders, a panic attack is likely to be the most frightening to the person experiencing it,

perhaps more so than persons experiencing the other anxiety disorders. In speaking about anxiety, President Roosevelt was quite right: "The only thing we have to fear is fear itself." Your fear is the fear of your own fear—but you can overcome your fear. Drugs to mask the anxiety are only a stopgap measure; they do not address the *cause* of the problem.

An animal's or person's natural response when confronted with anxiety is to withdraw or avoid, which lowers the anxiety, but ensures that the fear is perpetuated. If you respond to your fear of flying by not flying (naturally you have no fear when not flying) and take Xanax for the next twenty years, you will still have an anxiety response to flying when you try it again. You have done nothing to learn responses (e.g., relaxation) that are incompatible with an anxiety response to the feared stimulus. Many of the approaches psychologists have learned to treat anxiety come under the heading of "counterconditioning," the learning of a new response in the presence of the old feared stimulus. These approaches are based on science and not sorcery; therefore, they are not as popular for some people as are drugs.

Mary:

When you switched from Paxil to Lexapro did you have to wean from Paxil and wait before starting the Lexapro? Or is it possible to just switch midstream? I am new to the antidepressant field and my doc has suggested maybe Lexapro may be better for me. I was just wondering if you would have any imput on making the switch. Thank you.

Mary, you are new to the game, but I worry you will become a seasoned veteran in no time.

I'm on week 3 with Lexapro 10 mg. I was taking 20 mg for a few days, but I almost ran out of my script so I had to cut back both dosages. I could feel no differences in my OCD . Some days are good and some days are bad. It comes and goes, but I don't know if the Lexapro is helping at all. I'm going to wait at least 2 months before letting my doc know that it doesn't seem to work anymore.

If just waiting were a good technique to solve problems, I think you would be well on your way to a great cure.

Just wondering what you are taking Lexapro for? You mention anger – is this caused by anxiety and that's why you are taking the medication? If so, a higher dose may be in order. If that doesn't work, call your doctor and get on a different drug that works for you. Good luck.

You sound like you've been well conditioned by a current generation psychiatrist. If the drug doesn't work, the first step is to increase the dose.

Robert,

I really hope the Lexapro works well for you. I take Wellbutrin now and I read that you had an increase in appetite right away...me too!!! Most people notice a decrease in appetite and lose weight. I have not lost any weight. I was thinking about trying Lexapro, but I don't know if it is available in Canada yet. Also, I had side effects when I took Celexa, and I don't want that to happen. Luckily the Wellbutrin is good for that.

What about trying Paxil, has your doctor left that out?

Barry,

I have GAD and my anxiousness translates into anger as well, especially yelling at my wife and kids. This was one of the symptoms that told me and my doctor, that I have an anxiety problem.

Lexapro has really helped me with this. Things don't get "under my skin" like they used to. In fact, I moved up to 20 mg two weeks ago for this very reason and it has really helped me. It gives me enough control over the situation to think twice about "is this really worth it to get upset over?"

This is very interesting theory that yelling at your wife and child is due to anxiety. Have you also tried to blame it on bad genes; that's another good rationalization I have found. The most important thing you can do to solve the problem is to take *personal* responsibility for it—you (and not someone else) are responsible for your abusive behavior. At the end of your message you do, however, use a *cognitive* strategy that implies taking some personal responsibility: "Is this really worth it to get upset over?" Good advice. Take it.

Hi guys

I feel for you both. As a wife on the receiving end of that anger ... it sux!!! I am always tip toeing around ... I HATE it!!! I intervene when I think the kids are going to hear it!! ...my 9-year-old lost all authority with Dad because she looks at me for HELP when he is going off.

...they need love, not yelling. If you yell at my daughter now, she cries and gets anxious. She will even cry before the yelling starts. I am still taking Lex. I had a very bad week ... not sure if it is the med change ....or if 10 mg isn't enough ...or just one of those weeks???

It has been hell here ... running away seems like a good answer!!! A hotel to hide out in ...DREAMING

I realize you don't want to hear this, but your only effective solution in order to protect your children from your husband is to stop being a victim. There is no chemical solution to your very real marital problems. Placating a terrorist does not work. Doubling up on your pills will only protect you from the *knowledge* of the harm you are doing to your children.

Chat-line Survey

How many times have you switched SSRIs?

	Votes	*Percent*
I haven't switched	*9*	*10.84%*
2 different SSRIs	*31*	*37.35%*
3 different SSRIs	*20*	*24.10%*
4 different SSRIs	*10*	*12.05%*
5 different SSRIs	*9*	*10.84%*
more than 5 different SSRIs	*4*	*4.8%*

From my experiences in surveying these drugs in several benefit plans, the above is quite representative. There are a number of people who always try the newly approved antidepressant drug.

Started on Elavil (to help sleeping first off), then it helped with depression. Felt like a happy zombie so switched off. Paxil 20 mg. felt like Superman! Had every single side effect while on it, so decided to try Zoloft: 50 mg up to 100 mg. Slight

decrease in side effects but felt like I was on speed – nothing could knock me out at night, so I switched back to:
Paxil: went from 20 mg to 40 mg [after heart surgery] on to Remeron, Best sleep ever. Felt drugged up during the days though, and packed on the pounds big time.
Switched to Serzone. Great night's sleep, great sex life, but very clouded thinking and motivation problems. Now trying Celexa ...

"Why can't the drug industry come up with the perfect antidepressant – one that will take away all my problems and leave me with only pleasant side effects?" Dream on.

I have tried the following drugs: Prozac, Wellbutrin, Paxil, Geodon, Serzone, Xanax, and now Lexapro. Lexapro seems the best for me yet.

Yes, you would be best sticking with one — fewer side effects.

Prozac, Celexa, Wellbutrin, Effexor, Trazadone, Klonopin – as of now. None of them seems to be worth the trouble they cause, though Effexor is working the best of any of them.

Would you tell me how good "is the best of any of them?"

I can't remember all of them but I've been on: imipramine, prozac, celexa, remeron, effexor, serzone. They've finally figured out I just don't seem to mesh very well with SSRIs. A couple of them gave me some sort of tremors, or too sleepy even if taking them at night and celexa turned me into a raging wild woman. I was so scared after one dosage of that med, with the fury I felt within, I actually barricaded myself in my room and then struggled the rest of the night fighting the desire to throw my 5 ft long bureau out the closed window. I'm not a violent person ...ever.

I'm now on wellbutrin, topamax, and trileptal ...being taken off topamax because it's causing my hair to fall out. I don't know how many meds are left for me to try ... I'm sure they will figure out something..?

I would not get hopeful about "I'm sure they will figure out something?" They won't. They will come up with more of the same. To get better–or at the very least to have a life free of side effects–you have to stop putting yourself and your health into the hands of someone else. Some might say your agitation with

the urge to kill is a side effect. Of course, your drug company denies it and attributes it to your problems—though it's out of character for you.

Hi, I suffer from OCD and I have been on prozac, zoloft, remeron, luvox, celexa, risperidal, neurontin, depakote, klonopin, trazadone, buspar, paxil, effexor, and now paxil CR and seroquel. I am still looking for the med that works the best. I feel my luck is running out.

Sometimes you have to give up your dreams, including the dream of finding the perfect pill. I don't like to be discouraging to people, but maybe that perfect pill is *not* out there.

The ones I can remember are:
Serzone – I was on it the longest worked great
Wellbutrin – Drove me over the edge
Celexa – Too many side effects
Prozac – Gained way too much weight
Paxil – Sexual side effects
Lexapro – I'm on 10 mg now
There are a bunch more, just can't recall.

Do you think maybe you need a completely new plan?

I've been on Paxil (took me off because of weight gain), tried celera, effexor and now am switching back to celexa. I sure don't know how they know which ones to try a person on. I'd have to agree with some that it's been so long since I've felt happy about life and not depressed that I don't think any pill is going to make me feel good. I mentioned I cried a lot to my doctor so that is why he switched me back to celexa, said this one works best for crying problems. Anyway, I think my system is too mixed up from trying so many things, what works best for me is a narcotic, like vicodin, makes me hyper, I can socialize and it makes me feel good, it wipes emotions and pain away from me, unfortunately, doctors watch how much of this we use for their pain (mine being knee arthritis pain).

I am sure it must seem like magic to "know which ones to try a person on." I am sure your prescriber will tell you it is based on science, but I suspect

rolling the dice to determine the drug would be just as effective. I hope you're not headed for the use of street drugs. I am sure your doctor will come through for you instead.

I just discovered today that my 80-year-old father has just started Zoloft. He got a starter kit ... 7 – 25 mg and 14 – 50 mg doses. I don't really think he knows what it is for .. just taking his meds as the doctor prescribed ...

Stan

Isn't it nice that he got his own little starter kit, but I have the idea that his little starter kit won't be the end of it.

I am on the verge of tears this morning...don't know why. I wrote down the things that I feel I need to tell my doctor but none of it makes any sense.

Sad for no apparent reason.

Self loathing/hate myself.

Tired beyond belief and go to bed at 8:30 p.m. and even find empty office at work to take naps in.

Think about weight problem 24/7 but when craving hits I justify and tell myself I don't drink, smoke or do drugs and this is the one bad habit that I enjoy, but then wake up and hate myself all over again and feel so controlled by food.

Feel craving is stronger than me, no control.

Hate myself and hate the way I look.

Just sleep, eat and try to exercise but eat so much will never help with weight.

Shrinks don't help, they just listen and use common sense.

I would suggest getting another shrink who does something more than "listen and use common sense." Or ask your doctor to give you a pill that will take away how you feel about your obesity. You say you don't do drugs?

Anyway this is my life and last week I was happy go lucky and just felt great but now I feel sad. Last week I was on the starter amount of 25 mg (Zoloft) with my usual WB, SRISO and now that have gone up 50 mg feel sad again. Weird ... My daughter (11 year old) takes 150 mg and I am on 50 mg but not happy for past several days.

In reviews of pharmaceutical data, it is not unusual to see a mother and daughter on antidepressants, often the same brand.

Oh God! I think you are still adjusting. You may have experienced a "natural high" when you started the Z just because you were finally on your way.

I know its tough, but it will take awhile for the Z to kick in. But it WILL. I've been told by a Dr. that family members do great on the same med. Meaning if it works for your daughter, chances are great that it will for you, too.

Big hug – Faith

I know, Faith, that you are trying to help, but you are not. Neither is your doctor.

Thank guys for your support. I ended up going back to a low dose of EFXR since it worked so well for me in the past. I am going to see about just taking a low dose of 37.5 for now coupled with my usual WBSR and see what happens...

Well if the E doesn't work out I will probably go back to Z and just be more patient.

That's a plan, but is it a *good* one? Actually, depression (if that is your problem) is self-limiting; i.e., you get better even without treatment. Drug taking can actually work against getting better.

From my experience you don't need to wean off. I went from Paxil to Wellbutrin, (I think Wellbutrin is awful stuff) and then to Zoloft with no problem.

I have been taking a combo of Zoloft and Wellbutrin SR for about 3 months. I am at 75mg of Zoloft and 400 mg of Wellbutrin SR. I will say that adding the Zoloft has made me very anxious. I can almost feel the electricity running through my body. The plus side is that my depression has moved ... pitch black to a dull gray.

Is the dull gray enough to keep you on your present path? Not to be a spoilsport, but it's not working.

Hi,

I've been off prozac for about 2 months now after being on it for 3 years, however even since stopping them I have felt really dopey and out of it, almost like being permanently stoned, however the good news is that I don't feel in the slightest depressed so I don't need to go back on them again.

However, I have my driving test next week and if I take it in the condition I'm in I will almost certainly fail yet when I was on Prozac I had no problem driving. My idea is to take a few prozacs the night before and hopefully I'll be like I was for the test and be able to pass, what do you all think?

Yes, but *should* you be driving a car — much less taking a driver's test?

Um...doesn't sound like the greatest idea to me but I am not an expert..ask your doctor?

Yes, most of us would agree that her plan "doesn't sound like the greatest idea to me." Sending her to her doctor is probably not good advice, though, because he was the one who put her on all those drugs in the first place. He might come up with a drug to take away her dopiness. No, we better not suggest that because he might add an amphetamine.

Have you considered strong coffee the day of the test? That's what I did for mine. I was alert and did everything perfectly (except signaling...who does in California?).

Good luck on your test.

Since coffee is not an approved drug, I doubt that her doctor would recommend it. I still suggest she should stop driving.

Hello everyone! I've been looking around the forum for side effects of pausing Prozac but the closest I came was to stopping it whole.

3 days ago I forgot to take my meds for the weekend and I haven't had my Prozac these last three days and my mood and attitude is completely messed up. I feel super shaky, highly irritable, very aggressive (feel like shoving or punching anyone who slightly disturbs my mood), easily angers, volatile...in short, I feel I am gonna blow up any second now and yell at the first person who slightly tries to bother me.

...I'm also kind of mad because I feel helpless without the Prozac.

I want to be a prozac-less person again...I feel awful and have lost a lot of hope of ever recovering.

I have a thought. How about starting Prozac Anonymous? You could have another Twelve-step program, the first step being withdraw from the Prozac. You seem to be going through withdrawal and having a rage reaction, although your drug company would deny these are side effects and would attribute them to your "condition."

....maybe consider going on something else.

No, I like my idea better.

My doctor is thinking of prescribing Prozac for my anxiety disorder (GAD). Will it effectively treat this problem for me?

No —but is that what you want to hear?

When I started on Prozac, I started because of depression but I also had a lot of anxiety and it helped mine. You just need to give it time 5-6 weeks at least. Good luck, Kate

How about five to six *years*?

Prozac increased my anxiety and paranoia extremely but helped the depression also extremely. No I'm not depressed but I'm anxious and paranoid.

What are you complaining of? One out of three's not bad. But the cure sounds worse than the disease.

Hi, as far as I know paranoia and anxiousness are bad side effects of Prozac, and should go away with time...if they haven't for you, maybe you should try another HD?

If paranoia and anxiousness are bad side effects of Prozac, maybe it should be withdrawn from the market.

I used to be quite anxious myself and the prozac had actually made me less anxious. I have been very lucky that way I guess.

I would say you are one of the luckiest ones I've come across.

Topic: Remeron's Anxiety Journey, My road to calmness. Well, as of this date, I have been on Remeron now 9 months – 5 months at 45 mg. Has helped tremendously for my depression and my insomnia – still have some bad nights but not on a nightly basis anymore. My main problem is daytime anxiety – added Paxil on 1/10/03 to combat this problem – 20 mg is way too much for me so I am back down to 10 mg ...Maybe 10 mg will work or I will add some buspar. Something to stop the obsessive worrying and anxiety without the sexual side-effects...what do all of you Remeron users take for anxiety?

Let's hear it from the Remeron users.

Your mention of anxiety caught my eye. Have you thought about lowering the dose to 30 mg? ...Remeron becomes stimulating at higher doses. To quote one source: ("higher doses of mirtazapine result in the blockage of the alpha-2 adrenergic receptor, which produces an alerting or arousal effect.")

Have you ever thought of going into psychiatry? I do commend you, though, for trying to at least do some research.

One is struck by the extent of the horrendous side effects that these drugs have on people, which is only exceeded by the capacity that many of those patients have to *tolerate* some of these side effects. These reported side effects of antidepressant users should be considered alongside the official doctrine that current generation antidepressants have a very low side effect profile.

I am not making light or fun of these individuals' personal misery with my remarks, but I am emphasizing our great capacity for self-deception and our tendency to maintain a belief in something despite a mountain of evidence that contradicts the belief. If you can remove yourself from the above stories, as the storytellers cannot, there is a mountain of evidence that the drug approach is ineffective. Still, for many of the above drug users, the belief in the pill seems to be maintained to the very end.

CHAPTER VIII

THE WIZARD OF OZ AND THE TREATMENT OF ANXIETY AND DEPRESSION

In the Wizard of Oz, Dorothy's traveling companions – the Lion, Scarecrow, and Tin Man — all begin with what we would call mental health problems in our sophisticated twenty-first century knowledge. Of course, *these characters* do not identify their problems as "mental health" problems just as patients suffering symptoms of anxiety or depression today do not. As you recall from the movie, the Scarecrow identifies his problem as the lack of a brain, the Tin Man as the lack of a heart, and the Lion as the lack of courage. These literary figures, and their problems, are not unlike patients of today with everyday stress/anxiety and mood/depression. The Oz characters are in search of the Wizard to obtain a magical gift or something external to the self to make them complete.

The Confusion of Origin

The Oz characters and many patients today look to *physical* as opposed to *psychological* explanations for what ails them. With some exceptions, patients today tend to identify their problems in terms of *physical* symptoms, headaches, difficulty breathing, chest pains, stomach upset, difficulty sleeping, fatigue, poor memory, disinterest in sex, and hundreds of other bodily symptoms, physical complaints or other bodily dysfunction. Some with anxiety or depressive symptoms do, on their own, relate their physical malaise to ongoing interpersonal conflicts or other environmental stresses in their life, but these people are rare. Most of us attribute our physical distress to a *physical* rather than a *psychological* origin, which is the cause of much inappropriate medical care today.

The Disease Model

As long as healthcare is drivcn by a *disease* reduction instead of a *prevention* model we are destined to have unaffordable and poor quality healthcare. Although many might reluctantly agree that the disease model is expensive, people credit the disease model with quality. The faith that patients and most physicians have in the excellence of our healthcare is not sufficient in itself to determine its quality. We have to measure quality against some standard. In order to do that we have to answer the fundamental question: "What is good and appropriate healthcare?"

To answer that question—what is good and appropriate healthcare? —we have to describe what it is we are treating and are we treating what we should be treating?

The Kroenke Study

Kroenke and Mangelsdorff (Kroenke, K, 1989) conducted one of the most important and most overlooked health studies in 1989. The researchers, a physician and a psychologist, studied 1,000 patients going through an internal medicine clinic whose diagnosis for presenting symptoms could *not* be determined on the basis of the clinical history or physical exam. Patients were excluded from the study if their presenting complaints were explicable on the basis of previously diagnosed conditions (e.g., Type II Diabetes, asthma), or if the physician during the clinical exam could make the appropriate diagnosis to explain the patient's presenting complaints (e.g., the flu).

The research subjects had various physical complaints (see below) that required a variety of laboratory tests and/or other diagnostic procedures to correctly diagnose the source or sources of their physical symptoms/presenting complaints. The laboratory tests/procedures were used to formulate the diagnosis in order to initiate proper treatment. The presenting complaints of these 1,000 patients consisted of reports of body pain/physical discomfort much like others who come to primary care physicians for diagnosis and treatment, patients whose current complaints are not immediately explicable on the basis of their health history or physical exam.

The researchers reviewed the presenting symptoms of these 1,000 patients and were able to classify these reports of physical pain/discomfort into the following 14 most frequently reported symptoms.

- Edema (Swelling)
- Chest Pain
- Fatigue
- Dizziness
- Headache
- Back Pain
- Dyspnea
- Insomnia
- Abdominal Pain
- Numbness
- Impotence
- Weight Loss
- Cough
- Constipation

Adapted and reprinted from The American Journal of Medicine, Vol. 86, Kroenke, K., & Mangelsdorff, D." Common Symptoms in Ambulatory Care: Incidence, Evaluation, Therapy and Outcome." 262-266, © March 1989 with permission from Excerpta Medica, Inc.

The above symptoms are considered "non-specific symptoms" as to origin, meaning the symptom itself is not specific for any particular disease—or mental health disorder. For our purposes, these fourteen symptoms tend to be the *same* whether the patient presents him or herself to a physician or a psychologist for diagnosis and treatment. Patients as a group, however, tend to view their physical pain/discomfort as arising more from "physical" disease as opposed to psychological factors. As a result these patients are more likely to consult a physician rather than a psychologist or some other mental health professional with these physical symptoms.

The researchers followed these 1,000 patients in terms of the diagnostic origin of their symptom(s) and their subsequent treatment. The researchers were interested in determining for each of the 14 non-specific symptoms how often the symptom arose from an *organic* disease, a diagnosable *mental disorder* (e.g., clinical depression or an anxiety disorder), or if the symptom arose from an "*unknown*" or undiagnosable disorder.

People in general tend to overestimate an *organic* disease as the *origin* of their physical complaints. I am referring here to "normal" people and not just hypochondriacs.

<u>We Thought Organic, Too</u>

For instance, in an unscientific test of public opinion, I asked my whole staff to consider each of the fourteen non-specific symptoms. Then, for each symptom, my employees were instructed to estimate the percentage of the time the symptom in the patient would have been found to have arisen from an *organic* disease (from 0% to 100%).

TABLE I				
Common Symptom	Estimated Organic Disease or Cause	Organic Disease Found	Estimated Non-Organic Disease	Organic Disease Not Found
Chest Pain	62%	6%	38%	94%
Fatigue	44%	9%	56%	91%
Dizziness	65%	9%	35%	91%
Headache	49%	5%	51%	94%
Edema (swelling)	93%	15%	7%	85%
Back pain	64%	3%	36%	97%
Dyspnea (difficulty breathing)	54%	29%	46%	71%
Insomnia	27%	0%	73%	100%
Abdominal pain	57%	11%	43%	89%
Numbness	61%	12%	39%	88%
Impotence	50%	15%	50%	85%
Weight loss	41%	0%	59%	100%
Cough	77%	13%	23%	87%
Constipation	73%	0%	27%	100%
Average	58%	9%	42%	91%

Adapted and reprinted from The American Journal of Medicine, Vol. 86, Kroenke, K., & Mangelsdorff, D." Common Symptoms in Ambulatory Care: Incidence, Evaluation, Therapy and Outcome." 262-266, © March 1989 with permission from Excerpta Medica, Inc.

I have presented this data from my staff in Table I above – their average estimates of organic disease for each symptom – and in the same table I have presented corresponding data from the Kroneke/Mangelsdorff study reporting the frequency found for organic disease for each of the fourteen symptoms.

Since my staff is involved in arranging *mental health* care, one might argue that the staff was biased toward the "non-physical" side of health issues and would tend to *over* rather than underestimate the primacy of mental health factors in overall health. In comparing the *staff* estimates of the frequency of organic disease found for the presenting symptom with the *actual* facts of the cases (only about 9% of the cases proved to have had an organic disease), one can observe a very wide gap indeed between belief and fact. There is a very widespread belief that usually an organic disease is responsible for our physical pain/physical distress when in fact that is not generally the case. Our healthcare delivery system, sharing the general public's overestimation of organic disease, is enamoured with the disease approach to medicine and the attempt to find an *organic cause* for any health problem.

Ruling Out Organic Cause Does Not Rule In Mental Problems

Dr. John's patient, Alyesha, complains of shortness of breath, dizziness, and difficulty sleeping. Certainly these are common healthcare problems and Dr. John's (like general medicine's) approach is not to efficiently diagnose and treat the problem but to rule out organic disease first. First, Alyesha's very likely anxiety disorder is made worse rather than better by putting her through an unnecessary and expensive cardiac workup. The cardiac workup has also made subsequent effective diagnosis and treatment for Alyesha's anxiety disorder more difficult.

When Dr. John tells his patient after all of her tests prove negative that she does not have heart disease, she is no closer to knowing what she *has* and what can be done about it. When Dr. John tells her she does not have a disease, he has in a sense made a *back door* mental health diagnosis. ***Since I find no evidence of organic disease, your problems must be mental.*** Many doctors say that to women without doing any lab or other tests. Such a back door diagnosis is not only incorrect but it is irrational; one cannot prove the *existence* of something by proving the *absence* of something. "Alyesha, I have proved to my satisfaction that you are not a carrot; therefore, you are a tomato." Dr. John should learn to live by the dictum: *"Absence of evidence is not the same thing as evidence of absence."* After the diagnostic workup he can only legitimately tell Alyesha that he found no evidence of heart disease -- not that she does *not* have heart disease or any other organic disease for that matter.

Diagnosis: Up Close and Personal

In general medicine today with regard to mental health problems the standard of care is nothing short of scandalous. The diagnosis of a mental health problem by the general physician is by exclusion or through the back door ("It is not this so it must be that."). What is worse, a treatment is prescribed (e.g., Prozac) without a diagnostic understanding of Alyesha and her problems.

Even with organic diseases the great English physician, Dr. Osler, said in effect that it is more important for recovery that the physician know the *person* who has the disease than knowledge of the disease itself. This truism for general medicine is especially true for the mental disorders. The diagnosis itself has limited value unless we know the psychological makeup of the person who *has* such a diagnosis. The diagnostician must know not only the psychological makeup but also the history and current life situation that the patient is encountering in life. We have to know what it is about Alyesha, her personality structure, her current life situation and environmental stresses/demands that give rise to *her* distressing symptoms before we can help Alyesha resolve these problems/symptoms. The diagnosis and successful treatment of Alyesha's problem is completely antithetical from her medical care thus far, the search for an *organic* cause for her distressing symptoms.

General physicians are trained to diagnose and treat organic disease, yet the Kroenke-Mangelsdorff study finds that of those patients with a possible organic disease only 9% were subsequently found to *have* an organic disease. A *diagnosable* psychological disorder was found in only 10% of the patients. Of the 58 symptoms considered of psychological origin, 26 were believed to be related to depression, 14 to stress, 13 to anxiety, and 5 to grief.

The authors did not conclude that unhealthy lifestyles or an unknown disease accounted for the symptoms of the 74% of the patients with one or more nonspecific symptoms classified as etiology (cause) unknown. Rather, the researchers surmised that many of the symptoms that were unrelated to an organic or a *diagnosable* "psychological" cause were related to various *psychosocial* factors or stresses.

Table II presents data for patients who were evaluated to determine an organic cause and the costs associated with discovering the organic cause.

TABLE II

Diagnostic Evaluation of 14 Common Symptoms

Symptom	Number (percent) Evaluated	Number of Organic Diagnoses Discovered by Testing*	Hit Rate	Estimated Cost (dollars) Per Evaluation	Per Organic Diagnosis*
Chest pain	80 (83)	5	6%	$272	$4,354
Fatigue	57 (70)	5	9%	130	1,486
Dizziness	34 (62)	3	9%	223	2,532
Headache	20 (38)	1	5%	389	7,778
Edema	26 (58)	4	15%	122	793
Back Pain	31 (76)	1	3%	234	7,263
Dyspnea	31 (84)	9	29%	209	720
Insomnia	6 (18)	0	0%	110	†
Abdominal pain	27 (90)	3	11%	202	1,816
Numbness	17 (65)	2	12%	160	1,364
Impotence	13 (54)	2	15%	161	1,046
Weight Loss	18 (100)	0	0%	325	†
Cough	15 (100)	2	13%	147	1,104
Constipation	7 (58)	0	0%	409	†
Total	382 (67)	37	10%	$218	$2,252

* Includes only those diagnoses not apparent after initial interview and physical examination.
† Indeterminate since no organic diagnoses discovered by testing.

Adapted and reprinted from The American Journal of Medicine, Vol. 86, Kroenke, K., & Mangelsdorff, D." Common Symptoms in Ambulatory Care: Incidence, Evaluation, Therapy and Outcome." 262-266, © March 1989 with permission from Excerpta Medica, Inc.

After the third column for each of the 14 common symptoms, I have added a column of "hit rates", the percentage of times an organic cause was found for the number evaluated. The hit rate percentage varies from 0% (constipation, weight loss and insomnia) to 19% for Dyspnea (shortness of breath). Only about 10% of the evaluations ended up with an organic cause, which is far from being cost effective. Some symptoms resulted in *higher* diagnostic costs than others. Evaluating 80 patients with chest pain yielded only 5 patients with an organic cause at a cost of $4,354 per diagnosed case. For headache, it cost $7,778 to find 1 patient out of 20 who had an organic cause for the headache symptom. Only 1 of 31 patients with back pain was found to have an organic cause for the symptoms at a cost of $7,263 per diagnosed case. The diagnostic hit rate for the 10 cases cost a total of $83,324. It would be much more cost effective to have these patients evaluated psychologically (and treated psychologically when appropriate) *before* medical diagnosis, since 90% of the cases were not found to have an organic disease.

As we have seen, the vast majority of these patients have psychological or psychosocial as opposed to an organic cause for their symptom(s). There is no need to routinely involve the psychologist (for diagnostic purposes) when the physician can establish an organic cause for the patient's non-emergency distress on the basis of the history, physical examination or routine laboratory work. However, if a functional or organic cause cannot be established, the patient should be referred to a psychologist for diagnosis and appropriate treatment when appropriate. You may say, "Dr. Ruthven, What about the 10% of the cases in the above who indeed *had* an organic cause for their non-specific symptom? What about them?"

Doctor, Would You Take Another Look at This Patient Medically?

Psychologists frequently ask for medical consultation when one or more of their patient's symptoms do not square very well with their diagnostic understanding of their patient. A "depressive" symptom may be so extreme in the individual case, e.g., excessive fatigue to the point in which the patient can hardly get out of bed, that a diagnosis of depression can simply not explain all of the patient's symptomotology. In such a case, the patient *is* depressed, but the array of symptoms and behaviors show something is missing diagnostically.

As we have seen, headaches rarely arise from an organic cause such as a brain tumor, but brain tumors *do* occur, and headache is a frequently occurring symptom. We know, however, that if *vomiting* accompanies headache then immediate medical intervention is needed and not behavioral health services. Most headaches are tension or stress related, but psychologists know that people are surprisingly consistent in their behaviors and in the ways in which their bodies show the effects of stress. A forty-five year old with *first time* headaches referred to a psychologist for stress management is very likely to have an *organic* cause for the headache since the patient had no history of responding to stress in this way previously.

What we have now in the vast majority of cases with non-specific symptoms is an expensive delay of *behavioral intervention* while the physician goes through a costly rule out of organic disease. Physicians often bring up a "red herring" in the form of liability risk if they fail to diagnose a patient's organic disease, which justifies in their mind extensive testing to protect themselves from liability. I am not at all sympathetic to this reasoning because the "problem" can easily be solved with a physician consensus on diagnostic standards. Such a standard is needed not only for more timely and more appropriate care, but more efficient diagnosis decreases the financial waste involved in unnecessary diagnostic technology.

An MRI (for scanning the brain or body) costs over $800 and 80% or more of these procedures are unnecessary. There is no need, for example, to use a CT Scan or MRI to diagnose Alzheimer's disease in a single, elderly patient with memory problems. The most effective and cost efficient way to make a diagnosis would be to have the patient evaluated by a neuropsychologist (a psychologist who specializes in brain-behavior relationships) rather than, as now, conducting all the costly and less powerful diagnostic procedures first and finding nothing, then referring the patient to the most powerful diagnostic procedure for brain damage (neuropsychological testing).

The Kroenke and Mangelsdorff study revealed an additional and important finding that should be mentioned. In the study, the researchers followed up all subjects to determine the eventual diagnosis, kind of treatment received and treatment outcome for all patients. First, those with a non-organic disease (55%) often received no treatment. The authors attributed the lack of follow-up treatment of these patients to a perception that therapy for these non-organic problems is ineffective or perhaps to a lack of enthusiasm for managing non-organic disorders. When these non-organic or functional problems *were* treated, it was not surprising that (being physicians) prescribing medication was the most common therapeutic modality, outnumbering non-pharmacological mcasures three to one.

The researchers found that these untreated functional (non-organic) symptoms tended to persist. When outcome was noted for these patients in follow-up, nearly half of the *treated* patients did not get better. Prognosis and outcome was favorable if the patient had an *organic* disease and was treated, but if the patient had a *psychological* or *psychosocial* problem the outcome was better if the patient was *not* treated than if the patient *was* treated!

TABLE III

Outcome of 14 Common Symptoms

Symptom	Number of Symptoms For Which Outcome is Known	Number (percent) Improved
Chest pain	57	37 (65)
Fatigue	43	20 (47)
Dizziness	27	16 (47)
Headache	26	10 (38)
Edema	25	16 (64)
Back Pain	21	13 (62)
Dyspnea	23	9 (39)
Insomnia	10	5 (50)
Abdominal pain	16	7 (44)
Numbness	17	9 (53)
Impotence	11	6 (56)
Weight Loss	15	6 (40)
Cough	10	8 (80)
Constipation	6	2 (33)
Total	307	164 (53)

Adapted and reprinted from The American Journal of Medicine, Vol. 86, Kroenke, K., & Mangelsdorff, D." Common Symptoms in Ambulatory Care: Incidence, Evaluation, Therapy and Outcome." 262-266, © March 1989 with permission from Excerpta Medica, Inc.

The above finding from the study is that if you have *mental health problems* you are much better off if your physician does *not* treat you then if he or she *does*. If antidepressants *were* effective in treating stress/anxiety and mood/depression then we should have *lower* rather than higher total pharmaceutical costs of those patients receiving these drugs. In one plan my company examined, 15% of all covered members were on antidepressants. These patients accounted for 37% of the plan's total drug bill. If these antidepressants *were* effective, patients on these drugs should have *lower* rather than *higher* pharmaceutical costs than their non-antidepressant using peers. Elsewhere I pointed out that in one study there was no expected reduction of medical claims in those whose depression was treated with drugs alone.

<u>The Seizure Disorder That Was Non-Existent</u>

I was in a case conference one time in which the pediatric neurologist was reluctant to make a diagnosis of complex partial seizures in a child because of the absence of *electroencephalogram* evidence of a seizure disorder. Now, the EEG is essential because pseudo-seizures that do not arise from electromechanical disruptions of brain wave activity fool many parents and physicians who make the diagnosis based on reports and descriptions by parents and others of the patient's "seizures." However, we had video monitoring of several of the child's seizures, which were quite stereotypical of *genuine* brain seizures. The other very experienced healthcare professionals saw the seizures as authentic. This patient's seizures *were* brain related. They were *behaviorally* associated with abnormal disruptions of normal brain wave activity. Seizure activity simply did not show up on the EEG *at the time* of the EEG monitoring, which is not unusual. The pediatric neurologist, however, was reluctant to make a diagnosis of complex partial seizures from the child's *behavior* alone because as yet there was no *EEG evidence* of such a diagnosis. Again, in general medicine behavior is often not considered to be "real."

Diagnosis: Hysteria Neither Organic Nor Depressive

Pseudo-seizures, which represent about 50% of the more "difficult" cases with episodes of seizure-type behavior, are considered to have an *hysterical* as opposed to a *brain* origin.

Sigmund Freud observed that some patients with a variety of physical disabilities of voluntary functions (paralysis, loss of hearing, visual loss and, in our case, "seizures") did not have organic disease connected to the sensory-motor systems. However, these patients seemingly converted *mental need* or *conflict* into a *physical* expression, perhaps in some cases for what is called "secondary gain." The hysterically blind person has a normally intact and functioning visual system but perhaps because of mental conflict, normal vision is *repressed* from consciousness, and the patient *behaves* as if blind and appears blind to others.

Hysterical phenomena must be distinguished from both hypochondria and malingering. Malingering refers to the *conscious*, deliberate attempt to fake an illness or disability (e.g., paralysis after an automobile accident) usually for financial gain. Hysterical conversion is an *unconscious* process, a dissociation of the intact sensory (or other) input from the self. For instance, the hysterically blind person has normal visual experience (e.g., he/she usually avoids hazardous situations) but the patient subjectively *experiences* complete blindness and he/she *appears* blind to many others.

As can be seen in this case, it is often not an easy task to separate those with genuine organic disease or disability from those with hysterical conversions. In psychoanalytic terms, the conversion is a defense or "resolution" of the repressed inner need or conflict.

In one case, a Catholic mother of six children, after her last birth, found herself unable to spread her legs apart, which precluded normal sexual relations. Her perception of her religion may have precluded the use of birth control or refusing her husband sexually and there existed fertile ground for hysterical conversion. The symptom enabled the patient to prevent further pregnancies.

For many years, I was frequently called upon by a variety of physicians to assess "problem" cases, those patients who were something of an enigma to the treating professionals.

A number of these patients had previously undiagnosed hysteria, yet they had been diagnosed and treated for the following problems: major depression, bipolar disorder, Alzheimer's disease, blindness, agent orange poisoning, obsessive compulsive neurosis, "seizures," a variety of anxiety disorders, low back pain, multiple sclerosis, and many others. The list of inappropriate healthcare services/procedures and treatments these hysterics received were horrendous as one could imagine.

Most of the patients had been on a variety of antidepressants, drugs for bipolar disorder (probably because of their emotional instability/lability), drugs for anxiety, atypical antipsychotics and others. In addition to numerous episodes of outpatient treatment, including referral to neurologists and many other diagnosticians, a number have had courses of electroshock treatment (ECT).

Hysterics May Act Depressed

Hysterics are very suggestible, and they are prone to pick up the latest disease or disability and assume the role of a patient with such a disease or disability. Since a number assume the role of a *depressed* person or one with Alzheimer's disease, I coined the diagnostic entities of "hysterical depression" (these patients are acting out a depressed role) and "hysterical dementia." A strong clue for the diagnosis occurs when a strongly extroverted, emotionally reactive person presents with seemingly classic depressive symptoms. The sensitive clinician picks up the strong contrast between the depressive *content* expressed by the patient versus the patient's more lively affects while expressing sad and depressed content.

Years ago I saw one such hysterical patient for psychological assessment for the State Department of Vocational Rehabilitation. The patient related to me a ten-year history of extensive psychiatric treatment, including ECT and psychiatric drugs. She said that, on her own counsel, she had stopped *all* psychiatric and medical treatment three years ago and *had been functioning* better since she stopped all treatment.

The problem of hysteria in the health care system is our failure to recognize it. Enormous financial burden ensues from this oversight in wasted healthcare resources. The next major problem with hysteria is when it *is* recognized and a professional attempts to "cure" it. Since Freud there have been and continue to be a sizable number of healthcare professionals who try to cure hysteria when there is no evidence that it is curable. Psychoanalytic and other types of dynamic-expressive therapies continue to try to resolve various child conflicts/trauma to "work through" repressed memories/trauma so the patient can "heal" and can now function normally. Until these patients are correctly diagnosed, and many times even after, these hysterics are consistent users of inappropriate and ineffective healthcare, using precious healthcare dollars that could be used more appropriately elsewhere.

The Therapy Approach

In the part of american psychology that deals with problems of a clinical nature, there have been two opposing and differing philosophical views about therapy. The one is a therapy model based largely on Sigmund Freud and other psychoanalysts. The other, from academic-experimental psychology, emphasizes how individuals learn and unlearn behavior. This type of therapy focuses on changing *behavior.* How we came to be as we are is very important in psychoanalytic psychotherapy, but non-analytic behavioral forms of treatment are less historically oriented and focus on the *here and now* of the patient's life.

The theory that current maladaptive behavior results from early emotional trauma is very beautiful sounding and the logic is very compelling. The only problem is that it does not seem to work, the patient either stays the same or more often gets worse with such therapy. I found in my own experience (I was taught one form of this expressive type of therapy) that this type of therapy did not work despite the fact that it was very intellectually and emotionally stimulating for both patient and therapist. Many of these therapists guard against this failure by telling the patient that the patient will have to get worse before getting better.

With these therapists there is always another issue to resolve, one more unconscious need/conflict for the patient to face before the patient can become "whole." These therapists never question the process itself, never attribute failure of the patient to the process itself. They look to factors other than the process itself to explain why the patient did not get better. Even if the patient complains of treatment failure, the therapist has a ready and unshakable explanation, i.e., the patient is showing *resistance* and fighting the therapist.

Ms. Browne, a clinical social worker was of this psychoanalytic school. Upon her retirement she transferred her patient, Thea, to me. Ms. Browne said Thea was functioning better but was *still in denial over having been sexually molested as a child.* Thea had no memory of sexual molestation as a child, but this therapist had made such a diagnosis based on Thea's particular complex of symptoms and behaviors. To take a patient's current pattern of maladjustment and, without any confirming evidence, to ascribe a specific, single cause for it is irrational thinking, but such thinking is quite popular in many mental health circles today.

Do not think that this is an isolated case because, unfortunately, it is not. This happens over and over to many patients with damaging results. Fortunately, Thea did not buy into Ms. Browne's belief that she had repressed her molestation, and she was less harmed than the many thousands of patients during therapy who had "recovered" memories of repressed physical abuse or sexual abuse as a child.

Cognitive Behavior Therapy (CBT) and the Wizard of Oz

Let's look at the non-analytic therapy of CBT as it has effectively treated depression, anxiety, and OCD. The average person's perception of psychotherapy is typically Freudian psychoanalysis, where free association uncovers and "resolves" unconscious conflicts from the patient's early childhood. CBT's premise is that *thought largely governs emotion.* This theory comes from experimental psychology. Its research concern has been with human learning, unlearning, and behavior change. The CBT concept is that there is an intimate connection between thought (cognition) and emotion (affect).

Core Beliefs Can Distort Life

The cognitive model of depression states that depressed patients have enduring assumptions or core beliefs (cognitive *schemas*) that come about through early learning. These core beliefs predispose people toward *negative* interpretations of life events. The negative interpretations are considered cognitive distortions or automatic thoughts (ATs), which propel one toward depressive behavior. CBT for depression includes therapist interventions, which focus on (1) publicly observable behavior, (2) dysfunctional automatic thoughts (ATs) and, (3) therapist-inferred cognitive structures or schemes of the depressed patient.

In CBT, the intervention could be self-directed (from directed readings) or therapist directed by way of direct therapy and homework assignments for the patient. More serious depressions usually require therapist interventions, but mild "depressions" might be correctable through directed readings for bright and motivated individuals. Either way according to CBT the distorted thinking or automatic thoughts (ATs) must be challenged and re-interpreted.

CBT moves in a progressive fashion. The therapist first focuses on behavior change, teaching the client to assess and correct situation specific distortions in thinking. Then, the therapist finally moves to the identification and modification of the more enduring depressive schemas. Typically the final phase is a relapse prevention process: the therapist teaches the patients to deal with situations when the identified negative thinking threatens to disrupt into depressive behavior. These depressive predisposing thoughts may never be completely cured, but attitudes and skills are learned to keep them at bay.

Several experts (Beck, A.T., et al., 1979) view the challenging/modification of the schemas as the core of treatment and the active change mechanisms. The treatment, however, is so multidimensional that a number of alternative explanations to account for its efficacy are possible. Two alternative (or complementary) explanations might be labeled the "activation hypothesis" and the "coping skills" hypothesis.

Activation Hypothesis

In the activation hypothesis, CBT may affect change by *activating* the patients which we have discussed previously. The therapist encourages the patient to become active again within the limits of their depressed mood and to seek available sources of pleasure, which psychologists call reinforcement. For example, the exercise of one's competency (e.g., going bowling in a league) is pleasurable for the non-depressed and depressed alike, which counters depression. In cognitive therapy, our major focus in treatment of depression might well be called "activation therapy." The therapist helps the patient re-establish behavior and activities that were positively reinforcing for the patient prior to the depressive episode.

Coping Skills

Another explanation for the effectiveness of cognitive therapy is a coping skills strategy. Through the therapy the patient learns to better cope with distressing life events or thoughts that might be considered "depressogenic." The learning of a new set of skills, along with behavior activation, may account for the alleviation of depressive behavior. There is a theoretical argument between those cognitive therapists who believe the cognitive distortions or automatic thoughts (AT) *must* be resolved to treat the depression effectively versus those who believe it is sufficient for the patient to learn effective *coping* skills with regard to the cognitive distortions – automatic thoughts (Jacobson, NS et al., 2002). This latter argument need not concern us further.

As one can see from the above, the various therapy procedures have definite relevance to the depressive disorder as I have described it. The therapy model has a much stronger connection to the disorder itself than the drug treatment model. The Seratonin model of depression that was so popular fifteen or so years ago had to give way when non-seratonin antidepressants proved just as effective (or ineffective as the case may be) as Seratonin based antidepressants. Moreover, the *behavioral* model of depression seems much more consistent with many of the facts of depression than the disease or drug model.

Adverse Events

Very few depressions spring up "out of the blue" as it were. We can usually see precursors of depression in adverse events from the patient's recent past. Some of these adverse events might appear harmless but when the adverse event is understood within the person's mental make-up, the connection between the adverse event and the developing depression becomes more obvious. Certainly one cannot *prove* the connection between the event and the developing depression, but it should be considered in our formulation of the problem and its treatment.

We have, then, a plausible explanation for the depression and the explanation gives us a treatment plan. Our treatment plan is not generic, e.g., antidepressant drugs or CBT, but it is directed to *this* depressed person and the adverse or triggering life event or events. For example, Ken, forty-five-years old, is laid off from a job after ten years, a man with limited education and perhaps, in his mind, limited prospects. Seeing his problem as a disease is not at all helpful. If we know something about people, we might think that any of us, in such circumstances and with similar personal characteristics, might well react depressively in such a situation. Some of us more than others are perhaps genetically predisposed to reacting with a depressed mood to many unfortunate circumstances, but any of us can react with a diagnosable depression under the "right" set of circumstances.

Ken may not be a person predisposed to depression, but he has become reactively depressed, nonetheless, to a situation that he is not equipped to handle. By "not being equipped," I do not mean that he had a mental disorder prior to his recent episode, he simply does not know how to cope effectively. Concentration camp inmates often respond with clinical depression to their dire situation, but does this fact mean these people were mentally abnormal prior to their incarceration? I think not. A return to personal freedom would have provided a quick cure for most of those imprisoned despite some expected long-term effects from the incarceration.

Common Symptoms of Depression

In our case example, does Ken have dysfunctional attitudes underlying his depression that requires resolution with CBT or will a job return him quickly to normal? Anyone in a depression, despite the external or internal source or sources, shares many things in common with all persons undergoing a depression. Depressed people worry, have difficulty getting to sleep, have difficulty feeling optimistic about the future and are, in short, depressed. Whatever their individual needs, depressed persons all need realistic hope.

Diagnosis Must Be Individual

Assessing Ken is more complex than simply reviewing and counting his symptoms to see if he meets criteria for a clinical depression. A general physician simply checking off symptoms does not have the training to understand Ken's depression and provide appropriate treatment. A cookie cutter approach (if this, then antidepressant drugs and if that, cognitive therapy) simply will not work with Ken or most depressed patients for that matter.

In a well trained professional, the diagnostic process comes down to one of clinical judgment (which improves with broad experience in diagnosing and treating many depressed patients). However, clinical judgment is far from perfect. Mistakes will be made in a particular case, but the professional will reformulate the case and select another approach to the patient's depression when the *initial* formulation does not work. If one takes a more comprehensive view of depression, that it is not a chemical imbalance, but it is a biopsychosocial disorder, we are better prepared to effectively treat *this* depressed person rather than treating all depressed patients alike with either drugs or cognitive therapy.

What Does it Mean in Oz?

In the Wizard of Oz, our three characters with mental health problems — the Lion, Scarecrow, and Tin Man — are not unlike many people who present themselves to psychiatrists or psychologists. Like many patients, the three characters reflect some serious symptoms (Why would they go in search of the Wizard if they were without problems?) combined with varying degrees of personal strengths. If one were to look at these characters as if they were patients, one could see how vulnerable each would be if exposed to a variety of therapists and theoretical orientations.

For example:

Gestalt therapy: " Mr. Lion sit in the hot seat, please."

Psychoanalysis: "Hmm."

Rogerian therapy: "you feel heartless?" or a dozen others.

Some therapists of varying persuasions would, if given a chance, turn these characters into lifetime patients, turning functional characters into dysfunctional ones.

The Wizard and The Psychologist

The Wizard of Oz makes the correct diagnosis of the Lion, Scarecrow, and Tin Man and formulates the correct treatment. He helps his patients redefine certain cherished but maladaptive beliefs each has about themselves. The Wizard's therapeutic approach is much like present day cognitive therapists when the therapist defines the core of the depression as residing in the patient's attitudes and maladaptive self-appraisals and not adverse life events or brain chemistry.

As I have mentioned before, a psychologist must understand the *source* of the depression in order to provide focused treatment. Does the depression arise from current adverse life events, toward which the therapy should be directed, or should the therapy be directed to the patient's inappropriate cognitions or both?

The Wizard correctly sees the source of his patients' dissatisfaction (we could probably not have diagnosed a full-blown depression for each character from the book) and like a skillful psychologist directs treatment to the *source* of the problems.

Sufficient, But Not Too Much

As mental health professionals we need sufficient intervention to provide help to improve the patient's quality of life and, as therapists, we can err on the side of giving *too little* or *too much* help. I have been critical of many therapists who seem to want therapy to *become* the patient's life rather than assisting the patient to have a more functional and fulfilling life *outside* of therapy. As a good therapist, the Wizard works with the patient's cognitions and quickly provides each patient with very effective behavior changing help. Earlier in my career I thought some patients required longer-term treatment, but I have long since changed my thinking. Over the past eighteen years, I have done a good bit of telephone assessment/counseling with a variety of patients with presenting problems and I continue to be struck by how much one can accomplish in just a few minutes' time with certain patients.

As an example of the effectiveness of short versus long-term treatment of alcoholics, one study (Edwards, G. et al., 1976) looked at *intensity* of treatment. One group of subjects had one telephonic assessment/counseling session and was sent self-help materials. A second group had outpatient counseling over a sixteen-week period. Subjects in the third group had a thirty-day inpatient stay followed by follow-up care. You guessed it; the subjects in the minimal treatment group did as well as subjects in the more intensive treatment groups. Also from the area of chemical dependency treatment, one study found the higher the staff/patient ratio the *worse* the outcome (Stinson, D.J., 1979). If we provide too much care, patient responsibility is undermined and the outcome poorer.

In looking at drugs versus therapy, one must keep in mind that unlike drugs, therapy generally has no adverse physical side effects. The one possible psychological side effect is from what I call victim-engendering therapy; in this type of therapy the patient becomes a lifetime patient who never gets better. These patients are comparable to patients who stay on antidepressant and/or anxiolytic drugs for a lifetime.

Satisfaction with Cognitive Behavioral Therapy (CBT)

Satisfaction surveys, if the responses are positive, are essentially testimonials and these surveys of course have limited scientific value. They do not compare very favorably with the results of placebo-controlled, double-blind studies. These surveys do, however, have some limited value and I would like to report some data here on satisfaction with CBT from cases at PMHM.

PMHM Survey

In my own firm, Preferred Mental Health Management, Inc. (PMHM), on a quarterly basis we survey all callers for services who received one or more face-to-face therapy sessions from one of our contracted providers (a psychologist or clinical social worker). We receive a 20 to 28% return on our surveys. The surveys are answered and are returned anonymously. The ratings refer to the quality (satisfaction) of the services received and not specifically with respect to the type of therapy provided. However, our providers are selected on the basis of their commitment to cognitive modes of therapy and we believe that in rating degree of satisfaction (a 4-point scale) we are indirectly surveying satisfaction with cognitive therapy approaches to problem resolution.

Figure I

Preferred Mental Health Management, Inc.
Outcome Research & Patient Satisfaction Information
Fourth Quarter 2002

During the fourth quarter of 2002, each patient who used a PMHM PPO outpatient provider was given an opportunity to rate the quality of treatment delivered through PMHM's assessment and referral system. *PMHM sent 664 surveys, and 153 were returned for a 23% response rate.*

The average is based on all responses to each question using a scale of 4 to 1. Calculated similar to a grade point average, every response was assigned a number - 4 being the highest rating (or most satisfied) and 1 being the lowest (or least satisfied). The total responses were then averaged.
The satisfaction rate for each question gives the percentage of the total who responded with either a 4 or 3 rating of satisfaction.

	Average	*Satisfaction Rate*
1. The person who first answered my call to PMHM was:		
very caring......not at all caring	**3.42**	**93%**
very knowledgeable......not at all knowledgeable	**3.40**	**94%**
very patient......impatient	**3.48**	**95%**
2. The PMHM psychologist who assisted with my referral was:		
very caring......not at all caring	**3.59**	**95%**
very knowledgeable......not at all knowledgeable	**3.58**	**96%**
very patient......impatient	**3.66**	**97%**
3. My first phone call to PMHM was answered:		
very quickly......after a long time	**3.53**	**93%**
4. The amount of time I was placed on hold by PMHM staff was:		
very reasonable......very unreasonable	**3.53**	**93%**
5. Would you recommend PMHM's referral services to a friend?		
definitely yes......definitely no	**3.55**	**91%**
6. The amount of time between my referral from PMHM and my first appointment with my local provider was:		
very reasonable......very unreasonable	**3.43**	**88%**
7. Overall, how would you rate the referral services you received through PMHM?		
excellent......poor	**3.47**	**90%**
8. The location of my provider's office is:		
very convenient......very inconvenient	**3.30**	**84%**

	Average	Satisfaction Rate
9. I was able to make follow-up appointments with my provider: *very easily......with great difficulty*	**3.58**	**92%**
10. When I came to appointments, I was usually able to see my provider: *on time......after a long wait*	**3.62**	**93%**
11. My provider was:		
very knowledgeable......not at all knowledgeable	**3.68**	**96%**
quite competent......not very competent	**3.68**	**94%**
easy to relate to......difficult to relate to	**3.60**	**88%**
very thorough......not very thorough	**3.53**	**90%**
12. I would recommend my provider to a friend: *definitely yes......definitely no*	**3.52**	**89%**
13. Overall, how would you rate your provider? *excellent......poor*	**3.54**	**90%**
14. The problems that I had when I called PMHM have: *greatly improved......become worse*	**3.20**	**88%**

15. How far did you go in school?

less than high school	**6%**	bachelor's degree	**30%**
some high school	**5%**	master's degree	**7%**
high school graduate	**15%**	specialist degree	**0%**
some college or technical school	**28%**	doctoral degree	**0%**
associate or technical degree	**9%**		

16. Please rate your progress in the following areas:

	Does Not Apply	Gotten Worse	Not Changed	Improved	Improved Greatly
The distressing symptoms have:	**7%**	**3%**	**20%**	**56%**	**14%**
The ability to handle daily life has:	**6%**	**2%**	**16%**	**64%**	**12%**
The personal/family life has:	**6%**	**5%**	**25%**	**52%**	**12%**
The mood/personal outlook has:	**3%**	**6%**	**18%**	**54%**	**19%**

Comments from all PMHM benefit plans:

- "We are very happy with our son's treatment."
- "Your hotline was so wonderful – Dr. ____(PMHM) so very patient and helpful and referral system acted with urgency."
- "I have only seen Dr.____ once. I really liked his onward and take action approach. That is what works for me. Thanks!"
- "We have a long way to go, but have made some progress."
- "The counseling did not help to salvage my marriage, but it helped me to accept that only he can make the necessary changes. I believe that I still need some counseling to continue forward in a positive way. Dr. ______ was excellent! My husband and I both related to her easily."
- "PMHM is excellent. I didn't have to go through an automated system. The lady I spoke to was very nice and patient. Dr. ______ has helped me realize a lot; my mood swings are becoming less. Overall, everyday is a challenge, but I know I'm not alone."
- "One day at a time. Some days better. Some days worse. Still too much stress."
- "We liked Dr. ______ very much. She is a very kind person. My daughter was not as receptive as I had hoped."
- "In 4 sessions we have made great strides and I feel much more positive about the future. My primary goal or objective was to be listened to and get things off my chest."
- "I was very impressed with the friendliness and ease with the referral process. My provider was impressed with the information they received from PMHM on the referral letters."
- "Dr. _____ has provided amazing insight into my behavior and how it impacts my family life. We still have a lot of work to do, but I am now sometimes able to see that I have the ability to make my life better."
- "_____spent whatever time it took to work through the problem. He was always available and really brought me back to what I could do as opposed to what I could not change."
- "PMHM is a wonderful company and you have helped me to get the help I need. Thank You!"

A review of Figure I shows that the callers using PMHM's assessment and referral services were generally pleased with both PMHM and the provider services received. As one can see the satisfaction rates were generally quite high, most being above 90%. About 45% of callers complain of anxiety or depression as their presenting complaint. Some callers ask for drug treatment, the caller often believing that drugs should be the primary treatment, but generally these patients accept referral to a psychologist or clinical social worker who will treat the problem and decide if drug therapy is needed.

PMHM Callers

For problems of stress or mood, PMHM and its providers rarely find that drugs are needed. When callers come to us already on antidepressants or anxiolytic drugs (or both) we tend to leave the drugs alone and focus on helping the patient to see the need for behavioral treatment, to learn coping skills to better master their stress or mood problems. It would not be productive for us to challenge the patient's beliefs about drugs and our approach is that we want to add something to assist the patient's problem solving.

Many people see psychotherapy or behavioral treatment as long-term, but here the confusion is with "psychoanalytic" types of therapy rather than the more modern types of therapy. In my company about 20% of the callers find resolution of their problem in one telephone consultation with a PMHM staff psychologist and those who require face to face therapy average between five and six sessions. Someone with a very severe depression may receive up to twenty sessions but about 80% of this more seriously impaired group have fewer than ten sessions.

One must keep in mind when looking at these figures that callers to PMHM have more serious problems, as a group, than those who are treated with drugs by primary care physicians. Even at that, half of those calling PMHM with complaints of anxiety or depression have difficulties that would *not* meet criteria for a diagnosis of depression or anxiety (See Figure 2). Nonetheless, these callers' stress and mood problems are *disabling* to their health and adjustment and these patients are candidates for appropriate treatment. On the other hand, primary care physicians are using antidepressant and anxiolytic drugs to treat primarily the so-called "worried well" among us, those without "physical" or "mental" disease who are reacting to various life stresses or whose problems are fueled by maladaptive cognitions.

Percent of Referrals from PMHM by Presenting Problem in 2002

59% of requests for authorization of outpatient treatment were for issues other than "mental illness"

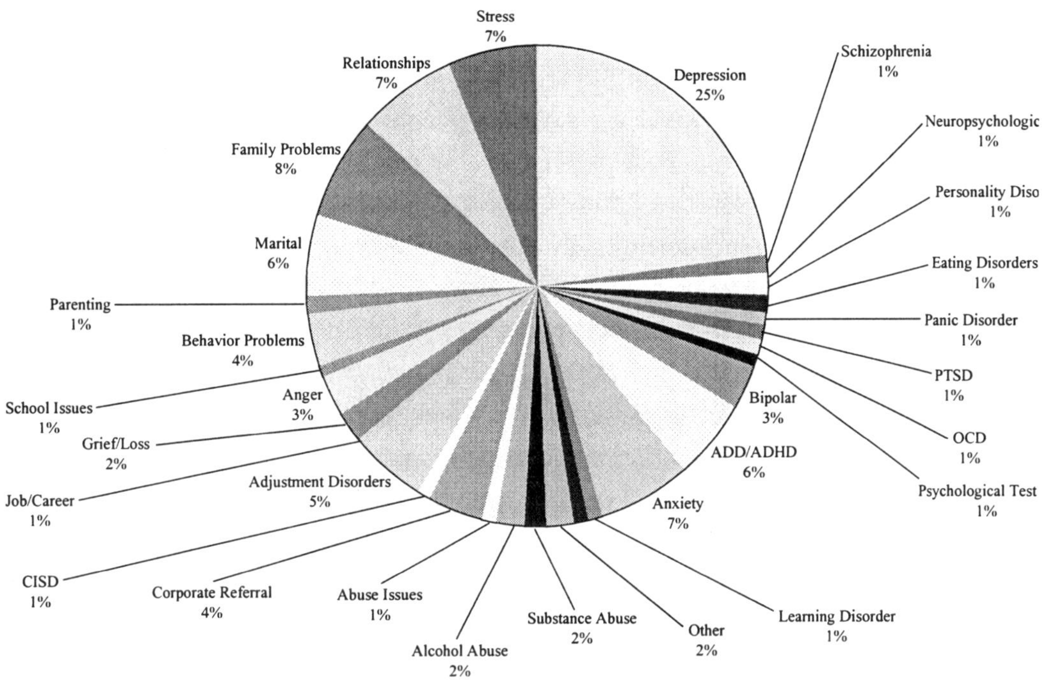

PMHM Costs

For focused treatment which PMHM arranges, the average cost per treated patient is under $400, which is only a fraction of the cost of treating these problems with drugs and primary care office visits. It behooves us to treat the "worried well" because of the high costs associated with the inappropriate medical care of these problems from physicians.

Benefit Plan Includes Switch to Non-drug Alternatives

PMHM has several benefit plans in which we provide plan members comprehensive employee assistance and mental health plan benefit services. In one plan the services for this group includes a program for those members on antidepressant and related drugs who call for consultation on non-drug alternative approaches to their problems. PMHM psychologists interface with those members with a history of taking these drugs (as the sole treatment of their problems) and those wanting to start on antidepressants. Reimbursement for an antidepressant prescription requires the member to call PMHM on an 800 number and to discuss their problems with a psychologist who offers information, education about alternatives to drug treatment and referral to a behavioral health specialist if the member is willing. Whatever the outcome of the call the psychologist gives the member authorization for the prescription.

The above is a very educational approach to the problem, but payers *could* use a variety of strategies or penalties to shape more appropriate treatment of these problems. For most depressive and anxiety disorders drug only treatment by general physicians is not even recommended by the American Psychiatric Association, and certainly not for pediatric treatment, but benefit plans routinely reimburse for these services by general physicians under the "medical" part of the plan. A payer could, for example, not reimburse for antidepressant or anxiolytic drugs unless the patient was being treated by a *behavioral health* professional addressing psychosocial factors involved in the patient's problems. A payer might also reimburse for these drugs at a reduced level if the drugs were only addressing the so-called *biological* problems of the patients.

Remedyfind Survey

A web site, called Remedyfind, had users of various medical/psychological services, including Cognitive Behavioral Therapy (CBT), rate the quality of the services received. In rating the CBT these patients received, 39 persons gave combined ratings on a ten point scale (0 = poorest to10 = best) for the whole group.

The 39 raters gave CBT an overall rating of 8.2; effectiveness 8.4; lack of side effects 8.6; ease of use 7.3; remains effective after long term use 8.4; and cost effectiveness 6.5. Overall, these individuals saw their therapeutic experience in a *positive* light. From their individual comments, a number *did* receive CBT, but a number received other types of psychotherapy, including "psychoanalysis" in one case.

However, not everything identified as CBT is CBT. For instance, I was asked to review an appeal in which a PMHM managing psychologist had denied further care for a patient from a psychiatrist who had been treating the patient with "CBT" for thirty-five sessions. Now, thirty-five sessions is very unusual for someone being treated with CBT. The progress notes made it very obvious to me that the patient was *not* receiving CBT. The patient was receiving emotional support and medication management — not CBT. I upheld the denial of further services from the treating psychiatrist and recommended termination and referral to another professional for CBT, which *was* the appropriate treatment for the patient.

It is not a simple matter to diagnose and treat depression or anxiety. When these problems *are* treated effectively the return to the patient, the family, the job and society at large is enormous. Taken together depression and anxiety is our number one health problem. It is ludicrous to think that a drug will solve this problem. Psychosocial more than biological factors are the most prominent in these disorders, and their alleviation requires *psychosocial* education. Though many may need CBT, not everyone now on a Prozac or Xanax-type drugs needs formal face-to-face CBT, but most need some form of behavioral intervention by a trained professional.

Some now on these drugs could resolve their problems through self-help groups, directed self-help readings, resolving some conflict in their life, talking to a psychologist briefly over the telephone, and, of course, face-to-face therapy when needed. Even when formal therapy is necessary, the treatment is, or should be, very *inexpensive*. Patients need to be given the tools and skills to solve their own problems so that they will no longer need a therapist. Patients when treated competently can become their own therapists. Long-term therapy tends to be dependency engendering much like dependency engendering parenting, which never allows the child or patient to function independently.

Some persons believe their problems are unsolvable, perhaps a woman married to an alcoholic or abusive husband. Our mental health is compromised by our feelings of powerlessness, and it is improved when we take charge of our life in a proactive way.

The Wizard does not change the reality that the Scarecrow, Lion and Tin Man are facing in their individual lives, but he helps each character correct and change his automatic thoughts, enabling a sense of empowerment and greater self-acceptance.

These are not placebo recoveries nor does the Wizard advocate a one-size fits all approach. He is actually a good psychologist who knows his subjects and knows how to bring about *self-healing*. The Wiz, a good cognitive therapist, is a good model for psychologists and mental health professionals to emulate.

While I have taken a long way to illustrate my point, the point is that appropriate treatment addresses and alleviates the problem rather than treating the myths of chemical imbalances or early trauma. Appropriate mental health treatment is time limited, recognizes and addresses the *core* problems giving rise to the distressing symptoms, gives patients the knowledge and tools to solve their own problems and allows distressed people to live healthier and more productive lives.

CHAPTER IX

BLINDED BY BELIEF: A CLOSE LOOK AT HOW "PROPONENTS" INTERPRET THEIR RESEARCH

A certain "blindness" often issues from deeply held beliefs that are maintained *despite any evidence to the contrary*. To these believers, however, these actions are logical and completely meritorious. Such beliefs, if held by only one person, do not have the staying power of beliefs that are shared by a sizeable number of people. A group of like-minded people with a shared belief system who reinforce each other strengthens the core belief system, whatever the belief might be. These unexamined beliefs, which seem to serve some very important basic needs of the believers, are frequently a cause for actions that are incomprehensible to observers who do not share the belief system. So it is with antidepressant adherents.

Much scientific data disproves such a belief system, yet the belief system is maintained despite this. Moreover, the presence of overwhelming contradictory evidence cannot convince its "proponents" to even *question* the veracity of their beliefs. It is as if the belief system and the evidence that contradicts it are on two different tracks; the believer in the one track may be aware of *some* of the contradictory evidence in the other track, but the cherished belief and the disconfirming evidence are never connected and viewed as a whole.

Let's look at some of the incomprehensible twists and turns, convolutions, perversions, deceptions, cover-ups, and willing blindness of the "proponents" as they try to make antidepressant drug therapy look like science instead of marketing.

Treatment of Depression – Newer Pharmacotherapies Review

The Agency for Health Care Policy and Research (AHCPR) arranged for a blue ribbon panel of experts, all researchers and practitioners, to review the literature on the newer drugs for treating depression. The panel as I mentioned previously selected 80 (from over 300) depression outcome studies using the present generation antidepressants (AHCPR, 1999). Remember, scientifically designed depression outcome studies are the *only* means to establish drug or treatment efficacy. The panel determined that the response rate (50% or more improvement) was 50% for the drug and 32% for inert placebo. We also have to keep in mind that response as determined by the antidepressant researchers is not *remission* but improvement.

Response or Remission

First, let's find out what the response rate really means. According to one researcher (O'Donovan, TR, 2002), approximately 1/3 of patients achieve a full remission, 1/3 experience a response and 1/3 are non-responders. Actually these numbers look better than they actually are. These were not *all* of the depressed subjects, but only those who *completed* treatment. The numbers do not include those who dropped out because of adverse drug side effects or those who dropped out earlier when they failed to respond. This could indicate that we have a drug-depression remission rate in reality of less than 20%.

In the above O'Donovan study, partial remissions included continuing symptoms of depressed mood, psychic anxiety, sleep disturbance, fatigue and diminished interest or pleasure, all fundamental symptoms of depression. We know that residual symptoms are powerful predictors of relapse. The patients in partial remission have a 3 to 6 times *higher* relapse rate than those who experience a full remission. Residual symptoms are also associated with more medical and psychiatric visits, increased public assistance, disability benefits and thoughts of and/or attempts at suicide. The risk of stroke and coronary events is also *higher* for patients with residual depressive symptoms, a finding demonstrating the influence that mental health factors play in disease.

"Proponents" Response

O'Donovan, after noting all of the negatives of a partial response to treatment rightly says that *remission* or recovery has traditionally been neglected in antidepressant trials. However, rather than saying "we need to find a better way than drugs to treat depression," he says, in effect, "the correct choice of initial antidepressant treatment should offer the greatest chance of achieving full remission." The "proponents" simply won't give up on the idea that there *must* be a *drug answer* to depression. Rather than tossing out the belief, we are told the "right" antidepressant was not selected or the "right" antidepressant for the patient is yet to be invented. If the *right* antidepressant were selected we would have had a full remission. The fact is that no one seems to come up with the *right* antidepressant after 40 or more years of trying and 20% or less of users have a full remission, an efficacy that would never be accepted in general medicine.

The conclusion drawn by the "proponents" from the above data on *partial* remissions is irrational. In their blindness they say the 3 to 6 times higher relapse rate of the partial responders means that depression is a chronic, relapsing disease that requires maintenance antidepressant therapy to address the biological origin of depression, rather than the depression was not competently treated *in the first place*. If we had an antibiotic that only achieved a partial response in treating an infection, would we say this *proves* that infection is a chronic, relapsing disease? Or course not.

If this thinking is transferred to general medicine, we immediately see the ludicrousness in the antibiotic example, but in the mental health area *any* absurdity seems to be acceptable to the "believers" and "proponents." In reality a partial response means that the depression has *not* been adequately treated. When something is not treated adequately, "relapse" is expected. "Proponents" pull out of thin air the concept of "a chronically relapsing disease" to cover the ineffectiveness of drugs in treating clinical depression.

Many psychiatrists and other physicians had believed that the SSRI and related antidepressants were more *powerful* than the earlier tricyclic antidepressants. Now, to the research panel's dismay, the panel's determination that the antidepressant drug response rate was 50% versus 32% for inert placebo showed that the newer, more expensive drugs were *no more effective* than the earlier drugs.

What inference did the research panel draw from this data, though? The panel concluded that newer antidepressants were as effective in treating depression as were the older tricyclics. Actually the results of 50% versus 32% means both sets of first and current generation drugs were only slightly more effective than an inert placebo response. One wants to say to the Blue Ribbon Panel: "*Look* at your data. How can you justify recommending *drugs* as a treatment for depression when your own data shows only marginal clinical value?" Obviously, the panel members were emotionally and intellectually committed to the drug treatment of depression. Of course, the panelists, who were mostly modern psychiatrists and only trained to use biological interventions, had no non-drug alternatives to offer. Again, if antibiotics were no better at treating infection than antidepressants are in treating depression, we would simply not have any antibiotic drugs.

However, when it comes to depression and mental health we can apparently accept a *lower* standard. A conclusion from the review study should have been that we must find something other than drugs to treat depression. The 18% differential improvement of drug over placebo means, as I have pointed out previously, that one would have to give antidepressant drugs to *six* depressed people to be sure that *one* of the six had something more than a placebo response! The antidepressant "proponents" have their blinders on. One would think that some of the facts, such as the above, would break through, but reality is safely ignored.

There was nothing wrong with the above review study. I am sure it was thoroughly objective and well executed. The fault was the panel's failure to look at the data and to draw unbiased, *scientifically* proper conclusions from the data. Moreover, the data was used to formulate depression treatment guidelines for general physicians and psychiatrists to treat depression.

All of the following examples issue from the "proponents" refusal to see the obvious, that is, that antidepressant drugs have little more than marginal value in treating depression. The review panel's report came out in February of 2002, but the basic facts were known and have been around for more than two decades. The problem is simply that the many antidepressant "proponents" and "believers" do not *want* to face the facts. In the past fifteen years, antidepressant use has exploded while more and more evidence has accumulated about the drug's ineffectiveness. The contradictory evidence seems to have had no effect on the drug's popularity and increasingly widespread use.

Cognitive Therapy versus Drugs

As we have seen elsewhere CBT is at *least* as effective as drugs in treating depression in the *acute* phase. CBT has a lower relapse rate than drugs, and there are many studies demonstrating its superiority to drugs. In many studies CBT alone appears as, or more effective than when combined with drugs. We have seen the "proponents" recommend CBT for antidepressant *relapse prevention*, not as the first line treatment. Now believers are promoting psychotherapy as an adjunct to drugs, not as a *primary* treatment but to increase drug compliance!

The first landmark study demonstrating the superiority of cognitive behavior therapy (CBT) over the drug treatment of depression was conducted by Rush and colleagues in the late seventies (Rush et al. 1977). That study showed that CBT was more effective than tricyclic antidepressant therapy in patients suffering from clinical depression. Further, a follow-up study (Hollon, 1991) twelve months post-treatment found relapse rates were *lower* among CBT patients (39%) versus those receiving antidepressant therapy (65%), although the difference was not statistically significant. Many other studies since that time have also concluded the superiority of cognitive therapy: (1) it effectively treats depression; (2) it is comparable, if not superior to medication treatment, and (3) it has an equal or lower rate of relapse in comparison to medication (Dobson, 1989: Hollon, 1981; Hollon and Beck, 1986; Hollon and Najavits, 1988; Hollon, et al., 1991, Miller – Berman, 1983).

<u>NIMH Treatment of Depression Collaborative Research Program</u>

It was against this background of impressive findings for cognitive therapy versus drug treatment of depression that NIMH funded two multi-site depression treatment outcome studies involving cognitive behavioral therapy (CBT), Interpersonal Therapy (IPT) and antidepressant treatment. In this multi-site study there were four treatment conditions: CBT, IPT, imipramine-clinical management (CM), and placebo plus CM (PLA-CM). The CM in the third and fourth groups included emotional support and minimal psychotherapy (including direct advice) for the antidepressant and the placebo groups.

Without taking severity of illness into account, there was no evidence that either CBT or IPT was superior to the other and *no* evidence that imipramine plus CM treatment was significantly more effective than either psychotherapy. Comparing each of the psychotherapies with the placebo-CM, there was limited evidence of the superiority of IPT over placebo but not for CBT. The latter was surprising in that CBT has *usually* been found more effective than interpersonal therapy in treating depression.

The findings are not controversial nor are they impressive for *any* of the treatments. What became controversial was NIMH's *interpretation of the findings*, that is, that *psychotherapy alone is appropriate for mild depression but moderate and severe depression requires drug treatment*. Such a recommendation was simply *not* supported by the research data. NIMH has always had a strong preference for drug treatment of all mental disorders including depression, and their bias was clearly demonstrated in their interpretation of the research being discussed. Many researchers who have examined the data do not believe that the data supports NIMH's interpretation or the policy that moderate and severe depression requires antidepressant treatment (Antonuccio, David, 1995).

Follow-Up Study

Moreover, the follow-up study (Shea, MT, 1992) does not support NIMH's conclusions. The follow-up studies were conducted at six, twelve, and eighteen months after assessment. The percent of those recovered and who *remained well* during follow-up did not differ significantly among the four treatments: 30% for those in CBT, 26% for those in IPT, 19% for those in Imipramine plus CM, and 20% for those in the placebo plus CM groups. These are hardly impressive findings for *any* of the treatments but the Imipramine and CM faired least well.

Also, the Imipramine group was not at all impressive in preventing relapse. Among patients who had recovered, rates of relapse were 36% for the CBT group, 33% for those in the IPT group, 50% for those in the imipramine plus CM group, and 33% for those in the placebo plus CM group. Again the Imipramine and CM group faired *least* well and even the minimal therapy with placebo group had a *lower* relapse rate than the antidepressant group!

Neither the basic study nor the follow-up supports the NIMH conclusion that psychotherapy is only appropriate for mild depression and that drugs should be the primary treatment for moderate and severe depression. When looking at patients remaining well after recovery for the four treatment conditions for severely depressed patients, we find 24% remained well (no relapse) in the CBT group, 18% in the IPT group, 23% in the Imipramine plus CM group, and 19% in the placebo plus CM group. No statistically significant differences between these groups were found. These data hardly speak well for the antidepressant effectiveness versus the placebo (23% versus 19%) in the severely depressed patients. The most telling statistic from the NIMH depression treatment outcome study was the *50% relapse rate* for the *antidepressant* group, the highest of the four treatment conditions!

"Believer" Response

These NIMH studies were used by NIMH to *uphold* its depression drug treatment agenda. To NIMH the study seemed to *support* its program of PCP treatment of depression and affirmed the necessity of drug treatment for moderate to severe depression. NIMH and perhaps the pharmaceutical industry, however, did not entirely overlook some of the negative drug findings in this research, especially the 50% drug relapse rate. Since these two studies, NIMH has been pushing drug treatment of depression as the first or primary treatment *followed* by psychotherapy (usually CBT) as a *relapse prevention* strategy! To come up with such a strategy one must throw out a vast literature of depression treatment outcome studies as well as throwing out all common sense.

Combine the Drug with CBT and it Works

A JAMA article (March, 2004) recently reported that in a multi-site NIMH supported study, combined treatment of CBT and Zoloft was *more* effective in treating Obsessive Compulsive Disorder than CBT alone, Zoloft alone or placebo. There was no CBT-placebo group, which was a failing in the study. Immediately after reporting that *combined* therapy was better than either alone, the writer of the article reported that Zoloft *was no better than placebo* in treating OCD! How can CBT plus Zoloft be better than either alone when Zoloft proved no better than placebo in treating OCD? Logically, it can't be, but I have noticed that drug "proponents" seem to have a logic of their own. The study, of course, questions the value of Zoloft in treating OCD.

Why Don't They Get It?

Why Patients Won't Take the Drugs

A layman might ask why prescribe a drug if the patient will not take it? There are dozens of these articles in the literature about the failure of patients to take antidepressants as prescribed, but no one has made the obvious recommendation to no longer prescribe these drugs. Rather, NIMH keeps funding million dollar research programs to find ways to help physicians to *keep their patients* on these drugs.

There are dozens of studies such as Lin's (Lin, EH, 1995) that show that it is extremely difficult to keep patients on antidepressants for adequate clinical trials, which are six to nine months. Antidepressants, unlike Xanax-type drugs that are active immediately, must be taken daily in order for the body to build and maintain a "therapeutic" level. Lin found that approximately 28% of antidepressant patients had stopped taking their medications by Week 4, and 43% had stopped by Week 9. At the end of six months, only 21.7% were still taking their antidepressants. Lin also reported that for a group of Medicaid patients prescribed antidepressants, there was a 28% dropout at week 4, 45% at Week 8, and 52% dropout at Week 12.

"Believer" Response

"Believers" usually attribute drug discontinuation to adverse side effects, which, I am sure, is partially correct. I am also quite sure that some drop out because (1) they are not getting better, and (2) some have had a "placebo" recovery. However, the "believers" focus on adverse side effects and fault the family physician for not doing the job of keeping his or her patient on the pills.

Often there are depression disease management programs in which nurses are called upon to telephone the patient to stay on the antidepressant, and to send literature explaining the rationale for staying on the antidepressant.

Geomatrix Technology

One study (Sheehan, D.V., 2003) demonstrates that drug compliance can be increased somewhat by decreasing side effects through the application of what is called Geomatrix technology. This technology provides a delivery system that controls the amount, timing and location of drug release, thus decreasing the *severity* of side effects. The researcher reported that Paxil was more effective in treating depression when Paxil was combined with the Geomatrix technology.

Figure 1 – Hamilton Depression Remission
Percentage of Patients Achieving Hamilton Depression Score < 7

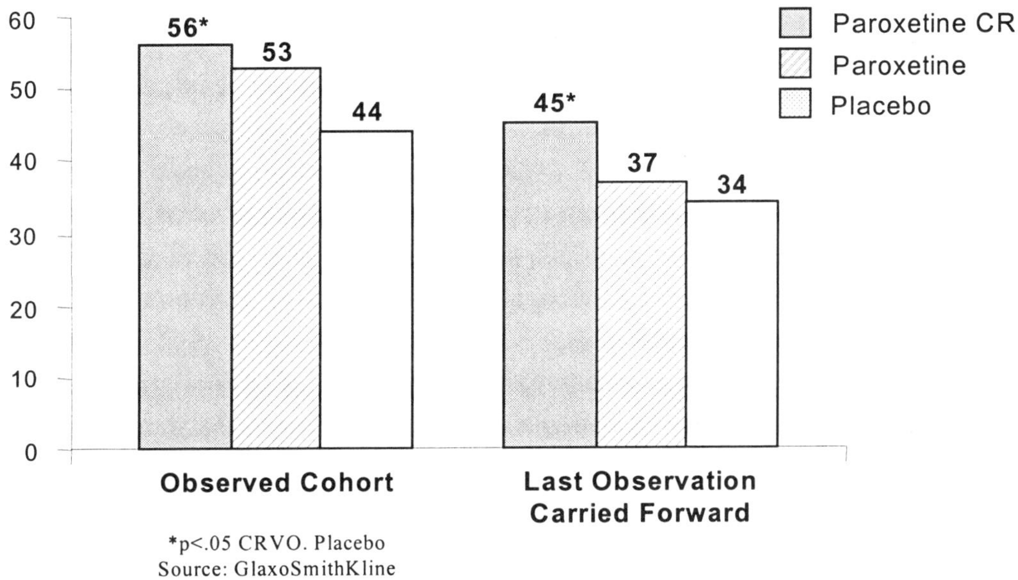

Adapted from and with permission: Sheehan, David V. "Improved Tolerability and Increased Length of Therapy." Supplement to Managed Care, Vol. 12, #7, 23-25, July 2003. Medimedia USA.

This technology (decreasing the intensity of the side effect) may improve apparent clinical efficacy (56% versus 53% reach improvement criteria), but from the data as a whole would you want to do it? (See Figure 1). I think not. First, the Paroxetine CR was not that much better than the standard drug (56% versus 53% and 45% versus 37%), and neither was substantially better than the placebo alone (even though there may have been a *statistically* significant difference between drug and placebo). At best there was a 12% difference in favor of the drug over placebo.

"Believers" and The Data

A "believer" looks at the above data and thinks of other ways to reduce side effects to improve drug compliance and to improve efficacy. A realist looks at the same graph and says, "We had better look for a better way to treat depression than with these drugs since these drugs are only a little better than placebo in treating depression." I worry many "believers" would not change their minds even if there was only a *1%* difference in favor of the drug.

Drug Company Proposal

One of my company's clients, a member of an employer health care coalition, asked me to review and comment upon a proposal of a drug company to provide coalition members with a *depression disease management* program. Anticipated to give the member companies a return on investment (ROI) the first year of 2.0 to 2.5, the return would be expected to rise to 6.2 to 8.7 after four years. The ROI means that each dollar invested in the program would return from 6.2 to 8.7 dollars, after four years, which if true, is quite a return.

These depression disease management programs are all basically the same: (1) give depression screening tests to patients of PCPs to increase the number of their patients diagnosed with MDD; (2) put these patients on antidepressant drugs, and (3) provide literature/telephone nurse coaching directed toward improving drug compliance. My review of the depression disease management program for PMHM's client was not encouraging.

Another Blinding by Belief Project – Antidepressant Algorithms

Many in psychiatric research have put much time and research money from the drug companies into establishing algorithms for drug treatment of depression, much like establishing algorithms for treating Type II Diabetes and other health problems. The algorithms, or medical formulas, attempt to focus the treatment process to produce no or minimal residual symptoms as an endpoint rather than just response.

The object is not just an antidepressant response (partial improvement or "better") but a complete *remission* of symptoms. This is a very laudable goal.

Elaborate Algorithms

Many of these depression algorithm projects are ostensibly directed toward improving cost effective treatment in the public sector. One such project reported per patient antidepressant treatment costs of up to $20,000 per case. The depression algorithm projects generally involve four broad types of antidepressants - (1) tricyclic antidepressants, (2) selective serotonin reuptake inhibitor antidepressants (e.g., Prozac), (3) selective norepinephrine reuptake inhibitor drugs (SNRIs such as Wellbutrin) and (4) dual drugs combining SSRI and SNRIs (e.g., Effexor). These antidepressant type drugs may in certain circumstances be used with other non-antidepressant "augmenting" drugs such as antianxiety drugs or other drugs such as Depakote, an antiseizure drug often used to treat patients with bipolar disorder.

Drug Schedule Primary

These algorithm projects typically only involve drugs and how various drugs are scheduled. The patient may start on an SSRI, then, if the patient improves to the point of remission (which is rare) he or she stays on the same drug. If there is no further improvement, perhaps the next step is a dosage increase on the same drug, the addition of a second type of antidepressant and or the prescription of an augmenting drug. From this one can see the vast number of combinations and permutations of drugs that can be used. In addition the physician must decide when to add, or not to add, augmenting or change to other drugs. The idea is that this system can be used by the practitioner for every case. Theoretically the system *should* bring about more effective and lower cost treatment for depression. Most of these projects are still in development, and I have not as yet seen any data on the end point, that is, the percentage starting treatment who actually *do* reach remission and for what period of time and at what financial cost. The goal of remission is laudable but in reviewing the algorithm system, the bottom line seems to increase drug company profits more than increase remission.

Problems with Algorithm Projects

There are a number of problems with these algorithm projects. These projects are grounded in drug treatment and there is simply no evidence that antidepressant drugs are more than marginally effective in treating depression. As an example of this, one depression algorithm project began with patients who have not responded adequately to a trial of *standard* antidepressants.

We know that tricyclic drugs are cheaper and are as effective as the more expensive, present day antidepressants; however, the researchers wanted to use the more *expensive* drugs first. This does not make sense when the goal is to control costs.

A part of the first problem is the fact that cognitive therapy, the most effective and cost effective treatment of depression, plays only a minor, if any, role in these depression treatment projects. These algorithms err in treating depression as if it were a simple "disease" that a general physician can treat using the guidelines to remission once the diagnosis is made. They suggest that treatment can be effective *without the treatment* being modified in any way *by psychosocial factors*. These projects treat "depression" but not *individuals with* depression.

Even if every patient going through the system *does* end up in complete remission, what have we proved? Let us say that *all* of the patients have remitted through drug treatment (none received psychotherapy). Have we proven that drugs, including augmenting drugs, effectively treated depression? The answer is no.

There are two reasons for this. The first is as we have seen (Kirsch, 2002), that about 85% of recovery with antidepressants is a placebo recovery. As depression is self-limiting, 32% of subjects recover with an inert placebo alone. Second, even if *all* patients have remission from their symptoms at the two year end point of treatment, was this outcome due to the drugs or due to the self-limiting nature of clinical depression? What about the "placebo" patient who *doesn't* improve? To follow the logic of the algorithm project, let's give this non-responding depressed "placebo" subject another drug. Will some of these patients on a *second* drug ("placebo") have a "placebo" recovery? These questions need to be answered to determine the meaning of such findings.

Have You Looked at the Cost of Antidepressant Therapy?

I don't think the "believers" have looked at the costs of drug treatment of depression and anxiety but I suspect some of the "proponents" have, and they are drooling. Lifetime rates for all of the anxiety disorders is 24.9%, with lifetime rates for depression at 17.1% (Kessler, 1996). Annual rates for treatment are approximately 17% for anxiety and 8% for depression, which is surprising to most people because depression gets most of the press. The combined 25% annual rate for both do not get treated during any one year and probably should not be. However, the National

Institute for Mental Health and the drug companies are trying to get *everyone* of these cases screened, diagnosed and treated with drugs.

In the above algorithm study, not surprisingly, 69.5% of all the drugs used were the Selective Serotonin Reuptake Inhibitor Antidepressants (SSRIs) such as Prozac, Paxil, and Zoloft. Almost 15% of the drugs involved antidepressants *other* than SSRIs, and 16% were for drug classes (e.g., Valium) other than antidepressant drugs.

The direct treatment costs of treating depression are staggering. In one study mentioned earlier (Terry, C.M., 1999), a total of 4,250 Patient Treatment Episodes (PTEs) were reviewed. All patients treated by *psychiatrists* were followed for a year because a PTE for major depression – by definition a chronic disease to many – is 365 days. In this large health plan study, there were 6.60 PTEs per 1,000 members (only those treated by psychiatrists).

TABLE III: OVERALL MAJOR DEPRESSION TREATMENT PATTERN

Average Covered Charges per PTE Diagnostic Cluster: Major Depression

Physician Specialty: Psychiatrists Age Category: 18-64 yr Severity of Illness: 1

Professional Services Charges Ambulatory-Outpatient Setting

Avg. Charge per PTE	Prof. Visits	Test	Lab/Path	Med/Surg	Rx	Prof. Inpatient Services
$2,287	34.7%	6.2%	3.6%	2.7%	35.3%	1.3%

Facility Charges		Other Charges	
Outpatient Facility (Visits)	Hospital Inpatient	Alternate Sites	Other Medical
4.7%	6.6%	1.0%	4.0%

PTE = Patient treatment episode; Rx = prescription

Adapted from and with permission: Terry, C.M., Thomas, S., and Cave, D. G. "Major Depression." of Managed Care Interface, Vol. 11, No. 11, 58-60, November 1998

TABLE IV: PROFESSIONAL SERVICES UTILIZATION

Ambulatory-Outpatient Setting: Prescription Drug Summary

Physician Specialty: Psychiatrists | Age Category: 18-64 yr | Severity of Illness: 1

	Percent (%) of all PTEs	Avg. Number of Rx's per PTE	Avg. Overall Charge ($) per PTE	Percent (%) Rx of Avg. Charge per PTE
Prescription Drugs Overall	100.0	16.3	2,287	35.3
No Rx Present	4.3	0.0	1,231	0.0
Single Rx Group	12.7	5.7	1,343	32.1
Two Rx Group	15.9	9.0	1,579	35.9
Three Rx Group	14.9	12.1	1,919	36.4
Four or More Rx Groups	51.6	23.7	2,920	36.7
Rx Present, No Group Code	0.6	15.2	3,214	23.2

PTE = Patient treatment episode; Rx = prescription

Adapted from and with permission: Terry, C.M., Thomas, S., and Cave, D. G. "Major Depression." Managed Care Interface, Vol. 11, No. 11, 58-60, November 1998

TABLE V: PROFESSIONAL SERVICES UTILIZATION

Ambulatory-Outpatient Setting: Single Prescription Drug Group

Physician Specialty: Psychiatrists | Age Category: 18-64 yr | Severity of Illness: 1

	Percent (%) of all PTEs	Avg. Number of Rx's per PTE	Avg. Overall Charge ($) per PTE	Percent (%) Rx of Avg. Charge per PTE
Generic Group	100.0	5.7	1,343	32.1
Single Drug Group Overall:				
Selective Serotonin Reuptake Inhibitors	69.5	6.0	1,425	36.5
Misc. Antidepressants	8.4	6.2	1,377	31.7
Tricyclic Agents	5.8	7.2	813	18.8
Other Single Rx Groups	16.3	3.6	1,164	12.4

PTE = Patient treatment episode; Rx = prescription

Adapted from and with permission: Terry, C.M., Thomas, S., and Cave, D. G. "Major Depression." Managed Care Interface, Vol. 11, No. 11, 58-60, November 1998

Terry's study found "Patients suffering from routine major depression received an average of 0.98 tests (i.e., allergy, imaging, functional and invasive), 2.62 laboratory/pathology services, and 0.50 medical/surgical procedures over the course of a one-year PTE. The average number of prescriptions was 16.29 per PTE. The next largest component, psychiatrist visits, average 10.64 visits per PTE."

The cost per PTE came to $2,287. Over 95% of these depressed patients treated by psychiatrists were treated with drugs. Thirty-five percent (35%) of the costs were for drugs and 35% were for psychiatrist outpatient visits. Also from the study, the charge per PTE for those treated *without* drugs was $1,231. When a single drug group was prescribed for 12.7% of the PTEs, the average cost was $1,343. *Fifty-one point six percent of the patients received prescriptions from four or more prescription drug groups*! This last statistic (50% of the patients received drugs from *four* drug groups) shows that psychiatrists are leading the way in the *polypharmacy* approach to treating depression. These data reflect the widely held belief among mental health professionals that psychiatrist treatment of depression – and anxiety disorders – is basically drug treatment (or drug management) rather than psychotherapy. At one time, psychiatrists and psychologists were actively engaged in delivering a variety of different types of psychotherapy. Today it is a rare psychiatrist indeed who has an active psychotherapy practice.

If Buzzing *One* Neurotransmitter Works, Why Not a Drug That Buzzes *Two* or *Three* Neurotransmitters?

There are a number of studies in the literature, many of which are underwritten by drug companies, which attempt to show that *dual* acting antidepressants such as Venlafaxine (Effexor) are more efficacious than *single* acting drugs such as the SSRIs. The SSRIs such as Prozac and others work on the serotonin system alone while others, such as Venlafaxine (Effexor), work on the serotonin *and* the norepinephrine systems. The rational is that if a drug corrects a chemical imbalance in the serotonin system, a dual acting drug that corrects a chemical imbalance in *two* systems would be more powerful. It should be, so I will report on one large study that *seems* to support such a belief.

Wait a Minute

However, let's look at a study comparing Venlafaxine, SSRI and Placebo on what is called depression-free days. In this study (Mallick, R., 2001) Venlafaxine (864 patients) seemed to compare very favorably against both the SSRI group (756 patients) and the Placebo group (450 patients). The SSRI group did statistically better than the Placebo group and the Venlafaxine group was superior to the SSRI group. The Venlafaxine group had an average of 19.8 DFDs (depression free days), the SSRI group 17.3 DFDs and the Placebo group only 14.1 depression free days. The researchers certainly seemed to be singing the praises (in a professional manner of course) of Venlafaxine.

Again, this was a very good study, but the researchers (the "proponents") failed to point out the most important conclusion from the study. The mean number of depression free days (DFDs) for each group was the number of days the patient was free of depression *during a fifty-six day period*. Therefore, the Venlafaxine group had, on average, 65% depressed days, the SSRI group 69% depressed days, and the Placebo group 75% depressed days.

From the above data you would not want to give depressed people placebos, but with the same reason (efficacy) you would not want to treat them with either SSRIs or Venlafaxine. These patients on antidepressants were *still depressed on well over half of the days* in which these patients were on the drugs. Again antidepressants, even Venlafaxine that is touted to be more effective than the others, is not much more effective than a sugar pill and the researchers *should* have called for a better way to treat depression than drugs or sugar pills.

Let's Compare One Antidepressant with Another

In one such study (Braconnier, 2003) the investigators compared Paxil and Anafranil in treating depressed youth even though it has not been demonstrated that antidepressants with depressed youth are any more efficacious then inert placebo. The authors concluded the two drugs have similar efficacy; however, from the data we do not know if either drug has *superior* efficacy over placebo. Moreover, if one looks at the data in the study, the use of either drug to treat depressed children should be questioned. Study discontinuations occurred in 41.4% of the subjects on the drug Anafranil and 31.8% of the patients discontinued while taking Paxil. The reasons for discontinuation included 2 suicide attempts and a subject who developed suicidal ideas. Of those who continued on the drugs, 86% on one drug and 74.6% on the other reported treatment-emergent adverse events.

Despite the above, the researchers failed to recommend the obvious: "Don't use these drugs on children with depression." Instead, the researchers believed the result supported "the serotonin hypothesis" in this age group but did not confirm it in the absence of a placebo control.

Each of these two drugs had FDA approval with at least two adult clinical trials in which these drugs were *superior* to placebo (unless they used a comparator), but there is no report of the *number* of other trials that were *not* superior to placebo. These drug to drug comparisons have little value without a placebo group.

Want to Change the Standards

Many psychiatrist-researchers are critical of the standards used in the FDA antidepressant clinical trials (as I am for different reasons), which they believe to be poorly structured to demonstrate the "true" power of these drugs in treating depression. Among other changes, these researchers want *longer* term periods to judge drug effectiveness, but rather than conducting research with an "improved" experimental design, these researchers want to abandon science.

In trying to explain away the slight advantage of the drug over placebo in these clinical trials, these "proponents" say that such differences are comparable to other areas of medicine. If it were true, that most areas of medicine were no more effective than drug treatment of depression, we should abandon medicine entirely but of course we should not. Antibiotics are much more powerful in treating infections than drugs are in treating depression.

Let's look at another area of medicine, antihypertensives and the reduction of blood pressure. High blood pressure is, as with depression, a biopsychosocial problem (Do you think stress is not a contributor to high blood pressure?). Let's look at a drug's effectiveness in treating high blood pressure.

In one study (Prichard, B.N. et al., 2002) the medication was found significantly superior in reducing blood pressure compared to placebo. After eight weeks of drug treatment, systolic blood pressure dropped from 166.2 to 141.2 (a 15% reduction) versus placebo controls from 162.5 to 161.3, less than a 1% reduction. If antidepressant drugs treated depression as effectively as this drug treats high systolic blood pressure, there would be no argument and no need for this book. But antidepressants in treating depression are in no way comparable to antihypertensives in treating high blood pressure.

Laughren: SSRI Induced Suicide

The debate on the question of antidepressant-induced suicide in adults heated up in a paper by Teicher (Teicher, M.H., et al., 1990). Teicher and his colleagues published a paper describing a series of 6 adult patients with depression who, in their view, became suicidal as a result of being treated with Prozac. Ever since this publication, the FDA, the pharmaceutical industry, NIMH and others have been involved in a rear guard action defending the safety of antidepressants.

At an FDA meeting a representative from NIMH gave that agency's perspective on this issue. The representative essentially made the point that depression is a serious disorder that is associated with suicide, and argued that the data did not support the view that antidepressants further increase the risk of suicide in this population. We must remember, however, that these six suicides did not occur randomly in the population (The suicide rate for all depressed persons is 15% over time) — these and other suicides that were investigated occurred *during* treatment, which we know should *lower* suicide potential.

The FDA's response to this most serious question of antidepressant induced suicide is typical of a memorandum written by Thomas P. Laughren, M.D., Team Leader of the Psychiatric Drug Products Division of the FDA (Laughren, 2004).

Dr. Laughren brings out the antidepressant "increased energy" argument to account for antidepressant drug early suicides and, at the same time, raises the conventional wisdom that long-term antidepressant drug treatment *reduces* suicide risk, but no data of such a relationship is presented. He believes it is quite possible for a drug to have an *opposite* effect over time; with regard to antidepressants, a suicide risk in the *early* stages of treatment and a *decreasing* suicide rate over time. He implies by the "increased energy" hypothesis that this may be the price we *have* to pay for effective treatment of depression. I suppose anything is possible, but a simpler view is more honest, that is, antidepressants either cause or do not cause suicide over the whole range of their use, including during the withdrawal stage.

Dr. Laughren, in reviewing antidepressant induced suicide in children, does look at the question of efficacy and admits that the overall success rate for positive drug antidepressant clinical trials is 20% (3 of 15 studies) is clearly of concern. He gives a number of plausible reasons why so many drug trials demonstrated no effectiveness, but the only logical conclusion from the data is that these drugs have extremely limited value in treating either child or adult depression.

How did the FDA handle the problem of limited or no efficacy of these drugs in treating depressed children? Well, if you don't like the results of the placebo-controlled clinical trials, the standard used throughout the industry to establish drug efficacy, then just set up a *different* standard.

<u>Randomized Withdrawal Design</u>

At the hearing, Dr. Thomas Laughren of the FDA staff and others recommended a "randomized withdrawal design" to better show the "true" efficacy of these drugs in treating childhood and adult depression. This "randomized withdrawal design" would strengthen the already existing drug bias that exists in the current FDA approved placebo-controlled "blinded" studies.

In this withdrawal design, all depressed patients who get better on the antidepressant are randomly switched with half the subjects changing to placebo and keeping the other half on the drug. In this design, efficacy is determined by measuring any differential *relapse rate* between those continuing on the drug versus those subjects switched to placebo. One must understand that those who remain on the drug *are not exposed to the drug withdrawal problems* associated with the discontinuation of these drugs. Withdrawal is known to produce problems for the user, and, knowing this, how can these "proponents" in good faith make such a proposal?

This design, which has absolutely zero scientific merit to it, insures that the subjects switched to placebo will do worse because they, unlike the non-switched, *will be undergoing drug withdrawal* while being observed for relapse. Also, by using inert placebo those switched from the antidepressant to the inert placebo are more likely to be aware of switching, and such knowledge is likely to be related to subsequent relapse.

It is true in these studies that the patients who continue on the antidepressant take longer to relapse into depression than those switched to inert placebo. However, this finding does *not* prove that antidepressants are effective in treating depression as the advocates would have us believe. It only shows that a *faulty* experimental design favors the drug over the placebo group.

The FDA staff is ensuring that the drugged (non-switched) subjects will do better than the placebo subjects, but the reason has nothing to do with drug effectiveness. Antidepressant drugs are addictive and when people are withdrawn from these drugs either abruptly or on tapered withdrawal these patients encounter a range of adverse side effects. Could this withdrawal play a role in the subsequent relapse? We will never know for sure because this proposed research design by drug "proponents" is flawed. The proposed FDA studies are poorly designed and appear to be self-serving.

Few Patients Satisfied with Antidepressants

The National Depressive and Manic-Depressive Association conducted an online survey of close to 1,400 patients who were taking or had received antidepressant treatment within the past five years. Women were 75% of the respondents, which is expected since this gender difference is typical for antidepressant use in any benefit plan.

Survey Results

Of survey participants prescribed antidepressants, 81% described their social adjustment as either "moderately" or "extremely" impaired. Depression continued to impair work performance in 72% and continued to affect the family life of those polled.

Adverse side effects caused 17% to stop taking medication, and 60% reported that the medication caused drowsiness. Patients also reported headaches, insomnia, agitation, nausea and other gastrointestinal symptoms, and sexual dysfunction as a result of antidepressant medication.

Overall, 61% described themselves as "somewhat" or "very satisfied" with treatment, while 25% reported no improvement in their symptoms; 45% reported no improvement in fatigue and loss of energy, and 35% reported no increase in ability to experience pleasure while on antidepressant treatment. A majority 66% of respondents reported a "less than satisfactory relationship" with their treating physician, and more than half said their physician did not understand them.

This was hardly a scientific survey, but it was a valuable contribution nonetheless since 1,400 antidepressant users responded to the survey. I am surprised that 61% reported *satisfaction* with their treatment (were some of these also receiving therapy?), but in general the survey results were certainly *unfavorable* for antidepressant drug treatment. The group as a whole reported substantial ongoing impairment of work performance and family relationships, 25% reported no improvement. Large numbers reported ongoing negative drug side effects, and large numbers reported no improvement of some of the more core problems in depression (45% reported no improvement in fatigue and 35% reported no improvement in the ability to experience pleasure).

The data taken together is a very strong indictment of the use of antidepressants in treating depression. Certainly many of the side effects are depression-engendering symptoms and probably interfered with the self-limiting nature of depression. Even without any other data, the survey results on satisfaction with antidepressants seriously question the efficacy of antidepressants in treating depression.

Interpreting Blindly

The blindness is not in the above data but in its *interpretation*. The Reuters article quoted a spokesman who, in commenting on the survey, said the survey findings underscore the need for effective antidepressant medications with minimal side effects. The survey data suggests to non-believers that at the very least that antidepressant drugs are simply not very effective in treating depression, and, secondly, we need to find something that works.

From the comments, the spokesperson was aware that the results were deplorable, but, rather than questioning the drug approach, *the spokesperson wanted to continue the research for better antidepressant drugs with fewer side effects, and blamed the providers for not finding the "right" drug for the patient.* The spokesperson noted that there are *thirty* different antidepressant drugs, the implication being that the patient (and the doctor) should search until the "right" drug is found.

Good luck, and I am sure the drug companies would also support such a recommendation.

New Research on the Evaluation of SSRIs' Sexual Impairment

Sexual impairment is a common symptom of depression; usually 40% of depressed men and 50% of depressed women report sexual libido/performance problems. Antidepressant-induced sexual dysfunction is a major problem in antidepressant treatment, which occurs from approximately 30% to 70% of those patients treated with drugs (Clayton, AH et al., 2002). With such a high rate of drug induced sexual dysfunction there is a major problem, of course, with drug compliance.

An Assumption of Effectiveness

Brannon's study compared two antidepressant drugs on the issue of treatment-emergent sexual dysfunction. It is a good study (Brannon, SK et al., 2003) that again provides insight into how antidepressant believers are *impervious* to the evidence right before their eyes. The researchers compared two antidepressants, Duloxetine (Cymbalta) and Paroxetine (Paxil) and found that the former, a drug yet to gain FDA approval, had *fewer* treatment-emergent sexual dysfunction problems than Paxil.

The researchers had data from a 4 eight-week, randomized, double-blind clinical trial comparing treatment effectiveness of Cymbalta, Paxil and Placebo treated depressed subjects. The researchers took the treatment responders in each group and looked at treatment-emergent sexual dysfunction, but one must not lose sight of the question of treatment efficacy, that is, the number of responders/non-responders in each group. In the Cymbalta group, of the 736 drug treated patients, 297 patients met the criteria for improvement (40%); in the Paxil group, of the 359 patients, 140 patients met criteria for improvement (39%), and in the placebo group, 129 of 371 patients met criteria for improvement (35%).

Still Haven't Made the Connection

The authors report these figures without comment and report drug differences on treatment-emergent sexual dysfunction and drug improvement differences. However, the authors fail to point out that, of the drug treated patients, 60% failed to meet their improvement criteria over the eight-week trial. Moreover, the placebo-treated patients did as well (or badly) as the two drug treated groups. The slightly lower percentage of improvement in the placebo group (35% versus 39% and 40%) was not likely to have been a statistically significant difference in improvement. There are dozens and dozens of such antidepressant studies in which the authors simply ignore data that is inconsistent with the need to believe in the power of antidepressants.

In the above research the question of which antidepressant had fewer sexual side effects was moot because based upon such low antidepressant drug response rates, rates which were no better than placebo, why would one give *either* of these drugs to a depressed patient? People who have a vested interest in antidepressants — not only lay person users, prescribers, pharmaceutical companies but scientific researchers as well — want to believe that these drugs work and simply *ignore* any evidence to the contrary.

Relapse Prevention in the Treatment of Depression

Relapse means that the treatment, of whatever type, was not effective. Rather than searching for a better treatment, which would be the logical thing to do, the focus has been *adding* treatments during the maintenance period to *reduce* the drug relapse rate.

The National Institute of Mental Health, knowing the very high relapse with drugs in treating depression, has funded numerous studies both to evaluate relapse and to prevent or reduce it. In the following I will briefly mention some of these studies, all of which to varying degrees reflect the blindness of belief. These researchers dealing with relapse and the relative ineffectiveness of drugs in treating depression need to look at the outcome research on cognitive therapy. However, despite all evidence to the contrary the antidepressant believers remain committed to a drug first if not a drug exclusive approach.

<u>Cognitive Therapy in Whisman Study</u>

A number of these NIMH drug relapse prevention studies include cognitive therapy among other *relapse prevention* strategies. I am always a little skeptical of these studies that use cognitive therapy for relapse prevention because, as mentioned, cognitive therapy is appropriate for *some* depressed patients but not for others. In the drug approach, one makes the diagnosis of major depression and then prescribes the drug or in a research study randomly assigns the patient to the antidepressant or placebo or therapy condition.

For controlled research purposes one *has* to have a cookie cutter approach, random assignment to a drug condition or to a cognitive therapy condition, for example. The drug and cognitive therapy (or interpersonal therapy) condition must be delivered rather inflexibly, at times not meeting the patient's needs. Even with this cookie cutter approach, cognitive therapy shows up very well when compared to antidepressants and has a much lower relapse rate than drugs. A research study will better explain what I mean.

One study (Whisman, 2001) involving depression treatment with antidepressant and behavioral treatment (interpersonal therapy, cognitive therapy, the antidepressant imipramine plus clinical management and placebo plus clinical management) found that poor marital adjustment at the end of treatment was found to be associated with greater severity of depression for an extended period of time after the end of treatment. Not unexpectedly an improvement in marital adjustment was associated with a *decrease* in depression severity over the course of treatment.

When you have a depressed person with a bad marriage do you treat the depression (with drugs or cognitive therapy, for example) or do you treat the marital problem? At this point we need a diagnostician to evaluate the patient to determine the origin of the patient's depression. The need is for good clinical judgment to determine what is the best way to proceed. Will fixing the marriage problems cure the patient's depression? And if not, how is it best to proceed?

<u>Continuation Phase — Cognitive Therapy (CBT)</u>

One study (Jarrett, R.B., 2001) looked at patients with reoccurring depression (these had been treated with drug therapy previously) who are noted for having a very high rate of relapse.

These 84 patients, patients who had responded to treatment with cognitive therapy during the *acute* phase of treatment (they reported no treatment failures on cognitive therapy) were assigned to receive ten sessions of either continuation-phase cognitive therapy or evaluation only as a control procedure over a period of eight months. None of the patients received any psychotropic medication over the period of the study. Subjects were evaluated for sixteen months after the end of the eighth month continuation phase. Recurrence was defined as the return of symptoms reaching criteria for a major depression. Not unexpectedly, patients not receiving continuation cognitive therapy relapsed more frequently than the controls (31% versus 10%).

In this study, risk of relapse was associated with (1) initial depressive episode occurring at an earlier age and (2) unstable remission during the acute cognitive treatment phase. For the earlier onset depressions, those not receiving maintenance cognitive therapy were more likely to relapse than those receiving maintenance cognitive therapy (67% versus 16%), which is a marked difference. For the remission unstable patients, those *not* receiving maintenance cognitive therapy had a higher relapse rate than those who did receive it (62% versus 37%).

This is an interesting study and shows that even depressed patients with a poor prognosis who received appropriate cognitive treatment had a relapse rate of only 10%, which is very impressive in comparison with antidepressant treatment of similar patients. A weakness of the study was that cognitive therapy in the *acute* phase (helping patients acquire skills to reduce symptoms) did not include (as in the continuation phase) *coping* strategies to deal with anticipated vulnerabilities. Coping strategies, of course, lower the risk of relapse. It is no wonder that those with unstable remissions were more vulnerable to relapse. They had not been exposed in the acute phase to *coping skills* training to learn the skills needed to prevent relapse.

In another similar study (Fava, 1998) of CBT or medication management following pharmacotherapy, there was a differential relapse superiority of CBT (35%) over medication management (70%), which again points to the weakness of drug treatment. This and other studies raise serious questions about the efficacy of drugs in treating depression yet the researchers recommended "the stage-oriented model of psychotherapy of depression" in which successful pharmacotherapy is *followed* by psychotherapy.

There is no rational reason that a weaker treatment (drugs) should be employed first and then the more powerful treatment (CBT) second, especially to prevent relapse associated with the weaker treatment. The "believer" wants the *drug* to be able to treat the health problem (depression, high blood pressure, high cholesterol, etc.). Even though currently there are, in some cases, more powerful non-drug treatments, some believers retain hope that a *better* drug will come along one day.

At the close of a twenty-week treatment period, those receiving CBT had remitted from depression (25%) while only 13% remitted their depression under medication and clinical management. Remission of symptoms is a higher level of improvement (the patient is no longer diagnosable as depressed) than is just *partial* improvement. By the end of the 48-week follow-up period, patients receiving CBT had a lower relapse rate (29%) than those receiving drugs and clinical management (47%). In the CBT/antidepressant group 71% achieved and continued their remission while only 53% of the drugs alone group (plus medication management) achieved and sustained their remission.

A group of researchers (Murphy, Simons, Welzel, & Lustman, 1984) randomly assigned CBT *plus* nortriptyline (a tricyclic antidepressant), or CBT therapy plus active placebo. The placebo was designed to have mild sedative and anticholinergic effects (e.g., dry mouth) to simulate drug side effects and to make it more difficult for the patient (and the prescriber) to know these patients were on the placebo rather than the drug. Nine psychiatrists and three psychologists provided the CBT. The researchers used the Beck Depression Inventory and Hamilton Rating Scale for Depression to assess improvement. All patients improved on the two measures of the study. Cognitive therapy alone was as effective as the antidepressant drug, and there was no additive effect of the combined treatment (therapy plus drugs).

The patients in this study were followed for one year after treatment termination (Simons, Murphy, Wetzel, & Lustman, 1986). Patients who had received cognitive therapy, whether or not they received the antidepressant as well, were less likely to relapse. Those who had antidepressants alone did worse and those with antidepressants *and* CBT were immediate in terms of relapse. These results suggest that medication treatment not only seemed to make relapse more likely but also actually may have *interfered* with the long-term efficacy of cognitive therapy.

The latter finding is contradictory to the very poplar notion that combined treatment (psychotherapy and drugs) is more effective than psychotherapy alone.

Electroconvulsive Therapy (ECT) and Relapse

There is a great deal of "blindness" about Electroconvulsive Therapy (ECT) for so called *intractable depression*. The term *intractable depression* is used quite frequently in the industry to justify certain kinds of non-traditional treatments of depression and, if you are a payer of health care, when you see this term "beware of your pocketbook" because you should look out for a big ticket item. ECT has been around for approximately seventy-five years. Its popularity waxes and wanes, and ECT seems to have been gaining popularity over the past fifteen years, perhaps because of the increasing exclusive use of drugs to treat depression. There may be some justification for ECT use but, in my experience, it is much overused. Proponents argue its use for "intractable depression," and when you pin a proponent down on the meaning of the term, it is when a depression has not responded to two courses of drug treatment. One could say that ECT is warranted when the patient's depression has not responded to two "placebo" cures. In other words, "proponents" believe ECT should be allowed even when depressed patients have not received psychosocial treatment by a behavioral health specialist trained in CBT, for example.

One study (Sackheim, H.A., 2001) involved 84 patients who had a substantial reduction in depressive symptoms in response to a series of ECT treatments. These patients were then randomly assigned to (1) a nortriptyline (an antidepressant) group, (2) a nortriptyline plus lithium group, or (3) a placebo group. Relapse rates were 39% for the antidepressant plus lithium group, 60% for the antidepressant alone group, and 84% for those receiving placebo. The authors of the study seemed to be aware that ECT is not a very efficacious treatment of depression. These researchers mentioned that without post ECT active treatment, virtually all remitted patients relapsed within six months of stopping ECT. The authors noted that relapse is most frequent in the period immediately following discontinuation of the ECT. Rather than questioning the efficacy of ECT in treating depression, which would certainly be a logical conclusion from their data, the authors recommended *tapering* the ECT, starting the patient on an antidepressant *before* concluding the ECT, and starting lithium *after* the final ECT session. Perhaps physician researchers have a problem saying anything negative about any "generally accepted" *medical* procedure, although in this study these researchers seem to be trying to salvage the effects of ineffective (ETC) treatment. One might say the researchers could have used CBT as post ECT treatment to reduce relapse, but it doesn't make much sense to use a questionable treatment before using a more proven and effective method.

The Blindness Continues – Loss of Antidepressant Effectiveness

"Believers" have a problem in that facts have a habit of just popping up over and over again, facts that challenge the belief system. One such fact that the antidepressant believer must deal with is what the believer calls "Loss of Antidepressant Effectiveness." In one study (Byrne, SE 1998), a review of randomized double-blind, placebo-controlled studies, the authors discovered that during maintenance (drug) therapy, recurrence of depression ranged from 9 to 33% (up to 57% when the use of lithium alone was examined). It is interesting that the authors also found that in published case studies (this is not the best evidence), there are fewer reports of relapse with tricyclic antidepressants (TCAs). To account for their relapse rate during SSRI maintenance, the authors suggest a number of possibilities beside noncompliance. Their explanations including the loss of placebo effect, acquired drug tolerance, increase in disease severity, accumulation of a detrimental metabolite of the drug, rapid mood cycling, and ineffective doses for preventing recurrence. These researchers never seem to say the obvious: "Perhaps the antidepressant was not a very good treatment for the depression in the first place."

This so-called *loss of antidepressant effectiveness* has kept both researchers and practitioners busy. Proposed strategies have run the gambit from increasing the dose, changing to another class of antidepressant drugs (e.g., SSRIs to TCAs), using an augmenting drug (e.g., lithium) or having the patient take a drug holiday.

Paxil (SSRI) For Long Term Treatment of Social Anxiety?

One study (Stein, DJ 2002) looked at social phobias following a one-week single-blind placebo run-in, a twelve-week single blind Paxil treatment phase, and a twenty-four-week double-blind, randomized, maintenance treatment phase for patients deemed *responders* in the acute treatment phase. Again the placebo washout period stacks the deck in favor of the drug, and the study does not compare drug versus placebo. Response was defined as a decrease by at least two points on a severity of illness scale but about 25% of total subjects treated did not meet this criteria and were terminated from the study. The number of non-responders suggests the drug is not very powerful in treating social anxiety. Drug treatment subjects during the maintenance phase relapsed less frequently than those on placebo (14% versus 39%) and at the end of the study Paxil treated patients were rated "much improved" or "very much improved" at a higher rate than the placebo group (78% versus 51%).

Certainly this study suggests that Paxil has a much *lower* relapse rate than maintenance placebo, but it would seem more appropriate to compare the drug to CBT (rather than placebo) in treating social anxiety. Moreover, this study is flawed by not taking into consideration the Paxil withdrawal effects, which is a problem with all of these drug switching to placebo studies. There is often a *rebound* effect following drug withdrawal. In this last study, as in many others, one should ask when there is drug switching to placebo, is the poorer placebo response due to the lack of active drug or due to withdrawal effects from the drug phase? Moreover, in the Stein study 25% of the subjects did not meet improvement criteria and were dropped from the study, which again demonstrates the drug's weakness.

Brown Update

The Brown University Psychopharmacology Update reported findings from an investigation showing that the SSRI Luvox is "well tolerated and effective for the long-term treatment of social anxiety disorder." Let's examine some of their data reported from the study.

In the study we are told that 300 patients diagnosed with generalized Social Anxiety Disorder (SAD) were randomized to receive Luvox (N=149) or placebo for 12 weeks (Westenberg, et al., 2004).

Severely SAD

As is typical of these antidepressant studies, assessment of these patients reflected a severe level of impairment, which must be used for the drug to *have* any chance of beating the placebo in these types of studies. After twelve weeks of treatment, patients in the Luvox CR group experienced a 37% reduction in (assessment device) scores compared to a 28% reduction in scores in the placebo group (P=0.02). A 37% reduction in SAD symptoms is hardly impressive and less so than typically found in drug depression outcome studies (50% reduction in symptoms).

Adverse Effects

More patients on Luvox withdrew due to adverse events (26%) than those on placebo (5%) in the first three weeks. Treatment emerging effects were nausea, insomnia and anxiety – all of which are symptoms that SAD patients want to get rid of! The reviewers commented on the side effect profile of Luvox, but never questioned the advisability of giving such a drug to anxiety ridden patients with such a high frequency of "anxiety" related side effects. The reviewers noted that the drug did not significantly affect sexual function, which is about the only thing that the drug would have in its favor.

Their Conclusion

The authors concluded from the study that Fluvoxamine (Luvox) CR is an effective, safe, and well-tolerated option for the long-term treatment of adults with generalized SAD. From such a conclusion, did I miss something? First, can we really say the drug was well tolerated when 26% dropped out in the first three weeks due to adverse side effects?

Forgot to Include in Conclusion

The investigators noted the 26% dropout rate, but they seem to have forgotten these patients in their conclusion, as if these dropouts had not existed. The investigators determined the differential drug-placebo response rate of those who were able *to stay on the drugs* or placebo, that is, the 74% who remained on the Luvox and the 95% who remained on the placebo. However, should efficacy of a drug (in a placebo-controlled trial) be assessed *only* on those who were able to continue on the drug or should efficacy be looked at in terms of the *total* group receiving the drug? The reader already knows my answer to this question.

We saw in the above that even when a restricted drug sample of patients was used (those who were able to tolerate the drug) the drug-placebo differential improvement was hardly very impressive (37% improvement versus 28% for placebo). In the real world we want to know how many people with SAD, if given Luvox, *will* get better. The question should not be, as in the study under consideration, how many will get better if *they can tolerate the drug*. The data from the study *really* says that for every 100 SAD cases given either Luvox or placebo, 27 would improve on the drug versus 27 would improve on the placebo. Even though the differential drug-placebo improvement rate was 37% versus 28%, the improvement rates should be applied to the *total* persons treated. Projecting the study data to the whole population of those SAD cases who might be put on Luvox or placebo, 27 of the 74 patients tolerating the drug would get better versus 27 receiving placebo (28% of 95 patients tolerating the placebo). Looked at in this more appropriate way, Luvox is no better than a placebo in treating SAD and we would have to find something other than *Luvox* or a *placebo* for that matter to treat SAD.

Again, the researchers doing these kinds of antidepressant drug outcome studies, most of which are partially or fully funded by the drug maker, are simply not looking at their data and not accepting the obvious conclusions from their own data. These drug "proponents" are emotionally committed to a *drug* answer to these problems and anything that is incompatible with this deeply held belief is simply ignored.

The maker of Luvox, who supported funding of the above research, will, of course, use the conclusions from the above study to market the drug to PCPs and psychiatrists. Typically drug makers not only fund such research as in the above but also pay researchers and other professionals to appear at conferences in which the supposed benefits of the drug are touted. These drug funded conferences on topics such as depression or SAD or others typically ignore any non-drug treatment alternatives and perhaps 98% or more of the presenters and attendees at these conferences are committed to a drug answer to all of these problems.

Brain Changes Associated with Antidepressant Drug Treatment—PET

Positron Emission Tomography (PET) is a tremendous research tool to evaluate brain-behavior mechanisms. The PET Scan picks up glucose as it is being metabolized by brain cells in various regions of the brain. During scanning, the researcher may ask the subject to solve a mathematical problem, for example, and the scan picks up the pattern of glucose utilization as the subject mentally solves the problem.

PET Appealing

The PET technology has been very appealing to the antidepressant believers who endorse the chemical imbalance theory of depression, and there has been increasing use of PET in antidepressant drug studies. Since there is a very strong relationship between brain and behavior, depressed people in their PET Scans have much less glucose metabolism going in their brains than non-depressed people. This reduction in glucose metabolism corresponds to the behavior of depressed persons in their day-to-day behavior. When depressed people get less depressed due to time, antidepressants, placebos or psychotherapy, their PET Scans light up more (i.e., brain glucose metabolism increases) than the PET Scans when the person was in a depressed state.

CBT Changes PET, Too

I used to hear from some psychiatrists that the PET research *proved* that depression was a biological disease (a chemical imbalance for some), but this kind of talk has decreased since there have been reports of PET changes following CBT of depressed patients as well.

In one PET study examining brain changes of depressed patients on either Prozac or placebo, 17 hospitalized depressed patients had six weeks of either Prozac or placebo. All patients received standard inpatient treatment, including group therapy but none received Cognitive Behavioral Therapy (CBT). All subjects were given the Hamilton Depression Scale at baseline and at the end of the six-week study period. Clinical response as usual was defined as having a 50% decrease in depressive symptoms.

The investigators were less interested in *efficacy* of drug versus placebo but were more interested in the PET brain changes of Prozac versus placebo. Of the placebo patients who got better (4 of 7), there were significant *regional* metabolic changes involving the pre-frontal, anterior cingulate, premotor, parietal, posterior insula and posterior cingulate, as well as with metabolic decreases involving the subgenual cingulate, hypothalamus, thalamus, supplementary sensory area insula and parahippocampus.

Moreover, Prozac produced similar PET changes found in placebo subjects with one noticeable difference, the Prozac patients had more limbic system metabolism than those on placebo. The limbic system, which is well below the level of the cerebral cortex, is a brain center involved in emotionality and is thought to be a more "primitive" brain center than the cerebral cortex.

Metabolic Consequences

The authors were not interested in the question of efficacy so much as in the metabolic consequences of the drug or placebo of those whose depression improved. At the end of the study when the investigators learned which of the subjects were on the drug and which on the placebo, 4 of 10 subjects improved on Prozac (40%) and 4 of 7 subjects on placebo (57%). We know from the study that increasing metabolism in the limbic system is not critical in the recovery from depression. That the placebo was more or just as powerful as the drug in depression treatment in these subjects did not cause comment at all, but it again shows the limited efficacy of the drug in treating depression and how "proponents" often ignore unfavorable data.

The Fantasy of the Polypharmacy Approach – The Prescriber World

PMHM did an analysis of psychotropic drugs in several plans including one I will discuss. We selected a sample of 16 high *drug using* patients receiving psychotropic drugs and the patient's psychotropic drug data were submitted to a board-certified psychiatrist for her review and comment. This psychiatrist in addition to conducting psychotherapy in her practice uses antidepressants and anxiolytic drugs as well, but I wanted to see her opinion about the *quality* of the prescribing of these drugs in the plan, drugs prescribed by both psychiatric and non-psychiatric physicians.

Prescribing Problems

A consulting board-certified psychiatrist reviewed a random sample of the data and found the following problems:

Patient A: a stimulant was prescribed, two antidepressants, as well as a sedating antidepressant. Was the sedating antidepressant prescribed to counteract the side effects of the stimulant?

Patient B: the patient was prescribed three mood stabilizers and an anticonvulsant, four benzodiazepines, two antipsychotics, three antidepressants, and one sedating antidepressant. Are random symptoms being treated, or is this patient being treated for a specific disorder?

Patient C: the patient was being treated with three benzodiazepines, three antidepressants and a stimulant. No specific diagnosis warrants treatment with these three very different classes of drugs.

Patient D: this patient was treated with an antianxiety medication, a mood stabilizer, a stimulant, an antipsychotic, a benzodiazepine, an antidepressant, and a sedating antidepressant. This patient has been treated with all classes of psychotropic medications.

Patient E: this patient was prescribed a benzodiazepine, an anti-convulsant, two antidepressants, a sedative antidepressant, and an anti-psychotic.

Patient F: this patient was prescribed a stimulant and a sedative. Is this sedative being used to counteract the side effects of the stimulant?

Patient G: this patient was prescribed three benzodiazepines, two antidepressants, a sedative antidepressant, and two anticonvulsants.

Patient H: this patient received four antidepressants and was treated with a benzodiazepine. One would question whether a major depressive syndrome was being treated or a dysthymic disorder was present that would be non-responsive to antidepressants.

Patient I: a short-acting and a longer-acting benzodiazepine were prescribed as well as a serotonergic antidepressant. One would question whether a mood or anxiety disorder is being treated.

Patient J: two different strengths of two different antidepressants were prescribed. Had this patient had an adequate trial prior to change dose/medication?

Patient K: this patient was prescribed a short-acting benzodiazepine, four different antidepressants of different strengths, one with sedative qualities. Is the sedating antidepressant being used to counteract the side effects of the more activating antidepressant, are they being used together, or are antidepressants being used to treat a sleep disturbance?

Patient L: the patient was prescribed a benzodiazepine, mood stabilizer, stimulant, two antidepressant agents, a sedating antidepressant, and an antianxiety agent. What disorder this patient is being treated for?

Patient M: the patient was prescribed an antianxiety medication and four different antidepressants. Had adequate trials of one medication been tried prior to adding or switching to another?

Patient N: this patient was prescribed three mood stabilizers, four benzodiazepines, an anticonvulsant, an antipsychotic, and two antidepressants. What diagnosis is this patient being treated for?

Patient O: this patient was treated with various classes of drugs, benzodiazepines, antidepressants, and stimulants. Are these medications being used to treat various symptoms or a specific disorder?

Patient P: this patient has been prescribed an antianxiety medication, a mood stabilizer, an antipsychotic, two antidepressants, and a stimulant. Are these medications being used to treat various symptoms or a specific disorder?

In summary, the consulting psychiatrist said, "Primary care and other physicians appear to be prescribing psychotropic medications in a polypharmacy approach. In most cases, antidepressants, benzodiazepines and sedatives are being prescribed together. Aren't antidepressants *supposed* to ameliorate symptoms of anxiety and sleep disturbances?"

I am afraid the above cases of psychotropic drug misuse by general physicians and others are pretty typical for most benefit plans. The patients with the more serious problems, those who are less likely to respond to a placebo recovery, are the most likely ones to become badly managed with multiple drug treatment. Obviously, the above patients were not responding to drug therapy, but rather than referring the patient to a specialist, these physicians continued to chase symptoms (and probably drug side effects as well) with other drugs. The only entities that come out ahead of these prescribing practices are the prescribers and the drug companies.

One of the worst cases I have seen of inappropriate prescribing was conducted by a psychiatrist on an ex-alcoholic (at the time diagnosed incorrectly as depressed) patient who remained in the hospital for twenty-nine days. In my review of the hospital chart to evaluate questions of therapeutic necessity, I counted twenty-one different psychiatric drugs the patient was prescribed during his hospital stay. In my clinical opinion, the patient was not a candidate for *any* drug therapy at all much less twenty-one different drugs.

Novel Approaches to Treatment Resistant Depression

I am sure the reader has seen on the television news and read in the newspaper stories about "novel" approaches in patients with so called "treatment resistant" depression. First, who are these treatment resistant depressed patients? Typically these patients are depressed patients who have not responded to drugs and should be better described as those not responding to drugs, which is certainly a big population, but not necessarily "treatment resistant depressed patients." At least one of these novel approaches had gained approval by the Federal Drug Administration and there are others to follow. When you see the word "novel" in this context you should substitute the word *expensive*, which is the common denominator for what all of these approaches share.

Vagus Nerve Stimulation

Neurologists have actually used this surgical procedure with some success for treating some intractable seizure patients. Someone got the bright idea to try it with so called treatment resistant depressed patients, and perhaps there are thirty to forty depressed patients (the number will be growing) around who have had an electrical device implanted in their neck to electrically stimulate their vagus nerve. As I recall the device itself cost $12,500 (I am not sure how long a period it lasts) and with a hospital stay, the neurosurgeon's fee and the follow-up care, we are probably looking at perhaps $50,000 or more. I doubt any of these patients had ever been treated by anything more than drug therapy. Advocates of this procedure are the believers in antidepressant treatment, and they recommend VNS when drugs fail. If we used this procedure when drugs fail in treating depression, our health care costs would double. When I attended a workshop presentation on VNS, I was polite and did not ask the question, "How does this procedure fit in with your *chemical imbalance* theory of depression?"

TMS

Another esoteric novel approach to treatment resistant depression is Transcranial Magnetic Stimulation (TMS), which is a device that is implanted in the brain to provide the brain with additional electrical stimulation. These types of procedures make intriguing nightly television news stories including an interview with a bright-eyed surgical patient extolling the benefits of the procedure. Of course, these are not controlled studies (the use of unstimulated implant patients) and we only have testimonial "evidence." As I recall only about 30% of these and other implanted patients were described as improved. For $50,000 a case, one could provide quality mental health services for those needing services in a town with a population of about 15,000. Unfortunately, society through many health plans is paying for such "treatment" and I suspect these various procedures will gain increasing popularity.

Smoke and Mirrors--MRI

Magnetic Resonance Imaging (functional MRI), a very useful brain imaging tool for neurological diagnosis and for research into brain-behavior relationships, has been taken to the bosom of the antidepressant believers and marketers to support their case. We see the *before* image of the depressed person's brain, dull and not much going on in their brain (and also in their behavior I might add), and the *after* brain image (after six to eight weeks of antidepressant X) is lit up like a Christmas tree. Lo and behold another "victory" for the chemical imbalance theory. These ads don't tell you, however, that the depressed person's brain image also "lights" up during and following CBT or in many cases lights up without treatment.

The above study on brain imaging (Davidson, 2003) compared before and after MRI brain images on antidepressant treated patients versus normal subjects. I am sure this was not the intention of the authors, but it was more of a marketing study in that the depressed antidepressant subjects were compared not to placebo-treated depressed patients but to emotionally normal subjects. A double-blind, placebo-controlled study would have been much more useful. I think the MRI is a tremendous research tool in mental health, but *behavior* is the proof of the pudding in mental health and *not* a brain scan. Depression shows itself in *behavior* and not most directly in a brain image.

More Smoke and Mirrors--SYMBYAX

In 2004 Eli Lilly got FDA approval for SYMBYAX, the first and *only* FDA-approved treatment for *bipolar* depression, according to the Eli Lilly product announcement. There are several drugs approved for treating bipolar disorder but none for *bipolar depression*, which is a diagnosis that does not as yet exist in the DSM-V. However, let's not let a little thing like that keep us from opening up a new market. I thought depression was depression but not according to Eli Lilly. The next thing you know Eli Lilly will come out with a "new" cancer depression drug or a diabetes depression drug, but thus far we only have a *bipolar depression* drug.

What is this new wonder drug for treating bipolar depression? Well this new wonder drug is a combination of Prozac and olanzapine (Zyprexa), the latter being an atypical antipsychotic used to treat schizophrenia and bipolar disorder but not, according to Eli Lilly, *bipolar depression*. In the clinical trials submitted to the FDA, SYMBYAX was compared to placebo and olanzapine alone in an eight-week trial with depressed bipolar cases. SYMBYAX proved superior to placebo over the eight-week trial but olanzapine also was *not* superior to placebo. Of course the important condition was left out, that of Prozac alone, to see if SYMBYAX had any advantage over Prozac alone. What we *do* know is that olanzapine alone is *not effective* in treating "bipolar depression" and why add it to Prozac?

I am sure the answer to this would be found not in the science department at Eli Lilly but in the *marketing* and *finance* departments. Prozac's patent has run out, but SYMBYAX is now offered at a higher unit cost than Prozac. Combination drugs should not gain approval unless the combination *is* substantially superior to the individual ingredients alone. In the case of SYMBYAX we have no evidence of its superiority to Prozac alone and we now have a drug on the market with an expanded adverse side effect profile.

Believe it or Not

One psychiatrist (Niculeson, 1999), recognizing that hospitalization for general medical problems can engender anxiety or dysthymia in the patient, recommended routine *prophylactic* treatment of depression and anxiety with low doses of SSRI antidepressants for *all* hospitalized patients. I applaud his recognizing that hospitalization *is* a major stress for patients, but his solution reflects the physician model, "If there is a health problem, let's find a pill for it."

When in a state of stress *anything* that gives pleasure will allay fear and strengthens the immune system. We *know* how to allay fear and it is *not* by giving an SSRI. The fear experienced by a pending surgery patient causes more bleeding during surgery and delays recovery as a consequence of the anxiety. These consequences are reversible for the most part with *behavioral* intervention techniques. These techniques, however, are outside the physician model of health care and go unimplemented except for research studies from time to time.

The above psychiatrist recommending *prophylactic* antidepressant treatment obviously had a disease model of depression and anxiety, and his recommendation was quite consistent with that model. To us his recommendation is not only *not* supported by research but it is ludicrous.

Patients Can Be Blinded by Belief About Antidepressants, Too

Not only are *prescribers* subject to various kinds of strange inconsistencies concerning depression and its treatment but so are many users of antidepressants. The following are case examples of callers to PMHM experiencing various problems and emotional distress who took the promised pill cure rather than doing something constructive about their problems.

Examples

- One individual is taking Prozac to treat his "sexual addiction" to computer porn.
- A 12-year-old girl whose parents sought help for her due to her difficulty adjusting to having to move to a new town and leave behind her friends is currently on Effexor XR 150mg capsules (prescribed dosage unknown).
- A 17-year-old child (at the time of the contact) whose parents sought assistance through the EAP for his acting out, drug use, and disrespect is now on Celexa.
- One individual who called for help with bereavement is now on Celexa, while another who called for bereavement is on Clonazepam, Trazadone, and Ambien.
- One caller wanted help with his cocaine addiction. He had a long history of Alcohol, Cannabis and Hallucinogen abuse. He called back seeking a different referral when he learned that the psychologist could not prescribe medications. He refused to go to therapy and is now on Remeron and Effexor.
- A caller who requested assistance with "parenting skills" is taking Celexa.
- There were three cases of clearly addressable anxiety issues: panic, agoraphobia, public speaking, low grade anxiety, claustrophobia. One is on Clonazepam, another is on Alprazolam and the third is taking Celexa and Ambien. There is no indication that any of the three followed through with EAP or therapy.
- One individual called and received three separate authorizations to use the EAP for marital counseling, but never followed through. That individual is now taking Effexor.
- A couple both called and received their own authorization to use the EAP for marital therapy. It appears they continued in therapy after the EAP. One is now taking Celexa while the other is taking Hydroxyzine Pam.

Some physicians have told me they prescribe these drugs when requested by the patient because if they do not do it, another physician will. I have never bought this rationalization.

The magic pill is sought as an instant fix. It requires no changes in behavior of the person. Moreover, we don't have to understand the situation — the person, their behavior and important individuals in their lives — we just need to get the right pill to the person and everyone will be happy. Reality is far from simple. Reality, like people, is complex. There are no quick and easy solutions to complex problems.

Cardiac Rehab or A Pill

For instance, cardiologists for many years strongly recommended an extensive exercise program in their patients undergoing cardiac recovery. A high risk factor for heart disease has been a sedentary life style and it stands to reason that exercise would be very good for those who have had a heart attack.

A newspaper article referred to the fact that many cardiologists are no longer recommending exercise for their heart attack patients. This recommendation was not modified by any new scientific evidence discounting the health benefits of exercise in recovery (there continues to be hard evidence of its critical importance in recovery). Rather, the recommendation was withdrawn because so few (25%) cardiac patients were following the exercise recommendation! Apparently the cardiology group felt that since so few patients followed the exercise recommendation it was putting added stress on those who would not comply.

Here we have a situation in which there are known benefits of exercise in cardiac recovery, the vast majority of heart attack victims fail to follow the recommended exercise program and this is a dilemma that is ripe for a solution. The "rational" solution, of course, is to find a better way of encouraging compliance among these patients. The thinking may be "why tell these patients to exercise because they won't do it and if you tell them it will only add to their stress."

Crazy Like a Fox

These above case examples show "proponents" may not only be "blind" to some data, but at times crazy like a fox. In the following examples, unlike the others I've used, there are definitely ethical issues and self-serving economic needs involved.

Too Many Exclusions Compromise Data

In no other drug classification has the FDA allowed so many subject exclusions in clinical trials as in the antidepressant ones. Trials to determine the efficacy of antidepressants have historically evaluated only a small subset of depressed patients with what might be considered a specific and rather "pure" clinical profile. People not only with the milder forms of depression but patients with other types of psychiatric problems are excluded, including subjects who had ever been on any kind of psychiatric drugs including antidepressants in the past.

Not Severe

All FDA drug studies exclude certain subjects from a clinical trial even if the subject meets the criteria for the "disease" and such exclusions are inappropriate and *do* bias the results. However, if there are too many exclusions, we become extremely limited in our ability to apply the results of the clinical trial to the real world of persons with the "disease" or disorder. This fact does not deter the "proponents."

Attempt to Correct Placebo Error

One might think that by selecting the *severest* cases the drug company would be making its task more difficult in the clinical trials, but one must be aware that any drug in these trials must prove its efficacy over placebo. The drug companies who manufacture antidepressants have always known these drugs have limited effectiveness in treating depression. Less severe cases of MDD would be less likely to demonstrate superiority over placebo in treating depression.

There is no other illness or disease that is treated as is depression in FDA clinical trials. An infection *is* an infection irrespective of severity, diabetes *is* diabetes irrespective of severity, high blood pressure *is* high blood pressure and so on and so on. There is simply no justification to exclude many of those with *less severe* forms of depression from clinical trials. The drugs would not have gained approval if even the inert placebo had been compared with samples of all subjects meeting the criteria for Major Depressive Disorder.

Researchers looked at inclusion and exclusion criteria used in 31 antidepressant trials published from 1994 to 1998 in five psychiatric journals. Clinical trial researchers had excluded subjects with any psychotic features, those with a manic episode, anyone with a suicide risk, unstable medical illnesses, or a history of drug or alcohol abuse (Zimmerman, M. et al., 2002). Several also excluded subjects with eating disorders, obsessive-compulsive disorders or panic disorder or other anxiety disorders. These researchers at Brown University were not aware of any other medical condition in which subjects in clinical trials were excluded because they were not sick enough.

The antidepressant clinical trial data, in view of all the exclusions, could only apply to a small minority of depressed patients in the real world. The researchers evaluated depressed patients in a psychiatry outpatient clinic and found that 2/3 meeting the criteria of Major Depressive Disorder would *not* have been eligible for clinical trials and if *anxiety* was a cause for exclusion, 85% of these depressed patients would have been excluded from clinical trials. However, 90% of these subjects were *on* antidepressant drugs at the time of the study! To repeat, the clinical trial studies could not have been scientifically applied to their depressed population, yet 90% of these patients were on antidepressants!

The pharmaceutical industry knows that if a medicine seems to work on a highly selected group of depressed patients, physicians will use it for *all* patients. In physician offices all over the country, of the patients prescribed antidepressants, only about 15% of such patients would be similar to those selected in the clinical trials. In my own clinical experience, I suspect of those on antidepressants, perhaps 70% would not even meet criteria for Major Depressive Disorder, for which the FDA has granted the drug approval. In this the drug companies certainly deserve our "Craftiness Award."

More Than Creative Marketing

The FDA approved Xanax as a treatment for panic disorder partly because, at *four* weeks, Xanax was *twice as effective* as placebo in reducing panic attacks. But Upjohn failed to report in their advertising that at eight weeks, placebo patients were panic-free almost as often as patients treated with Xanax. At the end of the study (*Consumer Reports* 1993), there was no significant difference in the average number of panic attacks or in functioning at work, home, and social life between people taking Xanax and those who were taking placebo. This is more than a case of creative marketing; it is manipulative and dishonest. Upjohn also failed to report the "rebound effect." The Xanax group had averaged only 1.7 panic attacks (per patient) per week – and the placebo group 2.1 attacks a week - at the end of eight weeks of treatment. However, once the drug was discontinued, patients in the Xanax group went back up to 6.8 attacks a week – slightly worse off than these patients had been at the *beginning* of the study. By contrast, two weeks after the patients on placebo discontinued their "drug", these patients averaged 1.8 panic attacks a week.

Actually with such data as the above, the FDA should never have given approval for Xanax in the treatment of panic disorder. Such weak evidence of efficacy should not have overridden the fact that these benzodiazepine drugs are highly addictive and prone to abuse, especially in persons the drug was supposed to help, those with an anxiety disorder.

Women Only: Take Zoloft for Your (PTSD)

It is said timing is everything. About a month or so prior to the terrorist attacks on September 11, 2001, Zoloft gained FDA approval for treatment of PTSD. It was the first SSRI antidepressant to be approved for treatment of this disorder. First, Zoloft daily for twelve weeks has shown efficacy in *2 of 3* double-blind clinical trials. Again the magic number, 2 positive clinical trials. Response (improvement) rates were 53 and 60% for patients receiving Zoloft compared with 32 and 39% for patients receiving placebo in the two positive studies. Remember, in one of the 3 trials there was *no* drug-placebo difference. Did the marketing people fail to report that efficacy was only *limited to women* and efficacy in men was not clearly established (*Drugs and Therapy Perspectives 2001*)? Moreover, Zoloft also failed to show significant effects compared with placebo in 2 clinical trials conducted with patients who had predominately *combat* induced PTSD. Despite such weak evidence, Zoloft gained FDA approval to treat PTSD and I am sure it is the number one drug for Iraq veterans with diagnosed PTSD.

If the Diagnosis Does Not Fit Reality, Change the Diagnosis

When I talk about bipolar disorder (the modern term for manic-depressive psychosis), I usually preface my remarks by saying I believe in its existence. During graduate school in the early 1960s, I was doing part-time work at a state hospital and saw a dozen or more patients with manic-depressive psychosis, including these patients who were in a manic state. As a psychologist, I didn't think we had any definitive psychological treatment for these patients when they were in a manic state but, as the use of Lithium expanded in treating these patients, I saw a dramatic improvement in these patients' ability to function. It was as if the drug was addressing the core of the disorder, and the effects on the patients' ability to function were truly remarkable.

However, when a psychotropic drug is found effective in treating one disorder, psychiatrists have a habit of expanding its use to other disorders. To be diagnosed manic-depressive, the patient *must* have had at least one manic (psychotic) episode. These manic states are truly unique; there is nothing quite like them in all of psychopathology and they can be diagnosed fairly well retrospectively with the aid of a good historian. A patient was a candidate for Lithium only if the patient had experienced a manic state.

Expanded Diagnosis of Bipolar

Psychiatry did not want to be constrained by such limitations and the invention of an expanded diagnosis was the answer, bipolar I (for patients who had had a manic attack) and bipolar II, a "non-psychotic" form of the disorder. I don't think that science had anything to do with this expanded diagnosis, but I believe it was the need to expand the use of Lithium and the other mood stabilizers. The psychotic diagnosis restricted the drug developmentally (only adults) and could it be possible that other persons with expansive mood (e.g., used car salesmen) might have a milder from of the disease? Moreover, maybe the manic-depressive had the disease throughout their whole development but it never expressed itself until later life.

Preventive?

In the above kind of reasoning we are, of course, getting very far away from the facts, but I am afraid this is not a problem for the "believer." The next jump for the "believer" was to use mood stabilizers in a *preventive* sense, to try to identify "pre-manic" people and treat them *before* they had a manic attack, to in a sense head off the disorder at the pass. Making two forms of bipolar disorder (I and II) enabled psychiatry to expand the use of mood stabilizers to a wider range of patients, including those of infancy and childhood.

The above is analogous to an oncologist telling you that he or she cannot diagnose you with cancer, but he believes you have a genetic predisposition for it and he wants to give you chemotherapy as a *preventive* measure! An oncologist recommending *preventive* treatment like this would be laughed out of the medical profession, and rightly so, but somehow this thinking is quite acceptable in today's psychiatry. Several years ago I attended a workshop on bipolar disorder and one of the speakers, a world-renowned expert on bipolar disorder and its treatment, recommended such *preventive* treatment with mood stabilizers. Were there others in the audience of nine hundred or so mental health professionals who saw such a recommendation as harebrained? I hope so.

<u>Ludicrous</u>

Currently, the diagnosis of bipolar disorder has become nothing short of ludicrous. It has been expanded to so many disparate groups that it has lost all meaning. I suspect that 70% of those diagnosed as bipolar disorder do not have a disorder for which lithium or other mood stabilizers is appropriate or which will address the core of the disorder. When I hear of the diagnosis I am usually skeptical. In interviewing the patient (or a relative of the patient) with such a diagnosis I ask if the mood stabilizer resulted in a *dramatic* improvement in the patient's ability to function. Typically I hear, "Oh, a little bit better," which sounds more like placebo improvement. Without more science I don't see the justification of giving such drugs to children and infants, which unfortunately is the current standard of care.

I tell people that high energy, creativeness, ambition and the ability to do multiple tasks are traits of *normal* behavior – not psychopathology in themselves. I have also noticed that judges, entrepreneurs, or gung ho financiers, when these individuals get into trouble with the law, are often diagnosed as bipolar disorder. The examining psychiatrist tells us that with a mood stabilizer and psychiatric treatment the person will be able to conform to the straight and narrow path in the future. To this I say hogwash. The crook was *never* bipolar disorder. One notices that most of these cases one reads about in the newspaper come from the upper socioeconomic level and these persons are never an automobile mechanic or a carpenter.

Everyone and his buddy are now diagnosed with bipolar disorder. The diagnosis has lost all meaning or credibility.

Who Do We Blame for the Blindness?

I have not seen any evidence that American psychiatry has done anything to try to correct the public's erroneous view of depression as a disease and the mythical drug cure of these problems.

We have a situation in which psychiatric researchers and practitioners have their careers largely invested in the field of antidepressant drug therapy. We have the promoters marketing the supposed magic, and we have a society that wants to believe in the magic, a symbiotic relationship that is very powerful indeed.

The case examples illustrated above, e.g., the patient taking Prozac to cure his alleged computer porn addition, are examples of the magical power of cure that these pills have in the minds for large segments of society. I guess we really cannot fault people for wanting to *believe* in the power of antidepressants — especially those and their loved ones who have problems in need of solutions. If we did we would be faulting these people for being human. However, we can and *should* fault the promoters and practitioners who tacitly endorse such wishful thinking and profit thereby when they know as well as I do that these drugs have very limited efficacy at best.

Chapter X

WRAP-UP

The disease model of depression treatment with drugs by the family physicians has such an emotional appeal that it has become the driving force in the treatment of depression, anxiety and the more minor stress and mood problems that plague all of us from time to time.

Summary of Evidence

- The "evidence" presented by the antidepressant "believers" includes an interesting theory about the *biological* nature of depression, the so-called chemical imbalance theory, and a series of patient and provider satisfaction stories about the miracle nature of these drugs. Part of the folklore of these drugs is that the side effects are mild and tolerable, and that a physician relatively untrained in the mental/emotional disorders can treat these disorders very competently with drugs alone.
- Depression and anxiety, which are actually complex *biopsychosocial* disorders, are considered by the "believers" to be modifiable by the chemical manipulation of one or more neurotransmitters in the brain. Nevertheless, when a depressed patient fails to respond to an antidepressant (which occurs at least 50% of the time), or when an antidepressant responder relapses after drug termination, the drug's efficacy is still unquestioned by the believer. When the drug-treated patient fails to respond, the theory is offered that either the *right* antidepressant has not been selected, or the pharmaceutical industry has not yet discovered the *right* antidepressant that *will* address *this* patient's depression.
- To account for the high relapse rate following acute antidepressant treatment, the drug treatment theory brings in the tenant that depression is a *chronically relapsing* disease, much like chronic alcoholism, rather than the simpler theory that the drug did not correctly treat the problem in the first place. In a few cases, prescribers may add cognitive behavioral therapy (CBT) as an *adjunct* to the medication to decrease relapse, but the "believers" reject CBT as a *primary* treatment. The theory acknowledges that a minority of depressions are not responsive to present generation drugs, but it holds that patients who fail the

standard of care are good candidates for electroshock therapy, vagal nerve stimulation or brain implants for so called drug resistant intractable depression.

- Part of the appeal of the theory is its simplicity. The disease arises from one or more neurotransmitters, which need to be brought into balance so the patient can achieve or return to a non-depressed state. Even if the depressed patient *believes* that some of their down mood problems may arise from current adverse events in their life, that fact can be ignored or he or she can be told that the adverse life event is only a *symptom* of the chemical imbalance. Once the imbalance is restored, the adverse life event will be able to take care of itself.
- We have seen that this theory of depression owes its origin much more to propaganda and marketing than to science. What we know of depression and recovery from depression simply does *not* fit this theory.
- As we have seen from depression outcome studies, including the FDA submitted clinical trials, manipulating neurotransmitters with drugs has proven to have little more than placebo value. Not only do SSRI antidepressants *not* decrease the suicide rate of those treated, but in fact the clinical trial data suggests that the suicide rate of young people on antidepressants is substantially *higher* than those on a placebo.
- The promotion of these drugs as effective and safe treatments for both depression and the anxiety disorders by family physicians is a complete distortion of the clinical trial data, other outcome research and everyday practice. Moreover, we have seen that the drug companies, the FDA and other groups are intertwined in their respective goals. The FDA is not doing its job in regulating psychotropic or other drugs. There are many and powerful segments of society that have a vested interest in seeing that the drug companies realize their goal of selling more drugs. These entities are determined to maintain the status quo and want to see the further expansion of these drugs throughout society.
- These vested interests *have* to admit that these drugs are not very effective in treating depression. However, they hold out to the public the hope that *better* drugs are just around the corner and drugs will one day effectively treat *all* of our mental health problems.
- Litigation with regard to safety concerns may well continue to dampen the popularity of these drugs in the future. These lawsuits might consider asking for

punitive damages in malpractice cases when drugs are used as the *sole* treatment of these problems in lieu of referral to *specialists* for proven treatment of these problems.

- With only limited efficacy, we can tolerate little if any risk. With antidepressants we have a class of drugs with the worst of two worlds: limited efficacy and high and dangerous risks, including drug caused homicide and suicide. In looking at the scientific evidence of the efficacy of these drugs in treating depression (including the FDA submitted drug clinical trials), these drugs should never have gained FDA approval in the first place. The evidence is quite clear that these drugs should be taken off the market and the users helped to discontinue these drugs as safely as possible because of limited efficacy and dangerousness.

A Behavior, Not a Disease

- I and others like me see depression and anxiety as unlike schizophrenia and bipolar disorder. We hold that depression and anxiety are different in *degree* rather than *kind* from the stress and mood problems that all of us experience from time to time. We have *all* had bouts of depressed mood and anxiety. Most of us can easily understand what it might be like to be on one of the diagnosable extremes because we know and have experienced these two disorders at least in attenuated form.
- In the extremes of these disorders, we are dealing with a difference of severity, frequency, longevity and degree of social dysfunction from those with more minor emotional distress. All of the depression and anxiety disorders are *learned* disorders and successful treatment is a combination of counterconditioning of the stress-anxiety, problem resolution of the *causes* of the symptoms and modification of maladaptive patterns of thinking where needed to keep distressing symptoms from returning.
- Many of us learn to overcome irrational fears on our own without drugs or cognitive therapy as a part of normal development and learning. Many with severe reactions could master the anxiety or mood problem with professional help designed to desensitize the person to the feared situation or to learn to better cope with problems to restore normal mood. However, the DSM-V now lists many "diseases" such as social phobia, and the doctor now has a cure for all the ills that

are part and parcel of being human. The doctor now has a pill for us, one approved by the FDA, and we are told the pill cures our "disease." This is not true. Calling it a disease does not *make* it a disease, nor is it cured like one.

Magic Pill

There will be, of course, a better pill in the future that will relieve our depression, another for anxiety, one to roll back the health hazards from our sedentary lifestyle, a pill that will enable us to maintain normal weight and still eat all we want, a pill to compensate for our poor nutrition, and so on. When this all comes about it will truly be a great day for everyone, or so those who believe in the "magic" cure tell us.

The biologically-biased "believers" simply don't believe that people can or will change their injurious health behavior and "proponents" continue to search for the magic pill to address all of our health problems. We have mainly addressed the antidepressant drug promised cure, but as we have seen the desire to believe in the "magic health bullet" goes much deeper in society and keeps us from achieving better and more appropriate health care at affordable costs on the basis of *current* knowledge.

While we wait for this magic cure that will also reverse our injurious health behavior, we neglect to do what has been *proven* to prevent disease and improve our health, that is, to change our behavior or the way we live. The core problem in health care today — both the quality and cost — is the pursuit of better health through the path of chemistry. Currently we have some good drugs that do indeed address *causes* of our health problems, and we need more of these types of drugs, but what we *don't* need is drugs in the current market that only reduce *symptoms* and do not address *causes* of our health problems. However, we *know* taking *personal* responsibility for one's health risk behaviors is *the* way to better health, and we already have the technology available to assist people to change their behavior and to improve their health. We have to stop the current *disease* model of health care that tries to fix the health problem as if the body is a machine and to address both the biological *and* psychosocial aspects of illness.

The belief in the power of drugs to treat depression has such a strong emotional appeal that it completely overwhelms all facts and evidence to the contrary.

It is a question of facts and evidence going up against the power of belief, or more correctly, the *wanting* to believe. As one can see through history, belief has always been more powerful than the facts and often there is a resistance to face any facts that contradict the belief. Who wants to believe that drugs are very effective treatments of depression and anxiety? Many groups with vested interests hold on to the belief despite glaring contradictory evidence as we have seen.

Certainly economic greed may be operating to support some of the "blind" spots. The biological bias of many physicians and psychiatrists is also a problem. However, I suspect the much stronger motivation is the deeply held desire that a seemingly complex health problem can be solved by a simple solution, a drug from the family doctor. The simplicity of the drug solution by a family doctor is so emotionally compelling that it has pushed aside all evidence to the contrary.

We must remember how certain segments of society maintained for several hundred years the belief that the earth was the center of our universe despite the mountain of evidence to the contrary.

These beliefs that capture people's imagination often reflect a fixed world view and the way we *want* to see the world that is quite impervious to change. In the eighteenth century in the United States, Virginians and others believed that the *source* of the Potomac River, the site of the Nation's capitol, was either the Mississippi River or the Pacific Ocean. The thought that the Potomac was a *minor* river was not in keeping with the people's expectation of the future greatness of this country or the nation's capitol. This belief was supported by absolutely nothing, and there were many facts that were incompatible with the belief, but the belief continued for many years. It had a life of its own.

Some beliefs, of course, have *stronger* emotional appeal than others do. Emotionally compelling beliefs are more resistant to the facts and change in the belief system than beliefs that do not serve *emotional* needs. My mother-in-law, a very bright, well-read women in her eighties, read several chapters of this book prior to its publication. She seemed to understand my thesis but she suggested that I end the book with a paragraph saying that **we need to come up with an antidepressant that truly *is* effective**.

And after all, even Sigmund Freud once thought that he had come up with the magic drug, one that would cure all of his patients' mental health problems.

The name of Freud's magic drug was cocaine. Even the best of us are potential "believers" or "proponents" of a variety of myths and because of this we must not turn away from the science or facts that question our beliefs.

Another example of the power of belief was the popular idea in the 1960s and 1970s (and still today) that we can *learn* while we sleep, and technology was developed to transmit knowledge to us while we were sleeping. This belief is very much akin to the belief in antidepressants. No longer would we have to "waste" the night away — we could learn while we slept. The idea of eight hours of learning at night was so attractive and appealing that the belief captured the imagination of people, and the belief in sleep-learning took hold almost immediately. Psychologists, however, by hooking up sleeping subjects to an EEG, found that during the night these subjects learned while they were awake and failed to learn while the EEG was transmitting delta waves, i.e., when these subjects were asleep. Oops. No free lunch after all. Again, the belief in sleep-learning was so appealing to some that even today these devices are advertised and sold on television. Unfortunately, the *easy* way is the *preferred* way, even when it is not the *right* way.

If you as a reader shared the conventional wisdom about depression and its treatment before picking up this book, I hope that by reading this book your attitudes will have undergone some change. If they have changed, do not feel negative about yourself because you were taken in by the propaganda. After all, you have a *lot* of company.

Effective Methods

Questioning the efficacy and risks of these drugs will, I hope, assist antidepressant and future antidepressant users to look more closely at the benefits and risks of these drugs. In the process these persons will be able to make a more informed decision about their own mental health than others have in the past or presently.

The antidepressant drug treatment approach prevents and delays more appropriate treatment of these problems. Fortunately, we *do* have effective behavioral treatments, treatments such as CBT or IPT for treating anxiety and depression. Unlike a pill, these methods do not treat the patient as a passive victim. These behavioral therapy approaches require the patient to assume a *responsible* and *proactive* role in his or her recovery and the therapist must be *well trained* and astute to understand and address the *core* problems giving rise to the symptoms. We have seen that the power of the pill in treating depression is no more than the power of the placebo, but obviously the drug relapse rate requires that solutions to these problems be better than a placebo. As previously noted we already have effective and proven behavioral treatments for these problems even though the solutions are not magic or a quick fix.

We have examined the *science* of the antidepressant drug quick fix and found that the *magic* in the title of this book comes not from science but from the desire to *believe* in the magic.

NOTE TO ANTIDEPRESSANT USERS

Dr. Les would like to hear from you on your positive or negative experiences with these drugs, including those of you who have taken these drugs with or without therapy from a mental health professional. He would also like to hear from parents who have had a child prescribed these drugs by a pediatrician, family doctor, or psychiatrist with or without child/family psychotherapy.

Contact Dr. Les at antidepressants@pmhm.com

or

Dr. Les Ruthven
401 E. Douglas, Suite 300
Wichita, KS 67202

To order additional copies of this book visit:
www.antidepressanttruths.com

REFERENCES

Ackerson, J., Scogin, F., McKendree-Smith, N., & Lyman, R.D. "Cognitive Bibliotherapy for Mild and Moderate Adolescent Depressive Symptomatology." Journal of Consulting and Clinical Psychology, 66, 685-690, 1998.

Adapted from Hedlung & Vieweg. "The Hamilton Rating Scale for Depression" Journal of Operational Psychiatry, 10(2): 149-165, 1979.

American Psychiatric Association Press Release. "APA Opposes Implementation, Expansion of New Mexico's Psychologist-Prescribing Law." Arlington, VA., January 6, 2005.

Anderson, N. The Broken Brain: The Biological Revolution in Psychiatry. Harper & Row, 180-182, 1984.

Antonuccio, D.O., Akins, W.T., Chatham, P.M., Monagin, J.A., Tearnan, B. H., & Ziegler, B. L. "An Exploratory Study: The Psychoeducational Group Treatment of Drug-Refractory Unipolar Depression." Journal of Behavior Therapy and Experimental Psychiatry, 15, 309-313, 1984.

Antonuccio, D. O. and DeNelsky, G. Y. "Psychotherapy Versus Medication for Depression: Challenging the Conventional Wisdom with Data." Professional Psychology: Research and Practice, Vol. 26, No. 6, 574-585, 1995.

Antonuccio, D. O., Danton, W. G., DeNelsky, G. Y., Greenberg, R. P., & Gordon, J. S. "Raising Questions About Antidepressants." Psychotherapy and Psychosomatics, 68, 3-14, 1999.

Antonuccio, D. O., Thomas, M., & Danton, W. G. "A Cost-effectiveness Analysis of Cognitive Behavior Therapy and Fluoxetine (Prozac) in the Treatment of Depression." Behavior Therapy, 28, 187-210, 1997.

As reported in "Common Brain Changes Seen in Placebo and Antidepressants." Brown University and Adolescent Psycho-pharmacology Update 4(6): 1, 5-7, © Manesses Communications Group, Inc., 2002.

Ashton, C. H. DM.,FRCP. "Guidelines for Withdrawal of Antidepressant Drugs," January 2001. www.benzo.org.uk/ashtonad.htm accessed 11/18/2004.

Babyak, M., Blumenthal, J. A., Herman, S., Khatri, P., Doraiswamy, M., Moore, K., Craighead, E., Baldewicz, T., & Krishnan, K. R. "Exercise Treatment for Major Depression: Maintenance of Therapeutic Benefit at 10 Months." Psychosomatic Medicine, 62, 633-638, 2000.

Baldessarini, R.J. "Risks and Implications of Interrupting Maintenance Psychotropic Drug Therapy." Psychotherapy and Psychosomatics, 63, 137-141, 1995.

Bauer, M., et al. "Double Blind, Placebo-controlled Trial of the Use of Lithium in Augment Antidepressant Medication in Continuation Treatment of Unipolar Major Depression." American Journal of Psychiatry, 157: 1429-1435, 2000.

Beck, A.T., Hollon, S.D., Young, J.E., Bedrosian, R.C., & Budenz, D. "Treatment of Depression with Cognitive Therapy and Amitriptyline." Archives of General Psychiatry, 42, 142-148, 1985.

Beck, A.T., Rush, A.J., Shaw, B.F., and Emery, G. Cognitive Therapy of Depression. New York Giulford Press, 1979.

Beck, P., Cialdella, P., Haugh, C., Hours, A., Boissel, J.P., Birkett, M.A., and Tollefson, G.D. "Meta-analysis of Randomized Controlled Trials of Fluoxetine v. Placebo and Tricyclic Antidepressants in the Short-term Treatment of Major Depression." British Journal of Psychiatry, 176: 421-428, May 2000.

Bellew, K., McCafferty, J.P., Zaninelli, R.M. "Paroxetine and the Rate of Remission in the Treatment of GAD." Research presented at 54th Annual APA meeting, New Orleans, May 2001.

"Benefits of Fluovoxamine CR for Social Anxiety Disorder." Brown University Psychopharmacology. Vol.15, No. 2, 4, February 2004.

Blashki, T. G., et al. "Controlled Trial of Amytriptyline in General Practice." British Medical Journal, 1, 133-138, 1971.

Blatt, S. J., Sanislow, C. A., Zuroff, D. C., & Pilkonis, P. A. " Characteristics of Effective Therapists: Further Analyses of Data from the National Institute of Mental Health Treatment of Depression Collaborative Research Program." Journal of Consulting and Clinical Psychology, 64, 1276-1284, 1996.

Blumenthal, J.A., Babyak, M.A., Moore, K.A., Craighead, W.E., Herman, S., Khatri, P., Waugh, R., Napolitano, M.A., Forman, L.M., Appelbaum, M., Doraiswamy, P.M., Krishnan, K.R. "Effects of Exercise Training on Older Patients with Major Depression." Archives of Internal Medicine, 159, 2349-2356, 1999.

Boseley, S. "Drugs for Depressed Children Banned." The Guardian, Wednesday, December 10, 2003.

Bowers, W. A. "Treatment of Depressed In-patients: Cognitive Therapy plus Medication, Relaxation plus Medication, and Medication Alone." British Journal of Psychiatry. 156, 73-78, 1990.

Boyd, J. H. and Weissman, M.M. "Epidemiology." In Paykel, E.S. (ed.) Handbook of Affective Disorders. 109-125. New York, Guilford Press, 1982.

Braconnier, A., et al. "Paroxetine Versus Clomipramine in Adolescence with Severe Major Depression: A Double Blind, Randomized, Multicenter Trial." Journal of the American Academy of Child and Adolescence Psychiatry, 42(1): 22-29, 2003.

Brandes, L.J., et al. "Stimulation of Malignant Growth in Rodents by Antidepressant Drugs at Clinically Relevant Doses." Cancer Research, Vol. 52, Issue 13, 3796-3800, 1992.

Brannon, S. K., et al. "Comparison of Sexual Functioning in Patients Receiving Duloxetine or Paroxetine: Acute and Long-term Data." Program and Abstracts of the American Psychiatric Association 156th Annual Meeting: San Francisco, CA., Abstract NR477, May 17-22, 2003.

Brody, A. L., Saxena, S., Stoessel, P., Gillies, L. A., Fairbanks, L. A., Alborzian, S., et al. "Regional Brain Metabolic Changes in Patients with Major Depression Treated with Either Paroxetine or Interpersonal Therapy: Preliminary Findings." Archives of General Psychiatry, 58, 631-640, 2001.

Byrne, S.E. and Rothschild, A.J. "Loss of Antidepressant Efficacy during Maintenance Therapy: Possible Mechanisms and Treatments." Journal of Clinical Psychiatry, 59: 278-288, 1998.

Chilvers, C., Dewey, M., Fielding, K., Gretton, V., Miller, P., Palmer, B., et al. "Antidepressant Drugs and Generic Counseling for Treatment of Major Depression in Primary Care: Randomised Trial with Patient Preference Arms." British Medical Journal, 322, 772-775, 2001.

Clayton, A. H., et al. "Prevalence of Sexual Dysfunction Among Newer Antidepressants." Journal of Clinical Psychiatry, 63: 357-366. Abstract, 2002.

Conte, H. R., Plutchik, R., Wild, K. V., & Karasu, T. B. "Combined Psychotherapy and Pharmacotherapy for Depression: A Systematic Analysis of the Evidence." Archives of General Psychiatry, 43, 471–479, 1986.

Cotterchio, M., Kreiger, N., Darlington, G., & Steingart, A. "Antidepressant Medical Use and Breast Cancer Risk." American Journal of Epidemiology, 151(10): 951-957, 2000.

Coupland, N.J., Bell, C.J., & Potokar, J.P. "Serotonin Reuptake Inhibitor Withdrawal." Journal of Clinical Psychopharmacology, 16, 356-362, 1996.

Cucciare, M. A., & O'Donohue, W. "Integrated Care and The High Utilizer: An Explication of Medical Usage Patterns and The Role in The Healthcare Crisis." In N. A. Cummings, W. O'Donohue, & K. E. Ferguson (Eds.), Behavioral Health as Primary Care: Beyond Efficacy to Effectiveness (95-110). Reno, NV: Context Press, 2003.

Cuijpers, P. "Bibliotherapy in Unipolar Depression: A Meta-analysis." Journal of Behavior Therapy and Experimental Psychiatry, 28, 139-147, 1997.

Cummings, N.A. Advantages and limitations of disease management. In N.A. Cummings, W.T. O'Donohue, K.E. Fegason (Eds.), Behavioral Health as Primary Care; Beyond Efficacy to Effectiveness 31-44. Reno, NV: Context Press, 2003.

Cummings, Pallik, Dorken & Hinke. "Medicaid, Managed Mental Healthcare and Medical Cost Offset." In J.L. Thomas, J.L. Cummings (Eds.), The Value of Psychological Treatment, 324-335. Phoenix, AZ: Zeig, Tucker and Company Inc., 2000.

Dalfen, A.K. & Stewart, D.E. "Who Develops Stable or Fatal Adverse Drug Reactions to Selective Serotonin Reuptake Inhibitors? Canadian Journal of Psychiatry, 46, 258-262, 2001.

Davidson, R. J., et al. "The Neural Substrates of Affective Processing in Depressed Patients Treated with Venlafaxine." American Journal of Psychiatry, 160: 64-75, 2003.

Depression Guideline Panel, Clinical Practice Guideline Number 5: Depression in Primary Care, 2: Detection and Diagnosis. Rockville, MD: US Department of Human Services, Agency for Health Care Policy and Research; AHCPR publication 93-0551, 1993.

DeRubeis, R. J., Gelfand, L. A., Tang, T. Z., & Simons, A. D. "Medications Versus Cognitive Behavior Therapy for Severely Depressed Outpatients: Mega-analysis of Four Randomized Comparisons." American Journal of Psychiatry, 156, 1007-1013, 1999.

Dobson, K. S. "A Meta-analysis of the Efficacy of Cognitive Therapy for Depression." Journal of Consulting and Clinical Psychology, 57: 414-419, 1989.

Donovan, S., Madeley, R., Clayton, A., Beeharry, M., Jones, S., Kirk, C., Waters, K., Gardner, D. & Faulding, J. "Deliberate Self-harm and Antidepressant Drugs: Investigation of a Possible Link. British Journal of Psychiatry, 177, 551-556, 2000.

Drugs and Therapy Perspective, psychiatry.medscape.com/adis/DTP/2001/Vol.17.N16/dtp1716.01/dyst1716-01.01.html.

DSM-IV™, "Diagnostic and Statistical Manual of Mental Disorders." Published by the American Psychiatric Association, fourth edition, 394-395, January 1995. *Reprinted with permission from the Diagnostic and Statistical Manual of Mental Disorders, Copyright 2000. American Psychiatric Association.*

Edwards, G. et al. "A Controlled Trial of Inpatient and Outpatient Treatment of Alcohol Dependency." Lancet, 1, 555-559, 1976.

Elkin, I., Shea, M., Watkins, J., & Imber, S. "National Institute of Mental Health Treatment of Depression Collaborative Research Program: General Effectiveness of Treatments." Archives of General Psychiatry, 46, 971-982, 1986

Evans, M.D., Hollon, S.D., DeRubeis, R. J., Piasecki, J.M., Grove, W. M., Garvey, M.J., & Tuason, V. B. "Differential Relapse Following Cognitive Therapy and Pharmacotherapy for Depression." Archives of General Psychiatry, 49, 802-808, 1992.

Fava, G. A. "Holding On: Depression, Sensitization by Antidepressant Drugs, and The Prodigal Experts." Psychotherapy and Psychosomatics, 64, 57-61, 1995.

Fava, G. A. "Long-term Treatment with Antidepressant Drugs: The Spectacular Achievements of Propaganda. Psychotherapy and Psychosomatics, 71, 127-132, 2002.

Fava, M., et al. "Sexual Functioning and SSRIs." Journal of Clinical Psychiatry, 63 (suppl 5): 13-16, 2002.

Fava, R. C., et al. "Six Year Outcome for Cognitive Behavioral Treatment of Residual Symptoms in Major Depression." American Journal of Psychiatry, 155: 1443-1445, 1998.

Gould, R.A. & Clum G. A. "A Meta-Analysis of Self-Help Treatment Approaches." Clinical Psychology Review, 13, 169-189, 1993.

Green, B. "Persistent Adverse Neurological Effects Following SSRI Discontinuation (DANES)." Consultant Psychiatrist, Halton Hospital, UK and Hon. Geniso Lechnrer, University of Liverpool, UK, 2003.

Greenburg, P. E., et al. "The Economic Burden of Anxiety Disorders in the 1990s." Journal of Clinical Psychiatry, 60: 427-435, 1999.

Greenberg, P.E., Kessler, R.C., Birnbaum, H.G., Leong, S.A., Lowe, S.W., Berglund, P.A., Corey-Lisle, P.K. "The Economic Burden of Depression in the United States: How Did It Change Between 1990 and 2000?" Journal of Clinical Psychiatry, 64, 12, 1465-1475, 2003.

Greenberg, P.E., Stiglin, L.E., Finkelstein, S.N., & Berndt, E.R. "The Economic Burden of Depression in 1990. Journal of Clinical Psychiatry, 54, 405-418, 1993.

Greenburg, R.P., Bornstein, R.F., et al. "A Meta-analysis of Fluoretine Outcome in the Treatment of Depression." The Journal of Nerons and Mental Disease, 182, 547-551,1994.

Guthrie, E., Moorey, J., Margison, F. Barker, H., Palmer, S. McGrath, G., et al. "Cost-effectiveness of Brief Psychodynamic-interpersonal Therapy in High Utilizers of Psychiatric Services." Archives of General Psychiatry, 56, 519-526, 1999.

Hall, L. H. & Roberston, M. H. "Undergraduate Ratings of the Acceptability of Single and Combined Treatments for Depression: A Comparative Analysis." Professional Psychology: Research and Practice, 29, 269-272, 1998.

Hall, R.C., Popkin, M.D., Devaul, R.A., Fallaice, L.A., & Stickney, S. K. "Physical Illness Presenting as Psychiatric Disease." Archives of General Psychiatry, 35, 1315-1320, 1978.

Hallman, J., and Oreland, L. "Serotonergic Mechanisms and Psychiatric Disorders." Nordisk Psychiatrists Tedsskrift, 43, 53-59, 1989.

Haslam, C., Brown, S., Atkinson, S., & Haslam, R. "Patients' Experiences of Medication for Anxiety and Depression: Effects on Working Life." Family Practice, 21, 204-212, 2004.

Healy, D. "Conflicting Interests in Toronto: Anatomy of a Controversy at the Interface of Academia and Industry." Perspectives in Biology and Medicine, 45, 250-263, 2002.

Heinberg, R.G., Jester, H.R. "Cognitive Behavior Treatments: Literature Review In," Heinberg, R.G., Liebowitz, M.R., et al. eds. Social Phobia: Diagnosis, Assessment, and Treatment. New York: Guilford: 261-309, 1996.

"High Anxiety." Consumer Reports, 19-24, January, 1993.

Hiss H., et al. "Relapse Prevention Program from Treatment of Obsessive-Compulsive Disorder." Journal of Consulting Clinical Psychology, 62: 4: 801-808, 1994.

Hollon, S. D. "Comparisons and Combinations with Alternative Approaches." Behavior Therapy for Depression. Edited by L.P. Rehm, New York, Academic Press, 33-71, 1981.

Hollon, S. D., Shelton, R. C., & Loosen, P. T. "Cognitive Therapy and Pharmocotherapy for Depression." Journal of Consulting Clinical Psychology, 59 (1): 88-99, 1991.

Hollon, S. D. & Beck, A.T. "Cognitive and Cognitive-Behavioral Therapies." The Handbook of Psychotherapy and Behavior Change: An Empirical Analysis. Edited by SL Garlfield and AE Bergin, 2nd edition, New York, Wiley, 443-482.

Hollon, S. D. and Najavits, L. "Review of Empirical Studies on Cognitive Therapy." American Psychiatric Press Review of Psychiatry, Vol. 7, Ed. by A.J. Frances and R.E. Hales, Washington, D.C., American Psychiatric Press, 643-666, 1988.

Hopko, D.R., Lejuez, C.W., Ruggiero, K.J., & Eifert, G.H. "Contemporary Behavioral Activation Treatments for Depression: Procedures, Principles, and Progress." Clinical Psychology Review, 23, 699-717, 2003.

Hughes, E. "Depression: Living With and Treating the Disorder." American Medical Association, Chicago, 1996.

Hunsley, J. (in press). "Cost-effectiveness and Medical Cost Offset Considerations in Psychological Service Provision." Canadian Psychology.

Jacobson, N. S., et al. "A Component Analysis of Cognitive-Behavioral Treatment for Depression." Prevention and Treatment, Vol. 3, Article 23, posted June 2, 2000.

Jamison, C. & Scogin F. "Outcome of Cognitive Bibliotherapy with Depressed Adults." Journal of Consulting and Clinical Psychology, 63, 644-650, 1995.

Jarrett, R. B., et al. "Preventing Recurrent Depression Using Cognitive Therapy With and Without a Continuation Phase." Archives of General Psychiatry, 58: 381-388, 2001.

Joffe, R. T., et al. "Augmentation Strategies," Journal of Clinical Psychiatry, 57 (Suppl 7), 25-31, 1996.

Jorm, A. F. "Mental Health Literacy: Public Knowledge and Beliefs About Mental Disorders." British Journal of Psychiatry, 177, 396-401, 2000.

Journal of the American Medical Association. Vol. 283, No. 8, February 23, 2000.

Juster, H. R., Heinberg, R. G. "Social Phobia: Longitudinal Course and Long Term Outcome of Cognitive Behavioral treatment." Psychiatry Clin. North America, 18: 821-42, 1995.

Kessler, et al. "Lifetime and 12-month Prevalence of DSM-111-R Psychiatric Disorders in the United States. Results from the National Comorbidity Survey." British Journal of Psychiatry Supplement, 168 (supl.30): 17-30, 1996.

Kessler, R. C., Berglund, P., Berglund, P., Demler, Ol, Jin, R., Koretz, D., Merikangas, K. R., Rush, A. J., Walters, E. E., Wang, P. S. "The Epidemiology of Major Depressive Disorder: Results from the National Comorbitidy Survey Replication (NCS-R)." Journal of the American Medical Association, 289, 3095-3105. 2003.

Khan, A., Warner, H. A., & Brown, W. A. "Symptom Reduction and Suicide Risk in Patients Treated with Placebo in Antidepressant Clinical Trials: An Analysis of the Food and Drug Administration Database." Archives of General Psychiatry, 57: 311-330, 2000.

Kiev, A. & Feiger, A. "A Double-Blind Comparison of Prozac (Fluvoxamine) and Paxil (Paroxetine) in the Treatment of Depressed Outpatients." The Journal of Clinical Psychiatry, 58: 4, 146-152, April, 1997. Physicians Postgraduate Press. Adapted/Reprinted by permission.

Kirsch, J., Moore, T., Scoboria, A. & Nicholls, S. "The Emperors' New Drugs: An Analysis of Antidepressant Data Submitted to the U.S. Food and Drug Administration." Prevention and Treatment, Vol. 5, Article 23, posted July 15, 2002. Available on the World Wide Web: hhtp://www.journals.apa.org/prevention/volume5/pre0050023a.html

Kirsch, J., and Saperstein, G. "Listening to Prozac but Hearing Placebo: A Meta-analysis of Antidepressant Medication." Prevention and Treatment, Vol. 1, Article 0002a, posted June 26, 1998.

Koranyi, E. D. "Morbidity and Rate of Undiagnosed Physical Illnesses in a Psychiatric Clinic Population." Archives of General Psychiatry, 36, 414-419,1979.

Kroenke, K. & Mangelsdorff, D. “Common Symptoms in Ambulatory Care: Incidence, Evaluation, Therapy and Outcome.” Graft I and Tables I, II, III, IV. The American Journal of Medicine, Vol. 86, 262-266, © March 1989 Adapted and reprinted with permission from Excerpta Medica, Inc.

Kroenke, K, et al. “Similar Effectiveness of Paroxetine, Fluoxetine, and Sertraline in Primary Care.” Journal of the American Medical Association, 286: 2947-2955, 2001.

Langer, G. “Use of Antidepressants in a Long-term Practice” ABCNEWS.com Retrieved December 2001, from http://abcnews.go.com/onair/WorldNewsTonight/poll000110.html

Langhren, T. P. “Recommendation for Approval for Celexa (citalopram) for the Treatment of Depression.” Memorandum: Department of Health and Human Services, Public Health Service, Food and Drug Administration Center for Drug Evaluation and Research, Washington, D.C., March 26, 1998.

Langhren, T. P. (Houston Conference) 2000

Leber, P. Approval action on Forrest Laboratories, Inc. NDA 20-822 Memorandum: Department of Health and Human Services, Food and Drug Administration, Center for Drug Evaluation and Research, Washington, D.C., May 4, 1998.

Leuchter, A. F., Cook, I. A., Witte, E. A., Morgan, M., & Abrams, M. “Change in Brain Function of Depressed Subjects During Treatment with Placebo.” American Journal of Psychiatry, 159, 122-129, 2002.

Lin, E. H., et al. “The Role of the Primary Care Physician in Patients’ Adherence to Antidepressant Therapy.” Medical Care, 33(1): 67-74, 1995.

Lin, E. H. B., et al. "Relapse of Depression in Primary Care." Archives of Family Medicine, 7: 443-449,1998.

Louie, L. "A Prescription for Profits. Upside." Available on the World Wide Web: http://www.upside.com/texis/mvm/story?id=3b0964961

Mallick, R., et al. "Depression-Free Days and CGI-S: A Pooled Comparison of Venlafaxine, SSRIs, and Placebo." Proceeding of the American Psychiatric Association, New Orleans: Poster Presentation, 2001.

March, J. S., et al. "Combined CBT and Sertaline in Treating Obsessive Compulsive Disorder." Journal of American Medical Association (JAMA), 292, 1969-1976, 2004.

Martin, S.D., Martin, E., Rai, S.S., Richardson, M.A., & Royall, R. "Brain Blood Flow Changes in Depressed Patients Treated with Interpersonal Psychotherapy or Venlafaxine Hydrochloride: Preliminary Findings." Archives of General Psychiatry, 58, 641-648, 2001.

Mayberg, H. S., Silva, J. A., Brannan, S. K., Tekell, J. L, Mahurin, R. K., McGinnis, S., & Jerabek, P. A. "The Functional Neuroanatomy of the Placebo Effect." American Journal of Psychiatry, 159, 728-737, 2002.

McLean, P. D., & Hakstian, A. R. "Clinical Depression: Comparative Efficacy of Outpatient Programs." Journal of Consulting and Clinical Psychology, 47, 818-836, 1979.

McLean, P. D., & Hakstian, A. R. "Relative Endurance of Unipolar Depression Treatment Effects: Longitudinal Follow-up." Journal of Consulting and Clinical Psychology, 58, 482-488, 1990.

McLeod, C. C., Budd, M. A., & McClelland, D. C. "Treatment of Somatization in Primary Care." General Hospital Psychiatry, 19, 251-258, 1997.

Mental Health Works, First Quarter, 4-5, 2003.

Miller, R. C. and Berman, J. S. "The Efficacy of Cognitive Therapies: A Quantitative Review of Research Evidence." Psychology Bulletin 94 (1): 39-53, 1983.

Moncrieff, J. "Are Antidepressants Overrated? A Review of Methodological Problems in Antidepressant Trials." Journal of Nervous and Mental Disorders, 189, 288-295, 2001.

Moncrieff, J. "The Antidepressant Debate." British Journal of Psychiatry, 180, 193-194, 2002.

Moore, T. J. "Drug Safety Research: Special Report. Medical Use of Antidepressant Drugs in Children and Adults: 1998-2001." Paper presented at the Feb. 2, 2004 FDA Hearing on the Use of Antidepressants in Children. Accessed on the World Wide Web at http://drugsafetyresearch.com/downloads/med_use_antidep.pdf

Murphy, G. E., Simons, A. D., Wetzel, R. D., & Lustman, P. J. "Cognitive Therapy and Pharmacotherapy: Singly and Together in the Treatment of Depression." Archives of General Psychiatry, 41, 33-41, 1984.

Narrow, W. E., Regier, D. A., Rae, D. S., Manderscheid, R. W., & Locke, B. Z. "Use of Services by Persons with Mental and Addictive Disorders: Findings from the National Institute of Mental Health Epidemiological Catchment Area Program." Archives of General Psychiatry 50, 95-107, 1993.

National Institutes of Health, National Institutes of Mental Health, DHHS Publication No. (ADM) 91-1695, 1991.

Niculeson, A. B. Med. Gen. Med., December 30, 1999.

NIMH Consensus Development Conference Statement. "Mood Disorders: Pharmacological Prevention of Occurrences." American Journal of Psychiatry, 142: 469-476, 1985.

Nurnberg, H. G., et al. "Treatment of Antidepressant-associated Sexual Dysfunction with Sildenafil: A Randomized Controlled Trial." Journal of the American Medical Association (JAMA), 289-56: 56-64, 2003.

O'Donovan, et al. "Prevalence and Outcome of Partial Remission in Depression." Journal Psychiatry Neuroscience, 27 (4): 241-247, July 2002.

O'Meara, K. P. Insight Magazine, 10/16/2000, accessed on 11/24/2004 for the following: http://www.cspinet.org/integrity/nonprofits/national_alliance_for_the_mentally_ill.html

Pantalon, Lubetkin, & Fishman. "Use and Effectiveness of Self-Help Books in the Practice of Cognitive and Behavioral Therapy." Cognitive and Behavioral Practice, 2, 213-228, 1995.

Pardo, Jose V. et al. "Neural Correlates of Self-Induced Dysphoria," American Journal of Psychiatry, 713, May 1993.

Paykel, E. S., Hart, D., & Priest, R. G. "Changes in Public Attitudes to Depression During the Defeat Depression Campaign." British Journal of Psychiatry, 173, 519-522, 1998.

Paykel, E.S. et al. "Prevention of Relapse in Residual Depression by Cognitive Therapy." Archive of General Psychiatry, 56: 829-835, 1999.

Pomerantz, M.D., Jay M. "Viagra and Medical Necessity." Drug Benefit Trends, Vol. 14, No. 10, 33, 2003.

Preda, A., MacLean, R. W., Mazure, C. M., & Bowers, M. B. "Antidepressant-associated Mania and Psychosis Resulting in Psychiatric Admissions." Journal of Clinical Psychiatry, 62, 30-33, 2001.

Preskorn, S. H. "Clinically Relevant Pharmacology of Selective Serotonin Reuptake Inhibitors." Clinical Pharmacokinetics, 32 (Suppl. 1), 1-21, 1997.

Priest, R. G., Vize, C., Roberts, A., Roberts, M., & Tylee, A. "Lay People's Attitude to Treatment of Depression: Results of Opinion Poll for Defeat Depression Campaign Just Before its Launch." British Medical Journal, 313, 858-859, 1996.

"Psychiatric News." American Psychiatric Association, Vol. 39, Number 24, December 17, 2004.

Reuters Health Information, Nov. 30, 1999 www.drkoop.com/news/stories/november/antidepressant_unhappy.html

Robinson, L. A., Berman, J. S., & Neimeyer, R. A. "Psychotherapy for the Treatment of Depression: A Comprehensive Review of Controlled Outcome Research." Psychological Bulletin, 108, 30–49, 1990.

Robinson, P. "Implementing a Primary Care Depression Primary Care Pathway." In N.A. Cummings, W.T. O'Donohue, K.E. Ferguson (Eds.), Behavioral Health as Primary Care; Beyond Efficacy to Effectiveness, 69-94, 2003. Reno, NV: Context Press.

Rosenbaum, J. F., Fava, M., Hood, S. L., Ashcroft, R. C., & Krebs, W. B. "Selective Serotonin Reuptake Inhibitor Discontinuation Syndrome: A Randomized Clinical Trial." Biological Psychiatry, 44, 77-87, 1998.

Rush, A., et al. "Comparative Efficacy of Cognitive Therapy and Imipramine in the Treatment of Depressed Patients." Cognitive Therapy Res., 1: 17-37, 1979.

Sackheim, H. A., et al. "Continuation Pharmacotherapy in the Prevention of Relapse Following Electroconvulsive Therapy: A Randomized Control Trial," JAMA: Journal of the American Medical Association, 285:1299-1307, 2001.

Salerian, A. J. et al. "Sildenafil for Psychotropic-induced Sexual Dysfunction in 31 Women and 61 Men." Journal of Sex and Marital Therapy, 26:133-140, 2000.

Scogin, F., Jamison, C., and Davis, N. "A Two-year Follow-up of the Effects of Bibliotherapy for Depressed Older Adults." Journal of Consulting and Clinical Psychology, 58, 665-667, 1990.

Scogin, F., Jamison, C., Floyd, M., & Chaplin, W. "Measuring Learning in Depression Treatment: A Cognitive Bibliotherapy Test." Cognitive Therapy and Research, 22, 475-482, 1998.

Scogin, F., Jamison, C., & Gochneaut, K. "The Comparative Efficacy of Cognitive and Behavioral Bilbliotherapy for Mildly and Moderately Depressed Older Adults." Journal of Consulting and Clinical Psychology, 57, 403-407, 1989.

Seidman, S.N., et al. American Journal of Psychiatry, 158:1623-1630, 2001.

Seligman, M. Helplessness, Freeman, New York, 1992.

Seligman, M. G. P., Maier, S. F., and Geer, J. "The Alleviation of Learned Helplessness in Dogs." Journal of Abnormal Psychology, 73, 256-262, 1968.

Shapiro, M., Lehman, A. F., Greenfield, S. "Biases in the Laboratory Diagnosis of Depression in Medical Practice." Archives of Internal Medicine, 143: 2085-2088, 1983. Also abstracted in 1985 Yearbook of Psychiatry and Applied Mental Health, 155-156, Chicago: Year Book Medical Publishers, Inc., 1985.

Shea, M. T., Elkin, I., Imber, S. D., Sotsky, S. M., Watkins, J. T., Collins, J. F., Pilkonis, P. A., Beckham, E., Glass, D. R., Dolan, R. T., & Parloff, M. B. "Course of Depressive Symptoms Over Follow-up: Findings from the National Institute of Mental Health Treatment of Depression Collaborative Research Program." Archives of General Psychiatry,Vol. 49, 782-787, October 1992.

Sheehan, David V. "Improved Tolerability and Increased Length of Therapy." Supplement to Managed Care, Vol. 12, #7, 23-25, July 2003.

Silverstein, K. "An Influential Mental Health Nonprofit Finds Its 'Grassroots' Watered by Pharmaceutical Millions," Mother Jones Article, November/December 1999, http://www.cspinet.org/integrity/nonprofits/national_alliance_for_the_mentally_ill.html accessed 11/24/04.

Simon, G. E., Manning, W. G., Katzelnick, D. J., Pearson, S. D., Henk, H. J., & Helstad, C. P. "Cost Effectiveness of Systematic Depression Treatment for High Utilizers of General Medical Care." Archives of General Psychiatry, 58, 181-187, 2001.

Simons, A. D., Murphy, G. E., Levine, J. L., & Wetzel, R. D. "Cognitive Therapy and Pharmacotherapy for Depression: Sustained Improvement over One Year." Archives of General Psychiatry, 43, 43-48, 1986.

Sommers-Flanagan, J. et al. "Efficacy of Antidepressant Medication with Depressed Youth: What Psychologists Should Know." Professional Psychology-Research and Practice, Vol. 27, No.2, 145-153, 1996.

Smith, N., Floyd, M., Jamison, C., & Scogin, F. "Three-year Follow-up of Bibliotherapy for Depression." Journal of Consulting and Clinical Psychology, 65, 324-327, 1997.

Stein, D. J., et al. "Efficacy of Paroxetine for Relapse Prevention in Social Anxiety Disorder." Archives of General Psychiatry, 59:1111-1118, 2002.

Steinbrueck, S. M., Marvell, S. E., Howard, G. S. "A Meta-analysis of Psychotherapy and Drug Therapy in the Treatment of Unipolar Depression with Adults." Journal of Consulting and Clinical Psychiatry, 51: 856-863, 1983.

Stinson, D. J., et al. "Systems of Care and Treatment Outcomes for Alcoholic Patients." Archives of General Psychiatry, 36, 535-539, 1979.

Storosum, J. G., van Zwieten, B. J., van den Brink, W., Gersons, B. P. R., & Broekmans, A. W. "Suicide Risk in Placebo-controlled Studies of Major Depression." American Journal of Psychiatry, 158, 1271-1275, 2001.

Terry, C. M., Thomas, S., and Cave, D. G. "Major Depression," Managed Care Interface, Vol. 11, No. 11, 58-60, November 1998. Adapted/Reprinted by permission.

Thase, M. E. "Overview of Antidepressant Therapy," Managed Care Supplement, Vol. 10, No. 8; 6-9, August 2001.

Thase, M. E., Entsuah, A. R., et al. "Remission Rates During Treatment with Venlafaxine Or Selective Serotonin Reuptake Inhibitors." British Journal of Psychiatry, 178: 234-241, March, 2001.

Thase, M. E., Entsuah, A. R., et al. "How Should Efficacy be Evaluated in Randomized Clinical Trials of Treatments for Depression?" Journal of Clinical Psychiatry, 60 (Supplement 4), 23-31, 1999.

The Agency for Health Care Policy and Research (AHCPR), "Treatment of Depression-Newer Pharmacotherapies," 1999.

Viguera, A. D., Baldessarini, R. J. & Friedberg, J. "Discontinuing Antidepressant Treatment in Major Depression." Harvard Review of Psychiatry, 5, 293-306, 1998.

Wan, G. J., et al. "Are Venlafaxine and Venlafaxine XR Associated with Lower Hospitalization Costs in Depressed Patients With or Without Anxiety Compared to SSRIs?" World Assembly for Mental Health, Vancouver, Canada Poster Session, 2001.

Westenberg, H. G, Stein, D. J, Yang, H. et al. "A Double-blind Placebo-controlled Study of Controlled Release Fluvoxamine for the Treatment of Generalized Social Anxiety Disorder." Journal of Clinical Psychopharmacology, 24 (2): 49-55, 2004. Funding: Supported by Solvay Pharmaceuticals, Inc.

Wexler, B. E., & Cicchetti, D. V. "The Outpatient Treatment of Depression: Implications of Outcome Research for Clinical Practice." Journal of Nervous and Mental Disease, 180, 277-286, 1992.

Whisman, M. A. "Marital Adjustment and Outcome Following Treatments for Depression" Journal of Consulting and Clinical Psychology, 69:125-129, 2001.

Wilson, P. H. "Combined Pharmacological and Behavioral Treatment of Depression." Behavior Research and Therapy, 20, 173-184, 1982.

Xaton W., et al. "Distressed High Utilizers of Medical Care: DSM – 111 - R Diagnosis and Treatment Needs." General Hospital Psychiatry, 12:355-362, 1990.

Xaton W., et al. "Collaborative Management to Achieve Treatment Guidelines: Impact on Depression in Primary Case." Journal of the American Medical Association (JAMA), 273:1026-1031, 1995.

Zimmerman, M., Mattia, J. I., & Posternak, M. A. "Are Subjects in Pharmaceutical Treatment Trials of Depression Representative of Patients in Routine Clinical Practice?" American Journal of Psychiatry, 159, 469-473, March 2002.

Zimmerman, M., and Spitzer, R. L. "Melancholia": From DSMHI to DSMHIR. American Journal of Psychiatry, 146, 20-28, 1989.